Language and Motor Speech Disorders in Adults

Third Edition

Harvey Halpern, PhD
Emeritus Professor of Linguistics and Communication Disorders
Queens College of CUNY
Flushing, NY
and
Emeritus Professor of Speech and Hearing Sciences
The Graduate Center, CUNY
New York, NY

Robert Goldfarb, PhD
Professor and Program Director
Department of Communication Sciences and Disorders
Adelphi University
Garden City, NY
and
Emeritus Professor of Speech and Hearing Sciences
Lehman College and The Graduate Center
The City University of New York
New York, NY

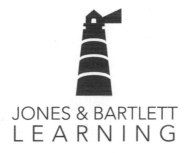

JONES & BARTLETT
LEARNING

World Headquarters
Jones & Bartlett Learning
5 Wall Street
Burlington, MA 01803
978-443-5000
info@jblearning.com
www.jblearning.com

Jones & Bartlett Learning books and products are available through most bookstores and online book-sellers. To contact Jones & Bartlett Learning directly, call 800-832-0034, fax 978-443-8000, or visit our website, www.jblearning.com.

Language and Motor Speech Disorders in Adults, Third Edition is an independent publication and has not been authorized, sponsored, or otherwise approved by the owners of the trademarks or service marks referenced in this product.

The authors, editor, and publisher have made every effort to provide accurate information. However, they are not responsible for errors, omissions, or for any outcomes related to the use of the contents of this book and take no responsibility for the use of the products and procedures described. Treatments and side effects described in this book may not be applicable to all people; likewise, some people may require a dose or experience a side effect that is not described herein. Drugs and medical devices are discussed that may have limited availability controlled by the Food and Drug Administration (FDA) for use only in a research study or clinical trial. Research, clinical practice, and government regulations often change the accepted standard in this field. When consideration is being given to use of any drug in the clinical setting, the health care provider or reader is responsible for determining FDA status of the drug, reading the package insert, and reviewing prescribing information for the most up-to-date recommendations on dose, precautions, and contraindications, and determining the appropriate usage for the product. This is especially important in the case of drugs that are new or seldom used.

Production Credits

Publisher: William Brottmiller
Acquisitions Editor: Katey Birtcher
Editorial Assistant: Teresa Reilly
Associate Production Editor: Jill Morton
Marketing Manager: Grace Richards
Manufacturing and Inventory
  Control Supervisor: Amy Bacus

Composition: Cenveo Publisher Services
Cover Design: Scott Moden
Cover Image: © Andrea Danti/ShutterStock, Inc.
Printing and Binding: Malloy Incorporated
Cover Printing: Malloy Incorporated

To order this product, use ISBN: 978-1-4496-5267-8

Library of Congress Cataloging-in-Publication Data
Halpern, Harvey.
  Language and motor speech disorders in adults / by Harvey Halpern and Robert Goldfarb.—3rd ed.
    p. ; cm.
  Rev. ed. of: Language and motor speech disorder in adults / Harvey Halpern. 2nd ed. c2000.
  Includes bibliographical references and index.
  ISBN 978-0-7637-7473-8—ISBN 0-7637-7473-1
  I. Goldfarb, Robert (Robert M.) II. Halpern, Harvey. Language and motor speech disorder in adults. III. Title.
  [DNLM: 1. Language Disorders—diagnosis. 2. Adult. 3. Speech Disorders—diagnosis. WL 340.2]

  616.85'5075—dc23
                    2011046405

6048

Printed in the United States of America
16 15 14 13 12   10 9 8 7 6 5 4 3 2 1

CONTENTS

CHAPTER 3   Aphasia   41

This introductory book provides an overview of the major neurogenically caused communication disorders in adults. Chapter 1 gives some definitions used in speech, language, and cognition, and introduces the seven major disorders. Chapter 2 reviews the neural basis of communication and touches upon the communication impairment that results from damage to the neural system. Chapter 3 contains a discussion of the language disorder associated with adult aphasia. Chapter 4 addresses the communication disorders associated with right hemisphere damage. Chapter 5 deals with the communication disorders associated with dementia. Chapter 6 presents the communication disorders associated with traumatic brain injury. Chapter 7 assesses the communication disorders associated with schizophrenia. Chapter 8 describes the motor speech disorders associated with dysarthria. Chapter 9 provides a discussion of the motor speech disorders associated with apraxia of speech.

Throughout the book, some professional terms are written in italics. These are defined and explained in a glossary which follows the chapters. Two appendices refer to a computerized version of Time-Altered Word Association Tests (TAWAT), which is based on our research over the past three decades. The online, interactive program permits responses to be entered, analyzed, printed, and emailed. Appendix A provides navigation instructions and a link to a website where the test is available for any device that has Internet access. Appendix B contains the manual for TAWAT, including theory, development, administration, and scoring. Included with this book is an access code to the website including TAWAT. Access can also be purchased separately.

We are daunted by the combined numbers we have accumulated: 100 years of university teaching and clinical practice; 50,000 therapy sessions provided to adults with neurogenic communication disorders; 10,000 undergraduate, masters, and doctoral students taught; 50 doctoral dissertations supervised as chair or committee member. It may seem glib to say that we have learned more from these individuals than we have taught them, but we are convinced that that is the case. We are grateful to them, as we are to our colleagues who reviewed earlier versions of this manuscript, to the remarkable professionals who guided us at Jones & Bartlett Learning, and, of course, to our families.

Harvey Halpern acknowledges the late Dr. Fred Darley, Professor Emeritus, Mayo Foundation, for expanding his view of neurogenic communication disorders in adults, and all his colleagues, students, and patients for providing the arena in which he learned a great deal of the subject matter.

Robert Goldfarb would like to thank Jacob Davidson for his assistance in writing the computer code for TAWAT.

Harvey Halpern is dedicating this book to Paula, Matthew, Lizzy, Kenny, Andrea, David, Annabelle, Juliet, Georgie, Maddy, Jake, and Abby. Robert Goldfarb's dedication goes to Shelley, Elizabeth, and Matt.

Nicole Bougie, MS, CCC-SLP
Adjunct Professor
Communication Disorders
Eastern New Mexico University
Portales, NM

Angela Hein Ciccia, PhD, CCC-SLP
Assistant Professor
Case Western Reserve University
Cleveland, OH

Colleen McAleer, PhD
Professor
Department of Communication Sciences and Disorders
Clarion University
Clarion, PA

Monica Gordon Pershey, EdD, CCC-SLP
School of Health Sciences
Cleveland State University
Cleveland, OH

Mary H. Purdy, PhD, BC-ANCDS
Professor
Southern Connecticut State University
New Haven, CT

M. A. Toner, PhD, CCC-SLP
Associate Professor
University of Arkansas
Fayetteville, AR

Robert Goldfarb, PhD, is Professor and Program Director of Communication Sciences and Disorders at Adelphi University; Emeritus Professor at Lehman College, CUNY; and former Executive Officer of the PhD program in Speech, Language, and Hearing Sciences at the CUNY Graduate Center. He has published more than 40 journal articles and book chapters in speech, language, and swallowing disorders of aphasia, dementia, and schizophrenia; edited *Ethics: A Case Study from Fluency* and *Translational Speech-Language Pathology and Audiology: Essays in Honor of Dr. Sadanand Singh*; and is also co-author of *Professional Writing in Speech-Language Pathology and Audiology*, *Professional Writing in Speech-Language Pathology and Audiology Workbook*, *Techniques for Aphasia Rehabilitation Generating Effective Treatment (TARGET)*, and *The Stocker Probe for Fluency and Language* (3rd ed.). An ASHA Fellow and Fulbright Senior Specialist, Dr. Goldfarb has received the Professional Achievement Award from the New York City Speech, Hearing, and Language Association and the Distinguished Achievement Award from the New York State Speech-Language-Hearing Association.

Harvey Halpern, PhD, is an Emeritus Professor in the Department of Linguistics and Communication Disorders at Queens College of the City University of New York; and Emeritus Professor in the Program of Speech, Language, and Hearing Sciences at the Graduate Center of the City University of New York.

He has worked as a speech-language pathologist at the Brooklyn College Speech, Language and Hearing Center, for the New York City Board of Education, and in private practice.

He has published numerous articles, several chapters, and was editor of the Pro-Ed series Studies in Communicative Disorders, to which he has contributed Adult Aphasia (1972), and Language and Motor Speech Disorders in Adults (1986; 2000).

He has participated in many professional panels, including delivering a number of mini-seminars and short courses. He was a postdoctoral fellow at the Mayo Clinic, and is a member of the Academy of Aphasia and the Academy of Neurologic Communication Disorders and Sciences.

He is a member of the New York City Speech, Language, and Hearing Association (NYCSLHA) from which he has received honors, and he is a member of the Long Island Speech, Language, and Hearing Association (LISHA).

He is a member with Licensure in Speech-Language Pathology and a past president of the New York State Speech, Language, and Hearing Association (NYSSLHA) from which he received honors. He is also a member with Certification in Speech Language Pathology, a former legislative councilor, and a fellow in the American Speech, Language, and Hearing Association (ASHA).

Introduction

The purpose of this text is to provide a clinically oriented, introductory framework for the major speech-language-communication disorders encountered by speech-language pathologists (SLPs) and other clinicians who work with adults with acquired neuropathologies. Specifically, this text will deal with the symptoms, etiology, diagnosis, and treatment of aphasia; the communication disorders associated with right hemisphere damage, dementia, traumatic brain injury (TBI), and schizophrenia; dysarthria; and apraxia of speech. The order is as follows: disorders of language due to focal brain activity, disorders of language due to diffuse brain activity, and motor speech disorders.

These communication disorders were chosen because they are the most frequent of the adult neuropathologies, and because they resemble one another in certain features. It is important to differentiate these particular speech-language-communication disorders from one another, because speech and/or language therapy might be similar, different, or not indicated at all. A glossary of professional terms can be found near the end of the text, along with two appendices for the computerized version of Time-Altered Word Association Tests (TAWAT), including data that show different patterns of responses for neurotypical adults (both older and younger) and populations of adults with aphasia, dementia, and chronic undifferentiated schizophrenia.

Throughout this text we will cite evidence-based practice guidelines established by the Academy of Neurologic Communication Disorders and Sciences (ANCDS). Each writing committee of ANCDS searched through electronic databases and conducted hand searches to complete exhaustive literature reviews. The purpose of each review was to assess levels of evidence, based on objective criteria agreed on by the committee, and to write guidelines based on the reviews and assessments of levels of scientific evidence. ANCDS then sought to make this information available to practicing clinicians and to determine areas where further research was needed.

Protocols for evaluating research related to interventions included reviewing some or all of the following (see, for example, Bayles et al., 2006, p. 14): the purpose of the study; characteristics of the participants; control of threats to internal, external, and content validity; characteristics of dosage of treatments, including frequency, intensity, and duration; measures of outcomes; results; and methodology.

In an early paper (Frattali et al., 2003), ANCDS identified the following five disorders as subjects of practice guidelines: dysarthria, acquired apraxia of speech, aphasia, dementia, and cognitive-communication disorders after traumatic brain injury. In the present text, the current authors will refer to more than 25 reports prepared by ANCDS writing committees.

Clinical practice recommendations reflect the level of the research evidence (Ehlhardt et al., 2008, p. 8):

Class I studies: prospective, randomized controlled clinical trials; masked outcome assessment; representative population with qualifiers

Class II: prospective, matched group cohorts; masked outcome assessment; representative population; lacking one criterion for Class I evidence

Class III: all other controlled trials where outcome assessment is independent of patient treatment representative population

Class IV: evidence from uncontrolled studies, e.g., case reports, expert opinion

Periodically throughout this text, we will refer to the International Classification of Functioning, Disability, and Health (abbreviated in the literature as ICF), developed by the World Health Organization (WHO, 2002). The purpose of the ICF is to establish a universally accepted set of terms for classifying health, as well as changes in body structure and function. "Function" applies to an individual's typical environment, as well as to one defined as standard, and accounts for environmental and personal factors.

There are three levels of functioning, according to the ICF: body or body part, person, and person in an environment or social context. ICF components of body systems include the following operational definitions:

Body structures refers to organs, limbs, and their components; in other words, the anatomical composition of the body.

Impairments refers to significant deviation or loss, caused by problems in body function or structure.

Activity refers to execution of an action or a task by an individual, who may have *activity limitations*.

Participation refers to involvement in a life situation, where the individual may have *participation restrictions*.

Environmental factors refers to the individual's physical and social environments, as well as attitudes toward these environments.

A document from the American Speech-Language-Hearing Association (2005) indicates that speech-language pathologists should know about and apply computerized and other technologies when working with individuals with cognitive-communication disorders. Among the cognitive process to be addressed are helping clients develop functional skills, compensatory strategies, and support systems. Accordingly, we have included a section on augmentative-alternative communication (AAC) in the chapter on apraxia of speech, and note that AAC is an appropriate intervention for many individuals with the other disorders discussed in this text. In addition, we provide a Web link, navigation instructions, and manual for the computerized version of Time-Altered Word Association Tests, based on our own research (see the appendices at the end of the text).

Following are some definitions of terms that will be used throughout the text. They are presented, along with some of the characteristics typically associated with each of the communication disorders, for the purpose of showing some of the similarities and differences among the disorders.

Definitions

A *communication disorder* (ASHA, 1993) is an impairment in the ability to receive, send, process, and comprehend concepts of verbal, nonverbal, and graphic symbol systems. It may be evident in the processes of hearing, language, and/or speech. It may range in severity from mild to profound and may be developmental or acquired. Individuals may demonstrate one or any combination of communication disorders. The communication disorder may be a primary disability or it may be secondary to other disabilities.

A *speech disorder* (ASHA, 1993) is an impairment of the articulation of speech sounds, fluency, and/or voice. An *articulation disorder* is the atypical production of speech sounds characterized by substitutions, omissions, additions, or distortions that may interfere with intelligibility. A *fluency disorder* is an interruption in the flow of speaking characterized by atypical rate, rhythm, and repetitions in sounds, syllables, words, and phrases. This may be accompanied by excessive tension, struggle behavior, and secondary mannerisms. A *voice disorder* is characterized by the abnormal production and/or absence of vocal quality, pitch, loudness, resonance, and/or duration, which is inappropriate for an individual's age and/or sex.

A *language disorder* (ASHA, 1993) is impaired comprehension and/or use of spoken, written, and/or other symbol systems. The disorder may involve the form of language (phonology, morphology, syntax). *Phonology* is the sound system of a language and the rules that govern the sound combinations. *Morphology* is the system that governs the structure of words and the construction of word forms. *Syntax* is the system governing the order and combination of words to form sentences, and the relationships among the elements within a sentence.

The disorder may involve the content of language (semantics). *Semantics* is the system that governs the meanings of words and sentences. It must be noted that a disturbance in the semantic aspect of language is probably the most common error found in all of the neurogenic adult language disorders. The disorder may also involve the function of language (pragmatics). *Pragmatics* is the system that combines the above language components into functional and socially appropriate communication. Pragmatics (Prutting & Kirchner, 1987) would involve eye contact with the listener, topic maintenance, turn-taking, modulation of loudness, proper decorum in the communicative setting, facial and bodily gestures that reflect the mood, proper use of register, and providing relevant information to the listener.

Cognitive functioning involves orientation, arousal, attention, speed of processing, memory, abstract reasoning, and visuospatial perception. *Orientation* is the ability to locate oneself in one's environment with reference to time (year, month, day, date, hour, etc.), place (thinking where one is at the moment), and person (the identification of self and other people). *Arousal* is an aspect of consciousness and is the next step above coma, which is a loss of consciousness.

Attention is attending to stimuli in space and the ability to hold objects, events, words, or thoughts in one's consciousness. *Selective attention* is the ability to zero in on selected visual or auditory stimuli despite a host of other, competing stimuli. It is the ability to pick out the figure from the background and maintain attention to that figure long enough to complete a successful response. For example, selective attention is a concern if someone is shown a strongly limned picture of a sailboat (figure) to respond to but instead the individual attends to some faintly drawn cloud in the distance (background) or to a number in the corner of the picture (background). (For a further discussion of attention, see the chapter on communication disorders associated with traumatic brain injury.)

Speed of processing refers to the amount of time it takes for a person to absorb information. It is especially apparent under timed conditions. *Memory* is the mental faculty or power that enables one to retain and to recall, through unconscious associative processes, previously experienced sensations, impressions, ideas, and concepts, and all information that has been consciously learned (*Mosby's*, 1994). (For a further discussion of memory, see the chapters on communication disorders associated with dementia and those associated with traumatic brain injury.)

Abstract reasoning is the process of looking at evidence, making inferences, and drawing conclusions. This reasoning allows one to draw inferences from experience and to find similarities among different but related phenomena (e.g., putting things in categories according to size, color, function, material, etc.). For example, someone looks at a picture of an old Ford Model T and another picture of a 2011 Ford automobile and puts both pictures in the category called "cars," despite the vehicles' obvious differences. Abstract reasoning is the ability to find the common thread (four wheels, a steering wheel, an area for the engine, an area for the driver and others, etc.) among things that appear superficially different.

Perception refers to the ability to organize incoming sensory stimuli by recognizing features and their relationships and then combining them with previous knowledge of these features (memory). Perception is the level above basic vision or hearing, and the level below reading or auditory comprehension. *Visuospatial perception* skills can include the ability to copy two- and three-dimensional drawings (e.g., circle, red cross, cube, cylinder, etc.), connect a series of numbers, draw on command a house or clock face, or reproduce figures that an examiner makes out of matches (Cummings & Benson, 1992).

Emotion includes mood and affect. Mood indicates the inner and subjective feelings of the patient, whereas affect is the outward expression of emotion. *Personality* is a third aspect of emotion, and refers to the total behavior over time and to the person's immediate emotional state (Cummings & Benson, 1992).

An adaptation of ASHA standards (2009) provides an overall view of the components of cognition, language, and speech involved in basic human communication. They are presented in schematic form in **Figure 1.1**.

Communication Disorders

The following communication disorders are discussed in this text.

Adult Aphasia

Adult aphasia typically has a sudden onset in middle and older age. The etiology is a brain lesion in the language-dominant hemisphere. The disorder is mostly chronic, with some cases of progressive aphasia. Typically, cognitive abilities are normal or near normal.

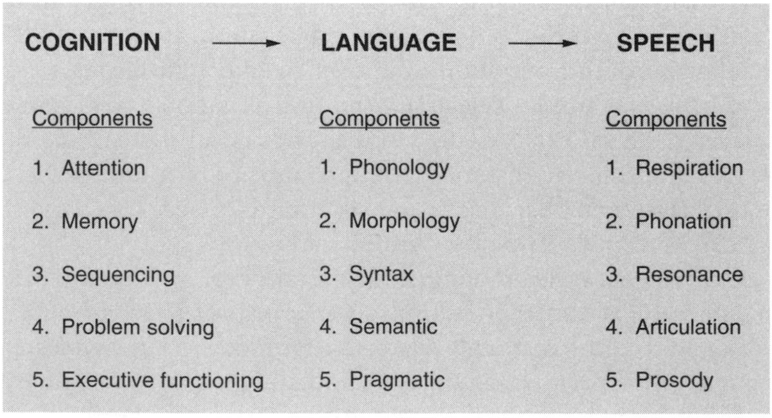

COGNITION	→	LANGUAGE	→	SPEECH
Components		Components		Components
1. Attention		1. Phonology		1. Respiration
2. Memory		2. Morphology		2. Phonation
3. Sequencing		3. Syntax		3. Resonance
4. Problem solving		4. Semantic		4. Articulation
5. Executive functioning		5. Pragmatic		5. Prosody

FIGURE 1.1 ASHA standards schematic.

The impairment can range from mild to severe, but the language components are affected regardless of severity. In many cases, the language components are affected unevenly; that is, some components are better than others.

The language impairment does stand out in relation to other abilities. Generally, the phonologic, morphologic, syntactic, and semantic components can be affected, with the pragmatic component mostly intact. Personality and behavior are typically normal or near normal. Therapy mostly involves a language stimulation approach.

Communication Disorders Associated with Right Hemisphere Damage

These disorders typically have a sudden onset in middle and older age. The etiology is a brain lesion in the right hemisphere (nondominant for language). The disorder is mostly chronic. Cognitive abilities can be affected, resulting in such problems as impaired recognition of faces (anosognosia) and left visuospatial neglect.

Language impairment, if present, is mostly in the mild range and does not stand out in relation to other abilities. The phonologic, morphologic, and syntactic components remain intact, while the semantic and pragmatic components may be affected. Personality and behavior may also be affected and can range from bizarre to near normal. Therapy mostly involves cognitive and executive planning approaches, with some language stimulation if needed.

Communication Disorders Associated with Dementia

These disorders typically have a gradual onset (although those accompanying vascular dementia can occur abruptly) in older age. The etiology is brain damage involving both hemispheres. The disorder is mostly progressive. Cognitive abilities involving thinking and recall are affected in direct proportion to the mild, moderate, and advanced stages of the disorder. Although deficits in lexical-semantic memory, and, to a lesser degree and in later stages, procedural memory are principle characteristics of dementia, we focus more on linguistic deficits in this text.

In *cortical dementia*, typically, the language components are affected according to the stage of the disorder. In the mild stage, the phonologic, morphologic, and syntactic components are all intact, while the semantic and pragmatic components begin to deteriorate. In the moderate stage, the phonologic component is intact, while the morphologic and syntactic components begin to deteriorate, and the semantic and pragmatic components further deteriorate. In the advanced stage, the phonologic component begins to deteriorate, along with a further deterioration of the morphologic and syntactic components, and a still greater deterioration of the semantic and pragmatic components. The language impairment does not stand out in relation to other abilities.

In *subcortical dementia*, typically there is no distinctive language breakdown. Language becomes restricted and simplified, and in the advanced stages there may be auditory comprehension and naming problems. Of the language components, the semantic and pragmatic aspects would most likely be affected. Speech can be dysarthric.

Personality and behavior are affected in both cortical and subcortical dementias. Therapy involves mostly cognitive approaches and, if necessary, the methods used for dysarthria.

Communication Disorders Associated with Traumatic Brain Injury

These disorders have a sudden onset and mostly appear in younger age (primarily in males) and in those older than 75 years. Typically, the etiology is brain damage involving both hemispheres. The disorder can be temporary or chronic. Cognitive abilities typically are affected in direct proportion to the severity of the disorder (mild, moderate, severe).

The language components are affected according to the stage of the disorder. In the mild stage, the phonologic, morphologic, and syntactic components are intact, but the semantic and pragmatic components may be impaired. In the moderate stage, the phonologic, morphologic, and syntactic components are intact, the semantic component may be impaired, and the pragmatic component is impaired. In the severe stage, the phonologic component remains intact, the morphologic and syntactic components may be impaired, and the semantic and pragmatic components are impaired.

The language impairment does not stand out in relation to other abilities. Personality and behavior are affected according to the severity of the disorder and can range from bizarre (severe stage) to near normal (mild stage). Therapy involves mostly cognitive and executive planning approaches.

Communication Disorders Associated with Schizophrenia

The cause of schizophrenia is not known, and the brain pathology is functional deficit (primarily in the frontal lobes) rather than structural deficit. Age of onset generally ranges from the teens to the late 30s. Cognitive abilities may range from severely impaired to exceptionally gifted, even in florid episodes of schizophrenia. There may also be extended periods of relative lucidity.

The language components are affected in a manner similar to those appearing in other disorders, making differential diagnosis crucial. In most cases, phonology and morphology are preserved, syntax may be intact or mildly impaired, the semantic component is often impaired, and the pragmatic component is most obviously impaired.

The effect of long-term ingestion of antipsychotic medication may be a form of dysarthria, accompanied by a movement disorder called *tardive dyskinesia*.

Personality and behavior are greatly affected, but the underlying symptom is a thought disorder. Speech-language therapy alone is not usually effective for the language disorder, but may be useful in treating symptoms of dysarthria.

Dysarthria

Dysarthria can have a sudden or gradual onset and can appear at any age. The etiology can be neurological impairment within the central nervous system (brain and spinal cord), or the peripheral nervous system (cranial nerves and spinal nerves). The site of lesion can be either focal, multifocal, or diffuse. The disorder can be temporary, chronic, or progressive. Typically, cognitive abilities are normal or near normal.

Dysarthria is a motor speech disorder involving motor execution problems within the neuromuscular system, and should present no language impairment. The affected speech components can involve respiration, phonation, resonation, articulation, and prosody in any combination. Personality and behavior are mostly normal or near normal. Therapy involves the re-establishment of the neuromuscular system's motor execution capabilities in the presence of an intact motor programming component.

Apraxia of Speech

Apraxia of speech typically has a sudden onset in middle and older age. The etiology is a brain lesion in the language-dominant hemisphere (focal). The disorder is mostly chronic. Typically, cognitive abilities are normal or near normal.

Apraxia of speech is a motor speech disorder involving programming problems within the neuromuscular system, and should present no language impairment. However, if accompanied by aphasia, as it often is, language will be impaired. The affected speech components involve articulation and prosody. Personality and behavior are mostly normal or near normal.

Therapy involves the re-establishment of the neuromuscular system's motor programming capabilities in the presence of an intact motor execution component.

A Note About Dysphagia

Swallowing disorders (*dysphagia*) are common consequences of stroke. Dysphagia may be manifested as aspiration, defined as the entry of food or liquid into the airway below the true vocal folds (Logemann, 1998). Videofluoroscopy, as opposed to bedside examination, is the current gold standard of evaluation of aspiration in acute stroke (Baylow et al., 2009). Frequently present during the acute phase of a cerebrovascular accident (CVA, or stroke), dysphagia can be a life-threatening complication because of its apparent sequela, aspiration pneumonia. Dysphagia with the co-occurrence of inadequate airway protection during swallowing has also been associated with the development of sepsis, dehydration, and malnutrition. Typically taught as a separate course, this important topic is not addressed as a chapter in the present text.

Organization of the Text

At the end of each chapter is a brief case or clinical description, representing people the authors have worked with or have known. Identifying information has been changed in order to ensure privacy. The case description is followed by 10 questions for discussion, 5 addressing theoretical areas and 5 therapeutic issues. Finally, there is a multiple-choice question on a topic addressed in the chapter, with 5 possible answers. Each option is explained. The authors recommend that the reader create a new multiple-choice question and explain each option, as a way of increasing mastery of the subject.

Goldfarb and Serpanos (2009) have noted that students are required to take multiple-choice tests from elementary through graduate school and beyond (Praxis II exam, ASHA special interest division continuing education quizzes), often from instructors who have had little or no formal training in preparing them. A multiple-choice item contains a *stem* and usually four or five *options*, or possible answers. The correct answer is the *key*, and the other options are *distractors* or *decoys*. Level I questions only assess knowledge, and require the cognitive behavior of remembering and understanding previously learned information. Level II questions are designed to test knowledge in context, and require the cognitive behavior of interpretation, that is, understanding the *why* and *how* of the situation. A question of this sort should present a problem to be solved by understanding a theory, principle, or technique. Level III questions assess evaluation and decision making. They require the cognitive behavior of synthesis of elements into a comprehensive whole. These questions may include hypothetical case information, in order to stimulate the process of designing or modifying treatment based on evidence. Standardized examinations, such as the Praxis II in speech-language pathology and audiology, mainly use Level II and III questions. Detailed information about multiple-choice test construction may be found in some professional writing books (e.g., Goldfarb & Serpanos, 2009).

References

American Speech-Language-Hearing Association. (2009). *Standards and implementation procedures for the certificate of clinical competence in speech-language pathology (Standard III-C)*. Rockville, MD: Author.

American Speech-Language-Hearing Association. (2005). Knowledge and skills needed by speech-language pathologists providing services to individuals with cognitive-communication disorders. *ASHA* (Supplement 25). Rockville, MD: Author. doi:10.1044/policy.KS2005-00078.

American Speech-Language-Hearing Association. (1993). Definitions of communication disorders and variations. *ASHA 35* (Supplement 10), 40–41. Rockville, MD: Author.

Bayles, K., Kim, E., Chapman, S., Zientz, J., Rackley, A., Mahendra, N., ... Cleary, S. (2006). Evidence-based practice recommendations for working with individuals with dementia: Simulated presence therapy. *Journal of Medical Speech-Language Pathology, 14,* 13–21.

Baylow, H. E., Goldfarb, R., Taveira, C., & Steinberg, R. (2009). Accuracy of clinical judgment of the chin-down posture for dysphagia during the clinical/bedside assessment as corroborated by videofluoroscopy in adults with acute stroke. *Dysphagia, 24,* 423–433.

Cummings, J., & Benson, D. F. (1992). *Dementia: A clinical approach* (2nd ed.). Stoneham, MA: Butterworth-Heinemann.

Ehlhardt, L. A., Sohlberg, M. M., Kennedy, M., Coelho, C., Ylvisaker, M., Turkstra, L., & Yorkston, K. (2008). Evidence-based practice guidelines for instructing individuals with neurogenic memory impairments: What have we learned in the past 20 years? *Neuropsychological Rehabilitation, 1,* 1–43.

Frattali, C., Bayles, K., Beeson, P., Kennedy, M., Wambaugh, J., & Yorkston, K. M. (2003). Development of evidence-based practice guidelines: Committee update. *Journal of Medical Speech-Language Pathology, 13,* 9–18.

Goldfarb, R., & Serpanos, Y. (2009). *Professional writing in speech-language pathology and audiology.* San Diego, CA: Plural Publishing, Inc.

Logemann, J. A. (1998). *Evaluation and treatment of swallowing disorders* (2nd ed.). Austin, TX: Pro-Ed.

Mosby's medical, nursing, and allied health dictionary. (1994). St. Louis, MO: Mosby.

Prutting, C., & Kirchner, D. (1987). A clinical appraisal of the pragmatic aspects of language. *Journal of Speech and Hearing Disorders, 52,* 105–119.

World Health Organization. (2002). Towards a common language for functioning, disability and health: ICF. Retrieved January 12, 2011 from http://www.who.int/classifications/icf/site/beginners/bg.pdf.

The Neural Basis of Speech and Language

Introduction

This section gives the reader a brief overview of what takes place neurally when a person starts a conversation by saying, "Hello. How are you? How was your vacation trip?" to another individual whom the person meets on the street. Simply put, the steps involved would be as follows:

1. Basic vision: seeing a person on the street
2. Visual perception: recognizing the person as someone the speaker knows
3. Cognition: the desire to speak with this person about a trip that the speaker may want to take in the future
4. Language: searching for the right sounds, syllables, words, and sentences, all presented in the right order, with meaning properly related to the greeting and the subject matter, to be expressed with a positive attitude
5. Motor programming or planning: readying the speech mechanism just prior to speaking so that the production is correct
6. Motor production or execution: speaking
7. Feedback: (1) from self: hearing and feeling oneself speak and then using that information as a guide for further appropriate speaking (e.g., usually we know when something said does not sound right, and we either repeat it or put it into different words); (2) from others: looking at and listening to another person speak to help determine what to say next (e.g., responding to questions from someone who looks and sounds angry as opposed to someone who does not).

Responding to auditory feedback from oneself or from others involves the hearing of sound (basic hearing). Recognizing that sound as speech and not some other environmental noise is auditory perception. Understanding what is said is language comprehension. All of the steps mentioned above, with the exception of cognition, will be commented on in the neural outline that follows. The neural basis for cognition (thinking and behavior) probably involves bilateral cortical areas (especially the frontal lobes) as the prime movers, assisted by subcortical and brainstem systems. Because of the widespread neural activity, localization of cognitive functions is quite difficult. However, cognition and defects of cognition are noted in other parts of this manuscript (e.g., the chapters dealing with right hemisphere damage, dementia, and traumatic brain injury).

The information in the following outline has been gleaned from Bhatnagar (2008), Duffy (2005), Kent (1997), Webb and Adler (2008), Webster (1999), and Zemlin (1998); the organization of the outline mostly follows that of Webb and Adler, with details from Bhatnagar. The reader is referred to these sources for further elaboration of any of the topics mentioned in the outline. In a number of places within the outline, examples are given of the speech and/or language problem that can occur if there is damage to certain portions of the neural system. Most of the speech and/or language problems given as examples are mentioned further in other parts of this text.

Definitions

The Neuron

The neuron, or nerve cell, consists of a cell body, dendrites, and an axon (**Figure 2.1**). The *cell body* (intracellular) contains a high concentration of potassium and low concentrations of sodium and chloride, compared to the fluids outside the cell body (extracellular). The concentrations

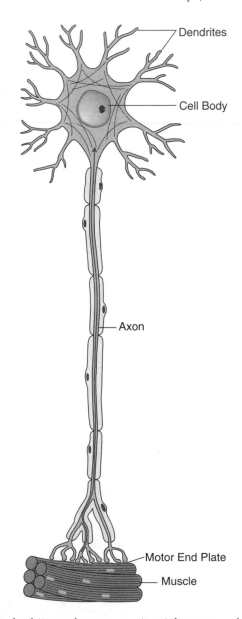

FIGURE 2.1 A neuron, with its cell body, dendrites, and axon, synapsing at the myoneural junction of the muscle.

are reversed in the extracellular fluids, thus creating an electrical current for transmission of neural impulses. *Dendrites* are numerous short projections that carry neural impulses to the cell body. The *axon* carries neural impulses away from the cell body. The neuron can transmit neural impulses to other neurons, glands, or muscles.

The juncture at which neural impulses are transmitted is called a *synapse*; neurochemical transmitters aid in moving the neural impulses along. *Myelin*, a fatty sheath that insulates the larger axons, is said to increase the speed of neural transmission and also to reduce interference with the neural message. There may be about 100 billion neurons in the human nervous system. Axons can produce anywhere from 1000 to 10,000 synapses, and their cell bodies and dendrites receive neural data from about 1000 other neurons. As a result, the number of synapses occurring in the brain may be about 100 trillion.

Nerve Cell Structure
Cell Body (also called *perikaryon,* or *soma*)
1. *Protoplasm* refers to the nucleus and cytoplasm.
2. *Cytoplasm* is composed of a watery substance and protein molecules, and is enclosed within the cell membrane. Microscopic structures in cytoplasmic materials include the following:
   a. *Neurofibrils* (which tend to become tangled in Alzheimer disease) serve as channels for intracellular communication.
   b. *Mitochondria* contain enzymes involved with cellular metabolic energy.
   c. *Ribosomes* are protein granules involved in the synthesis of RNA.
   d. *Lysosomes* contain enzymes that participate in intracellular digestion.
   e. *Golgi* complexes are responsible for protein secretion and transportation.

Axons and Dendrites
1. *Nerve fiber* means an axon and its covering sheath.
2. *Axons* are efferent (motor) structures that transmit information away from the cell body to other neurons. They depend on cytoplasmic proteins for survival.
3. *Axon hillock* refers to a cone-shaped region of the cell. Axons extend longer distances than dendrites. At their ends, they may branch into smaller multiple filaments, called *telodendria,* that include *synaptic knobs,* or end in a *terminal bouton (knob).* Both types of knobs contain neurotransmitters.
4. *Dendrites* are afferent (receptive) structures that transmit information to the cell body from other cells via synaptic sites. They tend to be short and have many branches. When they have spikes or spines, this increases the surface available for synapses with other nerve cells. Many of these spines atrophy from disuse as part of typical maturation. One theory of autism is based on an excess of especially short, stubby dendritic spines, although in Fragile X syndrome, also associated with autism, dendritic spines tend to be long and thin.

Myelin Sheath
1. *Myelin* is a multilayered lipid (fatty) material that insulates and protects the nerve fiber so that electric energy cannot escape during impulse transmission and speed of nerve impulses can be regulated. Intervals between the segments of the myelin sheath are called *nodes of Ranvier.*
2. *Oligodendroglial* cells produce the myelin sheath in the central nervous system (CNS). Myelin damage of unknown origin is associated with multiple sclerosis; a rare and

slowly growing neoplastic growth (glioma) may also occur (oligodendroglioma). In the peripheral nervous system (PNS), the myelin sheath is produced by Schwann cells that lie along the axons, and is sometimes referred to as the *sheath of Schwann* (also called *neurolemma* or *neurilemma*). A schwannoma or neurofibroma is a moderately firm, benign, nonencapsulated tumor resulting from proliferation of Schwann cells in a disorderly pattern that includes portions of nerve fibers (sometimes observed as an acoustic neuroma).

Synapse

1. The *knob*, or *bouton*, contains synaptic vesicles (subdivisions of embryonic neural tubes). They are filled with neurotransmitters.
2. The *synaptic cleft* is the space between the axon of the presynaptic nerve cell and the receptive ends of the postsynaptic cell. Nerve impulses do not cross the synapse, but are communicated through the neurotransmitter released from the bouton terminals.
3. The *receptive sites* of the connecting nerve cells are chemically activated to generate the electric impulses that stimulate the nerve cell body.

Nerve Cell Types

Multipolar cells have many dendrites and one axon. Most are in the CNS. The most common examples are spinal interneurons and cerebellar Purkinje cells.

Bipolar cells have two processes, one extending from each pole of the body: a peripheral process (dendrite) and a central process (axon).

Unipolar cells are T-shaped with one process that extends from the body and divides into central (axonal) and peripheral (dendritic) portions. Unipolar cells are found in spinal dorsal roots.

Golgi Cells

1. *Golgi type I* are nerve cells whose axons leave the gray matter of which they form a part.
2. *Golgi type II* are cells with short axons which ramify in the gray matter.

Neuronal Circuits

A *divergent circuit* amplifies an impulse when an impulse from a single presynaptic cell activates several postsynaptic cells.

A *convergent circuit* has two patterns of connections. In the first neuronal circuit of convergence, the postsynaptic neuron receives impulses from several diverged fibers of the same presynaptic nerve cell. In the second pattern, impulses from different nerve cells converge on one postsynaptic nerve cell.

In *lateral inhibition*, the signal or cellular message is sharpened by inhibiting the adjacent nerve cells.

The *reverberating circuit* is a self-propagating system between cells that, if activated, can discharge the signal continuously until its operation is blocked by an external source. In the reverberating circuitry, neurons are arranged in a chain formation. The incoming impulse activates the first nerve cell, which activates the second cell, which stimulates the third, and so on. Branches from the second, third, and fourth cells send impulses back to activate the previous nerve cell, forming a closed neuronal loop.

Neuroglial Cells

Glial (meaning "glue") cells support and protect the nerve cells. Found in the gray and white matter of the brain, there are 40 to 50 times as many glial cells as nerve cells. Glial cells do not generate or transmit nerve impulses.

Astrocytes function as connective tissue, providing skeletal support for the brain cells and their processes. They contribute to the *blood–brain barrier* by contacting capillary surfaces with their end feet and using tight junctions. This restricts the movement of certain substances from the blood to the brain through selective permeability.

Oligodendroglia cells form and maintain the myelin sheath in the CNS (see the section called "Myelin Sheath").

Ependymal cells form the inner surface of the ventricles. The choroid plexus, which secretes cerebrospinal fluid, consists of vascular pia surrounded by an epithelial layer of ependymal cells.

Microglial cells are multipotential, because they act sometimes as phagocytes (which remove dead neural tissue debris) and at other times as astrocytes or oligodendrocytes. They are the scavengers of the CNS.

After an injury to the brain, astroglial cells are important in recovery. In strokes (cerebrovascular accidents, or CVAs), the astrocytes, and microglial cells proliferate and migrate to the lesion site. Microglia phagocytose (engulf) cellular debris, leaving a cavity. For large lesions, astrocytes seal the cavity, which is called a *cyst*. In smaller lesions, astrocytes fill the space with a glial scar that is called *replacement gliosis*.

Nerve Impulses

Nerve impulses have a chemical component that underlies the electric potential of the cells. An *action potential* results from charged particles (ions) moving through the cell membranes. Nerve impulses activate the release of a neurotransmitter in a presynaptic neuron. The transmitter causes the adjacent postsynaptic receptors to open an ion channel.

When nerve cells conduct an impulse (and, to a limited degree, even when they do not), positive and negative ions on each side of a cell membrane are unequal (polarized). This membrane potential is maintained by an unequal distribution of positively charged sodium and potassium ions and negative charged chloride ions and proteins across the membrane. The negative ions are highly concentrated inside the cell, and the positive ions are in higher concentration outside the cell. Opposite ions attract, and identical ions repel. This tug of war forms an electrochemical gradient along the cell membrane, which is called the cell's *resting potential*.

Nerve Excitability

Excitability is a cell's response to various stimuli and its conversion of this response into a nerve impulse or action potential. The same stimuli that affect overall homeostasis in the body (e.g., chemical or temperature change, electrical pulsing) can affect action potential or intracellular potential. When the cell interior becomes more negative, it is hyperpolarized; in the other direction (depolarization), it triggers a large spike.

A change of at least 10 mV is required to trigger an action potential and depolarize a nerve cell. The resting membrane potential is arbitrarily defined as –70 mV inside the cell membrane. So a change which brings the cell interior from –70 to –60 mV is needed to trigger a nerve impulse or message.

Impulse Conduction

Nerve impulses are conducted on the basis of polarization. For example, passive impulse conduction for a short distance occurs when sodium enters the cell membrane. This makes the interior of the axon more positive than the adjacent area; the impulse allows positively charged ions to enter the cell membrane as it moves distally along the axon.

Similarly, polarization is the basis for exciting or inhibiting an impulse in the postsynaptic neuron. *Excitatory postsynaptic potential (EPSP)* refers to a lowered membrane potential in the postsynaptic neuron, which creates an environment for a new impulse. The opposite is true for *inhibitory postsynaptic potential (IPSP)*.

Neurotransmitters

Neurotransmitters are chemical substances released at a synapse to transmit signals across neurons. They help regulate brain mechanisms that control cognition, language, speech, and hearing, among other functions. For our purposes, *small-molecule* transmitters need particular study. They include acetylcholine and the following five monoamines, which are derived from amino acids: dopamine, norepinephrine, serotonin, glutamate, and γ-aminobutyric acid (GABA). *Large-molecule* peptides produce longer-lasting effects.

Most neurotransmitters have more than one receptor type and may have different effects on different synapses. Because more than one neurotransmitter may be secreted by a single terminal bouton, it is difficult to identify a specific behavioral effect of a given neurotransmitter at all times.

Acetylcholine

Acetylcholine is the primary neurotransmitter of the PNS and is also important in the CNS. Cholinergic neurons are concentrated in the reticular formation, the basal forebrain, and the striatum. Neurons in the forebrain supply the neocortex, hippocampus, and amygdala. Cholinergic projections from the forebrain are thought to participate in regulating levels of forebrain activity; those from the reticular formation to the thalamus are critical in the cycle of sleep and wakefulness. Actions of acetylcholine are slow and diffuse in the CNS, but brief and precise in the PNS.

Antibodies that interfere with the action of acetylcholine on muscle cells at the myoneural junction are found in the myasthenia gravis. Deficient cholinergic projections in the hippocampus and orbitofrontal cortex have been implicated in Alzheimer disease, but replacing acetylcholine has not been successful in alleviating or retarding progression of the disease.

Monoamines

Dopaminergic projections are located in the mesostriatal (midbrain and striatum) and mesocortical (midbrain to cortex) systems. We are more interested in the first group. Mesostriatal projections are dopaminergic cells from the substantia nigra to the putamen and caudate nucleus of the basal ganglia. Degeneration of the substantia nigra reduces production and transmission of dopamine and is associated with Parkinson disease.

Norepinephrine-containing (noradrenergic) neurons are in the pons and medulla, with most in the reticular formation. Noradrenergic neurons project to the thalamus, hypothalamus, limbic forebrain structures, and the cerebral cortex. Descending fibers project to other parts of the brainstem, cerebellar cortex, and spinal cord. Clinically, noradrenergic neurons are thought to be involved in generating paradoxical sleep and maintaining attention and vigilance. Drugs used for treating depression act by enhancing norepinephrine transmission.

Serotonin neurons are found at most levels of the brainstem, with terminals in the reticular formation, hypothalamus, thalamus, septum, hippocampus, olfactory tubercle, cerebral cortex, basal ganglia, and amygdala. Clinically, serotonin is concerned with overall level of arousal and slow-wave sleep. It contributes to the descending pain control system. Severe depression is thought to be associated with low serotonin, and a feeling of well-being is associated with higher levels of this neurotransmitter. Drugs such as selective serotonin reuptake inhibitors are used to control anxiety and panic disorders.

GABA, or γ-*aminobutyric acid*, is a major neurotransmitter for the CNS, just as acetylcholine is in the periphery. It serves as the inhibitory neurotransmitter from the striatum to the globus pallidus and substantia nigra, from the globus pallidus and substantia nigra to the thalamus, and from the Purkinje cells to the deep cerebellar nuclei. Clinically, GABA is implicated in Huntington disease.

The Human Nervous System

The human nervous system is made up of the central, peripheral, and autonomic nervous systems. The areas of the human nervous system that will be reviewed in the following pages are those that are vital for speech and language. The CNS contains the brain, spinal cord, meninges, ventricles, and blood supply. The PNS is composed of the spinal peripheral nerves and the cranial nerves (**Figure 2.2**). The autonomic nervous system (ANS) contains a sympathetic division and a parasympathetic division.

We have noted different myelin-forming cells: an oligodendrocyte, which myelinates many axons in the CNS; and a Schwann cell, which forms myelin exclusively for one internode of a peripheral nerve fiber. Composition of nerve fibers varies between the CNS and PNS.

Peripheral nerve fiber bundles are held together by connective tissue (*collagen fibers*, which compose connective tissue throughout the body, and in the brain form *fibroblasts* and other cells that form an *endoneurial membrane*). There is no such fibrous connective tissue in the CNS. The endoneurium wraps around a peripheral axon and merges with *neurilemma*, the most external layer of the multilayered myelin, which contains the nucleus of the Schwann cell. The neurilemma is important in the regeneration of injured axonal fibers in the PNS. Axonal shearing is discussed in the chapter on traumatic brain injury.

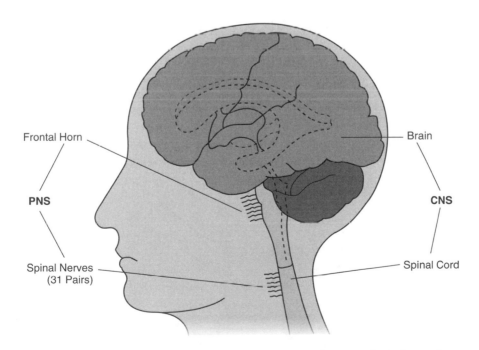

FIGURE 2.2 The CNS (brain and spinal cord) and PNS (12 pairs of cranial nerves and 31 pairs of spinal nerves).

The Central Nervous System

The central nervous system (CNS) consists of the brain, spinal cord, meninges, ventricles, and blood supply.

The Brain

The brain is composed of the cerebral hemispheres, the basal ganglia, the cerebellum, and the brainstem. The largest part of the brain is called the cerebrum and is made up of the two cerebral hemispheres and the basal ganglia. The cerebral cortex covers the cerebrum and is composed of many prominent sulci or fissures (grooves on the surface of the brain or spinal cord) and gyri (elevations or ridges on the surface of the cerebrum). Korbinian Brodmann (1868–1918), a German neurologist, established the numbering system for 52 areas of the cerebral cortex, which remains the universal standard (called *Brodmann areas*) used today.

Cerebral Hemispheres

The cerebral hemispheres are composed of a left and a right hemisphere and are connected by a mass of white matter called the *corpus callosum*. The purpose of the corpus callosum is to pass neuronal information from one hemisphere to the other. Medically directed severance of the corpus callosum has led to a good deal of "split brain" research. Included in the findings of this research is the observation that the left hemisphere serves a different purpose than the right hemisphere. Some of the functions of the left hemisphere are involvement in language and analytical and logical aspects, whereas the right hemisphere is involved with perceptual, spatial, intuitive, and holistic aspects (e.g., a lesion in a language area of the left hemisphere can result in aphasia, whereas a lesion in the right hemisphere can result in the patient's inability to draw information through inference that is arrived at by taking a holistic and intuitive approach).

The *longitudinal cerebral fissure*, which runs from the front to the back of the brain, separates the two hemispheres (**Figure 2.3**). The cerebral cortex in each hemisphere is partitioned

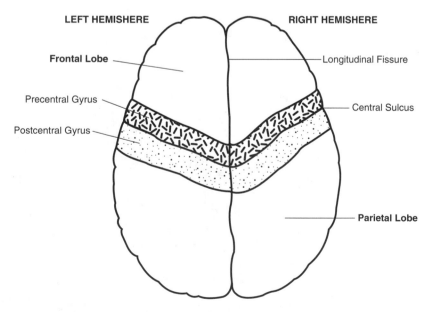

FIGURE 2.3 A superior view of the cerebral hemispheres.

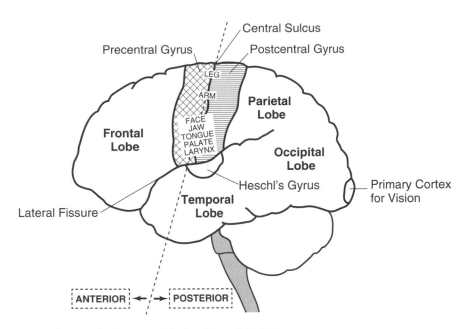

FIGURE 2.4 Lateral view showing the location of the four lobes of the brain.

into the frontal, parietal, temporal, and occipital lobes (**Figure 2.4**). Lying beneath the outer surface of the cerebral cortex is a fifth lobe called the *limbic lobe*.

The frontal lobe. The frontal lobe is bounded in the back by the central sulcus and below by the lateral fissure. The brain is divided into anterior and posterior regions by the central sulcus. Within the frontal lobe is the precentral gyrus, which lies immediately anterior to the central sulcus. The precentral gyrus is also known as the *primary motor cortex*, or "motor strip" area, and it controls voluntary muscular movement on the opposite side of the body (Figure 2.4).

The neurons within the primary motor cortex are organized in a pattern of a person ("homunculus," or "little man") standing upside down. Neurons devoted to motor movements in the face and neck area are closest to the lateral fissure, and neurons devoted to motor movements of the toes and leg are closest to the longitudinal cerebral fissure (Figure 2.4). Some parts of the body require fine motor movement, whereas other parts require less precise motor movement. There is a greater array of neurons devoted to the small muscles of the larynx, palate, tongue, jaw, and face than to the arm or leg. The number of neurons allocated for voluntary movement of a body part is typically not commensurate with its size. A lesion in the primary motor cortex within areas involving movements of the lips, tongue, or larynx can result in certain types of dysarthria.

Located in front of the precentral gyrus are the premotor and supplementary motor areas (**Figure 2.5**). These areas receive information from other regions of the brain, and their purpose is to integrate, refine, and plan or program motor speech output (e.g., a lesion in the premotor areas can result in certain types of dysarthria, or if in the dominant hemisphere, an apraxia of speech). Broca's area is in the third frontal gyrus of the dominant hemisphere (Figure 2.5). This important area plays a main role in motor speech programming and also connects to other parts of the brain involved with speech and language (e.g., a lesion in Broca's area can result in apraxia of speech in addition to the more commonly seen nonfluent aphasia).

The parietal lobe. The parietal lobe is bounded in the front by the central sulcus and below by the back end of the lateral fissure. Within the parietal lobe is the postcentral gyrus,

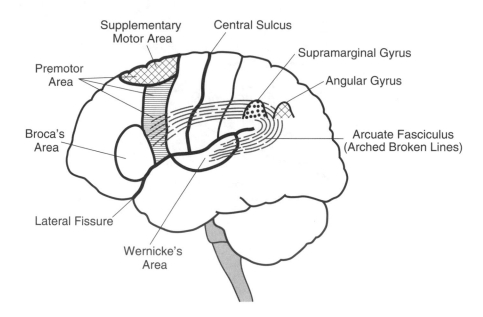

FIGURE 2.5 Lateral view of the left (dominant) hemisphere, showing the location of the language and motor speech programming (or planning) areas.

which is located in back of the central sulcus (Figure 2.4). The postcentral gyrus is a mirror image to the "motor strip" area of the frontal lobe and is a primary sensory cortical area ("sensory strip") having to do with temperature, pain, touch, and proprioception.

Proprioception (which includes the senses of movement, vibration, pressure, position, equilibrium, and deep pain) enables one to realize exactly where the individual parts of the body are in space, and the relationship of one body part to another (e.g., tongue in relation to the alveolar ridge in the production of lingua-alveolar sounds). This somatosensory cortex in the dominant hemisphere appears to play a part in motor speech programming, especially in the integration of sensory information in preparation for motor activity (e.g., a lesion in this area can result in apraxia of speech). In addition, Damasio (1994) has noted that the somatosensory cortex in the right hemisphere helps maintain reasoning and decision making, emotion, and feelings, with a special emphasis in the social and personal domain (see the chapter on communication disorders associated with right hemisphere damage for further discussion).

The parietal lobe in the dominant hemisphere also contains the supramarginal gyrus and the angular gyrus (Figure 2.5). The supramarginal gyrus curves around the back end of the lateral fissure and is responsible for the formulation of written language and possibly for phonological storage (e.g., a lesion in this area can result in aphasia). The angular gyrus lies directly behind the supramarginal gyrus and plays a major role in reading comprehension (e.g., a lesion in this area can result in aphasia with deep dyslexia).

The temporal lobe. The temporal lobe is bounded on top by the lateral fissure and in the back by the front border of the occipital lobe. Three important areas in the temporal lobe of the dominant hemisphere are Heschl's gyrus, Wernicke's area, and the insula (or the Island of Reil). Heschl's gyrus (or primary auditory cortex) is located on the lateral fissure, two-thirds of the way back on the upper surface of the temporal lobe (Figure 2.4). It is the cortical center for hearing, responsible for appreciating the meaning of sound (e.g., a lesion in this area can result in auditory processing problems, which can lead to an auditory comprehension deficit). Wernicke's area (an auditory association area) is located on the back part of the superior temporal gyrus (Figure 2.5) and plays a major role in auditory comprehension and other language abilities (e.g., a lesion in this area can result in aphasia). The insula, which can be seen if the two borders of the lateral fissure are pulled apart, is in the paralimbic area. The function of the insula is not clearly defined, but a lesion there can result in aphasia or apraxia of speech.

The occipital lobe. The occipital lobe is located at the back of the cerebral hemisphere. It is bounded in the front by the parietal and temporal lobes and in back by the longitudinal fissure. The primary visual cortex and visual association areas are situated in the occipital lobe. The primary visual cortex (Figure 2.4) is responsible for basic vision (e.g., a lesion in this area can produce degrees of blindness). The visual association area is needed for integrating and organizing incoming visual stimuli (e.g., a lesion here can result in visual perception problems, which in turn can influence reading comprehension).

The limbic lobe. The limbic lobe is situated on the medial surface of the cortex and contains the orbital frontal region, the cingulate gyrus, and the medial portions of the temporal lobe. The limbic system regulates emotions and behavior. For example, a lesion in this system can affect prosody, or possibly pragmatic abilities (see "Limbic System" in this chapter for further discussion).

The association areas. As mentioned previously, there are primary centers for motor, sensory, hearing, and visual functioning. These centers are connected to one another and to other parts of the brain by association areas. The association areas are responsible for higher mental functioning, including language, and are located in the lobes of each hemisphere.

The *frontal association* area is responsible for initiation and integration of purposeful behavior and for planning and carrying out sequences of volitional movement. The parietal association area, or somesthetic area, is responsible for the discrimination and integration of tactile information. The temporal or auditory association area is needed for the discrimination and integration of auditory information. The visual association area is responsible for the discrimination and integration of visual information. A lesion in an association area of the dominant hemisphere can result in aphasia, as can a lesion in a pathway connecting one association area with another, as in the case of the arcuate fasciculus (Figure 2.5), which connects the association area of the temporal lobe with that of the frontal lobe.

The Basal Ganglia (or Basal Nuclei)

In another part of the brain are subcortical structures called the *basal ganglia*. They are a mass of gray matter that lies deep within the cerebrum and below the cerebral cortex. The basal ganglia consist of the caudate nucleus, the globus pallidus, and the putamen; grouped together, these are called the *corpus striatum* (**Figure 2.6**). The globus pallidus and putamen are sometimes named together as the *lentiform nucleus*. The basal ganglia are responsible for controlling and stabilizing motor functions and for interpreting sensory information so as to guide and influence motor behavior (e.g., a lesion in the basal ganglia can result in dysarthria).

The Cerebellum

The cerebellum is located just behind the pons and the medulla at the base of the occipital lobe (Figure 2.6). The cerebellum contains right and left hemispheres that are connected by the vermis between them (**Figure 2.7**). These are the areas most involved in speech control. The cerebellum does not initiate motor movements, but through its connections to the spinal cord, cerebrum, pons, and medulla, it helps in coordinating the skilled, voluntary muscle activity produced elsewhere (e.g., a lesion in the cerebellum can result in dysarthria).

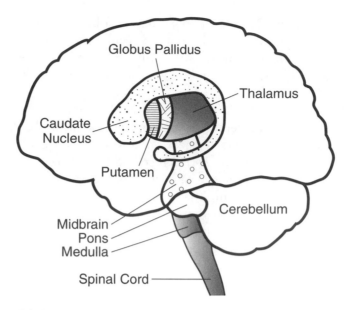

FIGURE 2.6 A sagittal section of the brain that shows the location of the spinal cord, brainstem, (medulla, pons, midbrain), thalamus, basal ganglia (caudate nucleus, globus pallidus, putamen), and cerebellum. A sagittal section is a vertical cut or slice which divides the body into right and left halves, producing two equal, mirror-image parts.

The Brainstem

The brain also contains the brainstem, which appears as an upward extension of the spinal cord and thrusts upward into the brain between the cerebral hemispheres. In ascending order, once the spinal cord enters the foramen magnum of the brain case, the brainstem consists of the medulla oblongata, the pons, the midbrain (mesencephalon), and two structures (diencephalon) called the *thalamus* and *hypothalamus* (Figure 2.6). Some authors include the thalamus and hypothalamus as part of the cerebrum.

The medulla and pons. The medulla contains nuclei for several of the cranial nerves, and ascending and descending tracts to and from the cortex that are important for the control of speech production. The pons contains nuclei for several of the cranial nerves, has major connections to the cerebellum, and has other connections to the cortex that are important for speech production (e.g., a lesion in a cranial nerve important for speech can result in dysarthria).

The midbrain, thalamus, and hypothalamus. The midbrain, or mesencephalon, serves as a way station in the auditory and visual nervous systems, and contains the corpora

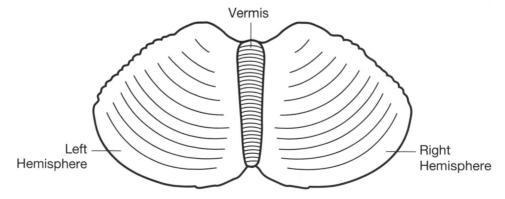

FIGURE 2.7 A superior view of the cerebellum showing the two hemispheres and the vermis.

quadrigemina (which means "the body of four parts"). There are synapses here for vision (two superior colliculi) and hearing (two inferior colliculi). The midbrain also contains the *substantia nigra*. The substantia nigra is responsible for the production of a chemical neurotransmitter called *dopamine*, which aids in motor control and muscle tone (e.g., a lesion in the substantia nigra can result in dysarthria).

The thalamus serves as a relay station for sensory information going to and from the sensory areas of the cortex, and has direct ties to cortical language and motor speech systems (Figure 2.6) (e.g., a lesion in the thalamus can result in aphasia). The hypothalamus controls aspects of emotional behavior (rage and aggression) and aids in the regulation of body temperature, food and water intake, and sexual and sleep behavior.

The Spinal Cord

In addition to the brain, the CNS also contains the spinal cord. The spinal cord extends from the skull through a large opening called the foramen magnum down to the lower back. The foramen magnum is the boundary between the medulla and the spinal cord. The spinal cord is encased in the vertebral column. A cross section of the spinal cord shows an H-shaped area of gray matter in the core of the spinal segment. The gray matter of the H shape contains motor and sensory neurons. The ventral or anterior portion of the cord conducts motor neurons, and the dorsal or posterior portion of the cord conducts sensory neurons.

The Spinal Nerves

Thirty-one pairs of spinal nerves (which along with the cranial nerves are part of the PNS) are attached to the spinal cord (Figure 2.2). The spinal cord, through these 31 pairs of nerves, relays sensory information from the receptor (e.g., skin) to the cortex for evaluation of the sensations of pain, temperature, touch, and vibration. The spinal nerves relay motor information from the CNS to the effector (e.g., muscles).

As with the cortex, the spinal cord contains gray and white matter. The gray matter contains the nerve cell bodies, and the white matter contains the ascending and descending nerve axon fibers. Ascending tracts carry sensory or afferent information, while descending tracts carry motor or efferent information.

The Reflex Arc

Occasionally, a motor response can avoid going through the higher centers of the cortex for interpretation; this shortcut is known as the *reflex arc* (**Figure 2.8**). For example, a receptor (e.g., skin) responds to pain or temperature and sends this information through an afferent

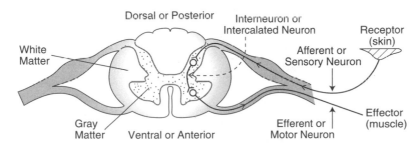

FIGURE 2.8 Cross section of the spinal cord showing the reflex arc.

(or sensory) neuron, which sends it to the dorsal (or posterior) horn (within the H shape) within the spinal cord. At this point, instead of ascending to higher centers of the cortex, the impulse travels through an interneuron (or intercalated neuron) within the spinal cord to the ventral (or anterior) horn (within the H shape). From there, the impulse descends through an efferent (or motor) neuron and into the effector (e.g., muscles), whose action will cause a hand to be removed instantaneously and without thinking from water that is too hot. This is a simplified version of a reflex arc taking place at the spinal cord level. There are different types of reflexes that can take place at different levels within the nervous system.

The Meninges

The brain and the spinal cord are protected and nourished by a system involving the meninges, ventricles, and blood supply. Protection of the brain and spinal cord starts with the hard bone of the cranium and the bony vertebral column of the spinal cord. Below the bone are three membranes called the *meninges* (**Figure 2.9**). In descending order the meninges are composed of the *dura mater* ("tough mother"), arachnoid mater ("spider mother"), and pia mater ("delicate mother").

There are several spaces that separate the meninges and provide a cushioning effect. Located between the outer bone and the dura mater is the extradural space. Located beneath the dura mater is the subdural space. Situated between the arachnoid mater and the pia mater is the subarachnoid space, which contains cerebrospinal fluid. (Physical trauma to the brain that tears or lacerates the meninges is identified as an open head injury, and can affect speech, language, or cognition.)

The Ventricles

There is a network of cavities within the brain called *ventricles* that are connected to one another by small canals and ducts (**Figure 2.10**). Cerebrospinal fluid, which is produced by the choroid plexus within each ventricle, fills all the ventricles. Through small openings in particular ventricles, cerebrospinal fluid fills the subarachnoid space of the meninges. The cerebrospinal fluid aids in the nourishment of nerve tissues, regulates intracranial pressure, removes waste products, and along with the meninges, cushions and protects the brain and spinal cord from physical trauma.

The ventricles involved are the two lateral ventricles, the third ventricle, and the fourth ventricle. Ventricular enlargement in babies not yet born is associated with in-utero stroke (Arroyo, Goldfarb, Cahill, & Schoepflin, 2010), a condition that occurs in about 1 in 4000 births. The lateral ventricle, which is paired (one in each hemisphere), is connected to the

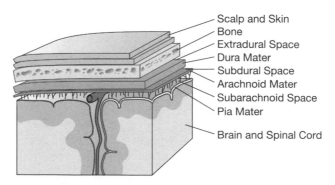

Scalp and Skin
Bone
Extradural Space
Dura Mater
Subdural Space
Arachnoid Mater
Subarachnoid Space
Pia Mater

Brain and Spinal Cord

Figure 2.9 The meninges that cover the brain and the spinal cord.

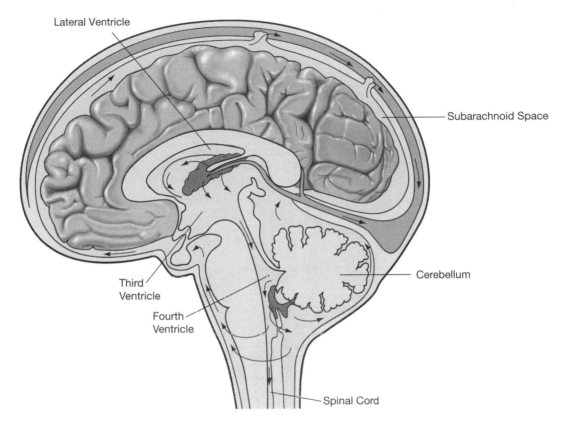

FIGURE 2.10 The ventricular system.

third ventricle through an opening called the *intraventricular foramen* (or the foramen of Monro). The third ventricle is connected to the fourth ventricle through the cerebral aqueduct (or the aqueduct of Sylvius). Congenital blockage of the cerebral aqueduct is associated with hydrocephalus in babies. The fourth ventricle leads into the subarachnoid space through the foramen of Luschka and the foramen of Magendi. Through this ventricular route, the cerebrospinal fluid flows into the brain and the spinal cord, and ultimately drains into the venous system for excretion.

The Blood Supply

Blood is composed of a liquid component called *plasma*, and solid components made up primarily of red corpuscles, white corpuscles, and platelets. Red corpuscles, which are produced in the bone marrow, are the cells that carry oxygen from the lungs to other parts of the body. For its proper nutrition and functioning, the brain needs oxygen and other elements carried by the blood. If the blood supply to the brain is stopped for five minutes or longer, cell death can occur.

Arteries carry blood away from the heart, veins carry blood toward the heart, and capillaries connect the arteries to the veins. The blood supply to the brain is as follows (**Figure 2.11**): The heart pumps blood into the aorta (major artery), which then branches off into four main arteries called the *two common carotid arteries* (one for the left side and one for the right side) and the two common subclavian arteries (one for each side). The two common carotid arteries ascend into the brain, where they divide into an internal carotid artery and an external

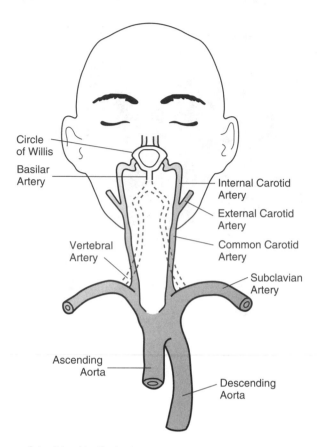

FIGURE 2.11 The major arteries supplying blood to the brain.

carotid artery on each side. The external carotid branch feeds the face area and is relatively unimportant for this review. The internal carotid branch further divides into the anterior and middle cerebral arteries (**Figure 2.12**). The anterior cerebral artery supplies the superior and anterior frontal lobes, corpus callosum, the medial surfaces of the hemispheres, and portions

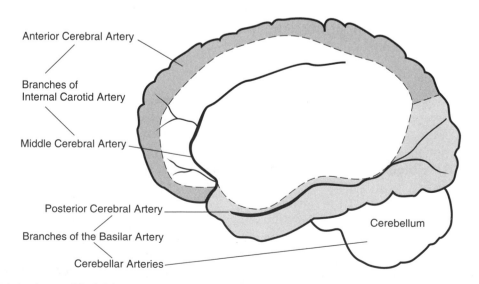

FIGURE 2.12 Lateral view of the left hemisphere showing the location of the anterior, middle, and posterior cerebral arteries.

of the subcortical areas. The middle cerebral artery supplies most of the lateral surfaces of the hemispheres and portions of the subcortical areas.

The two *common subclavian arteries* have branches called the *vertebral arteries*, which ascend into the brain. The vertebral artery branches (one from each side) join together to form the *basilar artery*. The basilar artery then ascends and divides into two *posterior cerebral arteries* (one for each hemisphere) (Figure 2.12), which supply the inferior lateral surface of the temporal lobe, and the lateral and medial surfaces of the occipital lobe. Through its branches, the basilar artery also supplies portions of the spinal cord, medulla, pons, midbrain, and cerebellum.

The circle of Willis (Figure 2.11) is formed in the brainstem by the joining together of the two internal carotid arteries and the two vertebral arteries. An interruption of the blood supply below the circle of Willis may not cause as much brain damage as lesions above the circle. The reason is that other undamaged blood channels can be utilized to feed all of the arteries below the circle. If an interruption occurs above the circle, alternative blood channels are not as readily available, and this can lead to more severe problems (e.g., a cerebrovascular accident above the circle of Willis in the middle cerebral artery can result in aphasia). Collateral circulation via the circle of Willis seems to work more efficiently in men than in women.

The Motor System for Speech

The neural motor pathways for the control of speech reside at all levels of the human nervous system and consist of the pyramidal system and the extrapyramidal system. The pyramidal system (or direct motor system) contains the corticospinal tract and the corticobulbar tract; both tracts are responsible for skilled voluntary motor movement (**Figure 2.13**). The function of the pyramidal system is primarily facilitative.

The Corticospinal Tract

The corticospinal tract, which controls skilled voluntary movements of the limbs and trunk, begins in the motor cortex or in the premotor cortex, which is a depository for information coming from various cortical and subcortical locations. The area primarily involved is the precentral gyrus (motor strip area) of the frontal lobe (Figure 2.4), and to a lesser degree, the premotor area of the frontal lobe (Figure 2.5) and the postcentral gyrus (sensory strip area) of the parietal lobe (Figure 2.4). The bilateral corticospinal tracts (Figure 2.13) descend from the cortex to a subcortical structure called the *internal capsule*, where they all converge. From the internal capsule, the tracts descend through the midbrain, the pons, and the medulla, and then to various levels of the spinal cord, where they synapse with the spinal nerves of the peripheral nervous system.

Before reaching the spinal nerves, about 85–90% of the corticospinal tracts cross over (decussate) to the other side of the body in a structure called the *upper medullary pyramids* (hence the name *pyramidal system*). (A lesion above the crossover decussation point of the medullary pyramids can result in paralysis of a limb that is contralateral [opposite side] to the site of the lesion. A lesion below the crossover point can result in paralysis of a limb ipsilateral [same side] to the site of the lesion.) The 85–90% of the corticospinal tracts that do cross over are called the *lateral corticospinal tracts*, and the 10–15% that do not cross over are called the *anterior corticospinal tracts*.

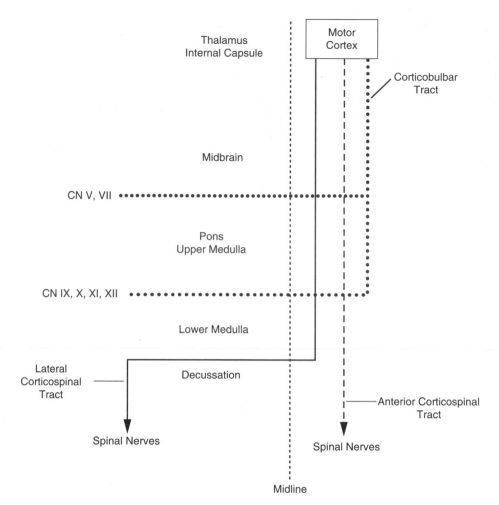

FIGURE 2.13 A schematic drawing of the pyramidal system in speech production, and the concept of the upper motor neuron (UMN) and the lower motor neuron (LMN). The pyramidal system (corticospinal and corticobulbar tracts) makes up the UMN. The cranial nerves (responsible for the innervation of the muscles used in phonation, resonance, and articulation) and the spinal nerves (responsible for the innervation of the muscles used in respiration) make up the LMN. CN = cranial nerve.

The Corticobulbar Tract

The corticobulbar tract ("bulbar," meaning "shaped like a bulb," is the old name for the medulla) controls the skilled voluntary movements of the speech muscles (except those used for respiration). The tract begins in the same area as the corticospinal tract and descends to the motor nuclei of the cranial nerves, which are located in the pons and the medulla (Figure 2.13). The corticobulbar tract has many ipsilateral and contralateral fibers, with crossover taking place at various levels of the brainstem. Because of the bilateral innervation that the corticobulbar tract produces, the majority of the midline structures work in bilateral symmetry (e.g., a unilateral lesion to the corticobulbar tract can result in a mild dysarthria because of help from the intact muscles of the other side).

The Extrapyramidal System

The extrapyramidal system (or indirect motor system) is made up of two major components— the indirect activation pathway and the control circuit areas.

The Indirect Activation Pathway

The indirect activation pathway (Duffy, 2005) consists of several short pathways that begin in the cerebral cortex and, through its connections, end in the spinal cord and in the cranial nerves. The indirect activation pathway is influenced by the basal ganglia and cerebellar control circuits, and through much of its journey it intermingles with the corticospinal and corticobulbar tracts of the pyramidal system. Its influence on the spinal nerves is more certain than its influence on the cranial nerves.

The function of the indirect activation pathway (Duffy, 2005) is that it helps regulate reflexes and maintain posture, tone, and other associated activities. This helps the direct motor system in accomplishing the appropriate speed, range, and direction of specific muscular movements (e.g., a unilateral lesion in the indirect activation pathway can result in a unilateral upper motor neuron dysarthria; bilateral lesions can result in a spastic dysarthria). The indirect activation pathway contains many tracts that are inhibitive in function.

The Control Circuits

The control circuits consist of the basal ganglia control circuit and the cerebellar control circuit (Figure 2.6). These control circuits do not have direct contact with the cranial nerve nuclei and the spinal cord, but rather have contact with the cortex, with portions of the pyramidal system and indirect activation pathways, and with themselves. The function of the control circuits is to provide information and sensory feedback to the pyramidal system and indirect activation pathways about the posture, orientation in space, tone, and physical environment in which timed and coordinated muscular movement will take place.

Motor disturbances associated with the basal ganglia control circuit are typically called *dyskinesias*, which means involuntary movement disorders. Within the dyskinesias are hypokinesia, which means too little movement (e.g., symptoms shown in hypokinetic dysarthria, associated with Parkinson disease), and hyperkinesia, which means too much movement (e.g., symptoms shown in hyperkinetic dysarthria, associated with Huntington disease).

Motor disturbances associated with the cerebellar control circuit are incoordination and hypotonia (a decrease in resistance when passive movement is performed) of muscular movements (e.g., a lesion in the cerebellar control circuit can result in ataxic dysarthria).

The Upper and Lower Motor Neurons

The Upper Motor Neuron

The upper motor neuron (UMN) pathways consist of the pyramidal system (or direct motor system), and a portion of the extrapyramidal system (or indirect motor system).

The pyramidal system contains the corticospinal tracts, which send motor impulses from the cortex to the spinal cord, and the corticobulbar tracts, which send motor impulses from the cortex to the cranial nerves located in the pons and the medulla (Figure 2.13). The portion of the extrapyramidal system that is a part of the UMN is the indirect activation pathway. The indirect activation pathway sends motor impulses from the cortex to the spinal cord, from the cortex to the cranial nerves, and from the cortex to the corticospinal and corticobulbar tracts.

The indirect activation pathway (Duffy, 2005) as part of the UMN (tracts that have direct input to the spinal nerves and the cranial nerves) is debatable because its anatomy and function are difficult to separate from the basal ganglia and cerebellar control circuits, and its input to the cranial nerves used for speech production is poorly understood. The control

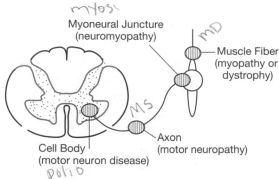

FIGURE **2.14** Lesion sites in the motor unit of the lower motor neuron: Site 1, cell body (motor neuron disease); site 2, axon (motor neuropathy); site 3, myoneural juncture (neuromyopathy); and site 4, muscle fiber (myopathy or dystrophy).

circuits do not have direct input to the spinal and cranial nerves, whereas the corticospinal, corticobulbar, and indirect activation tracts do have direct input.

The UMN pathways are contained in the CNS, and their function is to activate the lower motor neuron (LMN). Damage to the UMN can result in a spastic paralysis, which is primarily characterized by hypertonia (extreme tension of the muscles), hyperreflexia (an exaggeration of deep tendon reflexes), little or no atrophy (loss of bulk) of the musculature, and no fasciculations (fine muscle twitches). These characteristics can lead to decreased skilled movements, weakness, slowness, and reduced range of movement of the speech musculature (e.g., bilateral UMN damage can result in a spastic dysarthria).

The Lower Motor Neuron

The lower motor neuron (LMN) consists of the 31 pairs of spinal nerves and the 12 pairs of cranial nerves (Figure 2.2). The LMN pathways are activated by the UMN pathways, and then send motor impulses to the muscles for movement. The spinal nerves send motor impulses to the limbs, trunk, and the muscles used for respiration. The cranial nerves send motor impulses to the muscles of the speech mechanism (except those used for respiration).

Another name for the LMN is the *final common pathway* (FCP) because all motor activity must pass through it en route to the musculature. Damage to the LMN can result in a flaccid paralysis, which is primarily characterized by hypotonia, hyporeflexia, atrophy of the musculature, and fasciculations. Those characteristics can lead to weakness of the speech musculature. Lesions to the motor unit (**Figure 2.14**) of the LMN (spinal and cranial nerves) can occur in the cell body, in the axon leading to the muscle, at the neuromuscular junction, or in the muscle itself (e.g., bilateral damage to any portion of the motor unit can result in a flaccid dysarthria).

The Peripheral Nervous System

The peripheral nervous system (PNS) is composed of 31 pairs of spinal nerves and 12 pairs of cranial nerves (Figure 2.2).

The Spinal Nerves

The 31 pairs of spinal nerves leave the spinal cord and conduct sensory and motor impulses (functions) to and from other parts of the body (viscera, blood vessels, glands, and muscles). Each pair of spinal nerves contains a dorsal (posterior) root, which carries sensory messages through afferent fibers to the CNS, and a ventral (anterior) root, which carries motor messages through efferent fibers from the CNS.

The sensory messages (e.g., pain, touch, temperature) are passed to the thalamus, which in turn sends the messages to the sensory cortex (postcentral gyrus) for evaluation. The motor messages are sent from the CNS (corticospinal tracts) to the spinal nerves of the PNS, which in turn send the message to the muscles of the limbs and the trunk.

In descending order, the 31 pairs of spinal nerves consist of 8 pairs of cervical nerves, 12 pairs of thoracic nerves, 5 pairs of lumbar nerves, 5 pairs of sacral nerves, and 1 pair of coccygeal nerves. Portions of the thoracic division are responsible for the abdominal and intercostal muscles, and portions of the cervical division form the phrenic nerves, which are responsible for the very important diaphragm muscle. All of these muscles are involved in the respiratory component of speech production (e.g., bilateral lesions that produce significant weakness of the respiratory muscles can result in reduced loudness and reduced pitch variability, and can indirectly affect phonation [compensatory strained voice] and prosody [short phrases]).

The Cranial Nerves

There are 12 pairs of cranial nerves (one nerve of each pair on each side), although only the 7 pairs of cranial nerves most relevant for speech and hearing will be detailed here. The 7 cranial nerves involved leave the pons or the medulla and conduct sensory and/or motor impulses to and from the periphery and the CNS. Motor messages are sent from the CNS (corticobulbar tracts) to the cranial nerve nuclei located in the pons and the medulla, and then out to the musculature of the speech mechanism and other portions of the head, neck, shoulders, and the abdominal and thoracic viscera.

Sensory messages come from the periphery and go to the cranial nerve nuclei located in the pons and the medulla, from where they are forwarded to the thalamus. In turn, the thalamus sends the messages to the sensory cortex (postcentral gyrus) for evaluation. Of the seven cranial nerves most relevant for speech and hearing, only the cranial nerve responsible for hearing and balance does not follow this sensory route. The route for hearing and balance will be mentioned in another section.

Most of the cranial nerves receive bilateral neural innervation, some receive unilateral neural innervation, and some receive a mixture of bilateral and unilateral neural innervation (depending upon the branches of the cranial nerve) from the corticobulbar tract of the CNS.

A unilateral lesion affecting a cranial nerve receiving bilateral neural innervation will cause less severe speech problems than one receiving unilateral neural innervation. With bilateral tracts, the undamaged tract can compensate for the damaged one. Bilateral damage to bilateral tracts, and unilateral damage to unilateral tracts, will produce more severe speech problems.

Below is a brief outline of the cranial nerves (CNs), with expanded descriptions of those most relevant to speech production and hearing. Unless specified otherwise, sensory refers to the sensation of pain, touch, temperature, or vibration.

1. *Olfactory* (CN I; Special Sensory) functions in the special sense of smell (olfaction).
2. *Optic* (CN II; Special Sensory) functions to control visual information from the retina.
3. *Oculomotor* (CN III; Somatic Motor and Visceral Motor) functions to control muscles responsible for visual tracking or fixating on an object (somatic), and in reflexes associated with pupillary light (visceral).
4. *Trochlear* (CN IV; Somatic Motor) innervates the superior oblique muscle of the contralateral orbit, which helps in the precise movement of the eye for visual tracking or fixation.

5. *Trigeminal* (CN V; Sensory and Motor) receives sensory impulses from the jaw, lips, face, and tongue, and sends motor impulses to the jaw. Bilateral damage to the sensory function and/or the motor function can affect articulation and prosody (slow rate).
   a. *Ophthalmic nerve* carries sensory fibers from the cornea, conjunctiva, iris, lacrimal gland, upper eyelid, brow and front of the scalp, nasal mucosa, and vessels.
   b. *Maxillary nerve* conveys sensation from the lower eyelid, side of nose, upper lip, palate, upper jaw and teeth, part of buccal mucosa, nasal sinuses, nasopharynx, and from vessels and glands in its area of supply.
   c. *Mandibular nerve* carries sensory fibers from the lower jaw, teeth and overlying skin and mucosa, part of the skin and mucosa of the cheek; from the auricle and part of the external auditory meatus; from the temporal region, temporomandibular joint and masticatory muscles; from salivary glands from vessels in its area of supply; and from the anterior two-thirds of the tongue. Its *motor component* supplies muscles of mastication and tensors of the soft palate and tympanic membrane.
6. *Abducens* (CN VI; Somatic Motor) innervates the lateral rectus muscle of the ipsilateral orbit, which helps in the precise movement of the eye for visual tracking or fixation.
7. *Facial* (CN VII; Motor, Sensory, and Special Sensory) receives sensory impulses from the anterior two-thirds of the tongue (taste), soft palate (taste), and nasopharynx (taste), and sends motor impulses to the face, lips, and the stapedius muscle of the middle ear. Unilateral damage to the motor function can affect articulation (mild), and bilateral damage to the motor function can affect articulation (moderate to severe), prosody (slow rate), and facial expression (pragmatics).
   a. *Motor supply* to muscles of the face, scalp, auricle, buccinator, stapedius, stylohyoid, and posterior belly of the digastric; controls facial expression and assists in regulating movements required in speech and mastication.
   b. *Secretomotor* to the submandibular and sublingual salivary glands, to lacrimal glands, and to glands of the nasal and palatine mucosa.
   c. *Special sensory* taste fibers from the anterior two-thirds of tongue (via the chorda tympani) and soft palate (via the greater petrosal nerve).
8. *Vestibulocochlear* (CN VIII) contains a vestibular branch and a cochlear branch. The vestibular branch receives sensory impulses from the vestibular apparatus of the inner ear (responsible for equilibrium or balance) and forwards those impulses to the cerebellum and other areas to help maintain balance. The cochlear branch of this nerve receives sensory impulses from the cochlea of the inner ear (responsible for sound sensitivity) and forwards those impulses to the cochlear nuclear complex in the CNS.

After leaving the cochlear nuclear complex, most fibers then decussate and move to the superior olivary complex, which in turn sends the fibers to the medial geniculate body in the thalamus. The thalamus then sends the fibers to Heschl's gyrus (primary hearing center) in the temporal lobe of the cortex.

Unilateral damage that completely destroys the cochlea, auditory nerve, or cochlear nuclei will typically result in total deafness in that ear. Unilateral damage in the ascending auditory pathways and in the auditory cortex can result in impaired hearing but not total deafness because of bilateral auditory pathways. Hearing acuity problems can indirectly affect the speaker's loudness modulation, articulation, and prosody.

Unilateral or bilateral damage in Heschl's gyrus can result in auditory agnosia, a perceptual problem where the individual has difficulty recognizing and identifying sounds in the environment, including speech. Auditory agnosia is not due to hearing loss (hearing acuity is normal), nor aphasia (reading comprehension and oral and written expression are normal).

9. *Glossopharyngeal* (CN IX; Motor, Secretomotor, Special Sensory, and Sensory) receives sensory impulses from the posterior third of the tongue (taste and sensation) and from the pharynx, and sends motor impulses to the pharynx for dilation, contributing to the elevation and closure of the pharynx and larynx during the act of swallowing. CN IX works along with CN X, which has predominant control over laryngeal and pharyngeal sensory and motor function. Therefore, information concerning the effect on the speech mechanism is indicated under CN X.

   a. *Motor supply* to stylopharyngeus; may help innervate pharyngeal muscles.
   b. *Secretomotor* fibers promote parotid secretion and activity of mucous glands in territory of supply.
   c. *Special sensory* is the nerve of taste for posterior third of the tongue, including numerous taste buds in vallate papillae.
   d. *Sensory* fibers convey ordinary sensation from pharynx, pharyngeal part of tongue, fauces, tonsil, tympanic cavity, auditory tube, and mastoid cells. Chief nerve supply of carotid body and sinus.

10. *Vagus* (CN X; Motor, Sensory, and Special Sensory) receives sensory impulses from the larynx, pharynx, soft palate, and thoracic and abdominal viscera, and sends motor impulses to the larynx, pharynx, soft palate, and visceral organs. Unilateral damage to the motor function can affect phonation (reduced loudness, short phrases, breathiness, reduced pitch range, hoarseness, diplophonia), resonance (mild hypernasality, nasal emission), and prosody (short phrases). Bilateral damage can affect phonation (short phrases, reduced loudness, breathiness, aphonia, inhalatory stridor, hoarseness, reduced pitch range), resonance (moderate to severe hypernasality, nasal emission), articulation (weak pressure consonants), and prosody (short phrases, slow rate).

   a. *Motor* fibers innervate intrinsic laryngeal muscles and help to supply pharyngeal constrictors. Provide parasympathetic supply to heart and its vessels, to trachea and bronchi, to alimentary canal from pharynx almost to left colic (splenic) flexure and to its associated glands.
   b. *Somatic sensory* fibers supply meninges of posterior cranial fossa and parts of auricle, external acoustic meatus, and tympanic membrane.
   c. *Special sensory* fibers carry some taste impulses from epiglottis and valleculae.

The vagus is sometimes called a *vagabond*, because of its travels from the brainstem around the thoracic cavity. The anatomy of the vagus falsifies the neurochronaxic theory of phonation, introduced in 1950 by Raoul Husson (Weiss, 1959). According to this theory, a vibratory cycle is initiated by a separate nerve impulse to the vocalis muscle via the recurrent laryngeal branch of the vagus nerve. The frequency of one's voice would depend upon the rate of impulses delivered. Because the recurrent laryngeal branch has to loop around the aorta, it is longer on the left side, so bilateral innervation to the left and right portions of the vocalis muscle would be out of phase.

11. *Spinal accessory* (CN XI) contains a spinal and cranial root. The spinal portion sends motor impulses to the neck and the shoulder. Unilateral or bilateral damage to the motor function can cause neck turning and shoulder elevation problems, which may indirectly affect respiration, phonation, and resonance. The cranial portion sends motor impulses to the soft palate, pharynx, and larynx. CN XI works along with CN X, which has predominant control over palatal, pharyngeal, and laryngeal motor

function. Therefore, information concerning the effect on the speech mechanism is indicated under CN X.

12. *Hypoglossal* (CN XII) receives sensory and taste impulses from the tongue, and sends motor impulses to the tongue. Unilateral damage to the motor function can affect articulation (mild). Bilateral damage can affect articulation (mild to severe) and prosody (slow rate). Descending branch (not connected to hypoglossal nucleus) consists of fibers from C1, which join fibers from C2 and C3 to form ansa cervicalis; ansa supplies twigs to sternohyoid, sternothyroid, and omohyoid muscles.

The 12 cranial nerves, their general function, and, if damaged, their effects on the respiration, phonation, resonance, articulation, and prosody components of speech production are listed in **Table 2.1**. An old jingle to help remember the cranial nerves is "<u>O</u>n <u>o</u>ld <u>O</u>lympus'

TABLE 2.1

The 12 Cranial Nerves and, If Damaged, Their Effect on Speech Production

Cranial Nerve	Function	Effect on Speech Production
I Olfactory	s: smell	____
	m: ____	____
II Optic	s: vision	____
	m: ____	____
III Oculomotor	s: ____	____
	m: eye movement	____
IV Trochlear	s: ____	____
	m: eye movement	____
V Trigeminal	s: jaw, lips, face, tongue	Indirect—articulation
	m: jaw	Articulation, prosody
VI Abducens	s: ____	____
	m: eye movement	____
VII Facial	s: tongue, soft palate, nasopharynx	____
	m: face, lips, stapedius (middle ear)	Articulation, prosody, facial expression
VIII Vestibulocochlear	s: vestibular—balance	____
	s: cochlear—hearing	Indirect—loudness, modulation, Articulation, prosody
	m: ____	____
IX Glossopharyngeal	s: tongue, pharynx	____
	m: pharynx[a], larynx[a]	Phonation, resonance
X Vagus	s: larynx, pharynx, soft palate, thoracic and abdominal viscera	____
	m: larynx, pharynx, soft palate	Phonation, resonance, articulation, prosody
XI Spinal accessory	s: ____	
	m: spinal—neck, shoulder	Indirect—respiration, phonation, resonance
	m: cranial—soft palate[a], pharynx[a], larynx[a]	phonation, resonance
XII Hypoglossal	s: tongue	____
	m: tongue	Articulation, prosody

Note: s = sensory, m = motor.
[a]Along with cranial nerve X.

towering tops, a Finn and German viewed some hops." The first letter of each word represents the first letter of each name of the cranial nerves. Actually, the name change of CN VIII (from "acoustic" to "vestibulocochlear") means that the word "and" in the jingle above needs to be changed to a word beginning with "v." There is also a much racier version, which we will not print here.

The Neurosensory System

The neurosensory system is found in all the major levels of the human nervous system. Of vital importance for speech and hearing are the sensory pathways of general somatic functioning, the cranial nerves, vision and hearing, and the control circuits.

The General Somatic Pathways

The general somatic (pain, touch, temperature, and proprioception) sensory pathways dealing with the limbs and the trunk employ the spinal cord and spinal nerves. The somatic sensory pathways involved with the head and speech mechanism employ the cranial nerves (except for the process of respiration, which employs the spinal nerves). The sensory impulse from the periphery (e.g., skin of the arm or leg) is mediated and passed to the spinal nerves through the dorsal (posterior) portion of the cell body. From there, the sensory impulse moves through spinothalamic tracts to the thalamus, then through thalamocortical tracts to the internal capsule, and then onto the somatosensory area of the parietal lobe (postcentral gyrus, or "sensory strip" area). Sensory information about proprioception is needed so that adjustments and compensations can take place when necessary (e.g., speaking immediately after dental work, talking with food in your mouth, talking after biting your tongue or cheek, etc.).

The Vision and Hearing Pathways

The neurosensory system also contains special pathways used for vision and hearing. The visual system, under the mediation of the optic nerve (CN II), starts with the eye's absorbing light from an image, then sends the image through to the pupil. The image is then inverted and reversed as it travels into the lens. The lens focuses and projects the light onto the retina, which is a formation of nerve cells lining the inside of the eyeball. The retina sends the visual impulse to the optic nerve (this can be seen with an ophthalmoscope), which then sends it to the optic chiasma (a junction of the right and left optic nerves). At the optic chiasma, many of the fibers decussate and then move on to the lateral geniculate body of the thalamus, which then sends the fibers through the internal capsule. From there, the visual impulse is sent to the primary center for vision and the visual association areas of the occipital lobe. (Lesions of the optic nerve and the primary visual cortex can result in blindness. Lesions in the visual association cortex can result in visual perceptual problems [visual agnosia], and play a role in reading comprehension deficit [alexia].)

The neurosensory pathway used for hearing has already been noted in the section dealing with cranial nerves (under CN VIII). It is apparent that auditory and visual information is vital for the production of speech and language. The auditory system is crucial, and the visual system is quite important, in the acquisition of speech and language. The auditory system helps maintain these faculties throughout life.

The Control Circuits

The neural information that the basal ganglia and cerebellar control circuits give to the direct and indirect activation systems for their functioning rely on the masses of constant and instantaneous sensory information received from the periphery (e.g., proprioception).

The Autonomic Nervous System

The autonomic nervous system (ANS), which controls involuntary activity of the body, consists of a sympathetic and a parasympathetic division. The ANS is self-regulating and is present throughout the CNS and the PNS.

The sympathetic division is responsible for such activities as speeding up the heart rate, constricting the peripheral blood vessels, elevating blood pressure, raising the eyelids, redistributing blood, dilating the pupils, and decreasing contractions of the intestines. This division makes internal adjustments and alerts the body to cope with stress and crises (e.g., dilates the pupils of the eyes to allow more light to enter for better sight, distributes blood from the intestines to the skeletal muscles for strength, etc.).

The parasympathetic division is responsible for such activities as slowing down the heart rate, increasing contractions of the intestines, increasing salivation, and increasing secretions of the glands in the gastrointestines. This division is responsible for reducing internal activity and calming down the body (e.g., for digestion and bowel movement, sexual activity, etc.).

The ANS works along with the endocrine system (glands and other structures that release internal secretions called hormones) to maintain homeostasis (stability of the body's internal environment). All activity to maintain homeostasis is regulated by the hypothalamus in the CNS.

The ANS has an indirect effect upon speech and language, such as the nervousness (blushing, blanching, heart pounding, sweating, dry mouth, or jittery stomach) that one may feel before, during, or after certain speaking situations (e.g., speaking before an audience, a marriage proposal, playacting in a speaking role, social conversation during a blind date, etc.).

The Triune Brain

The triune brain is an integration–elaboration concept of neuroevolution. The brain, according to McLean (1978), is composed of *three* brains, only one of which, the neocortex, is responsible for human walking and talking behaviors. Each brain represents a major evolutionary stage and may be differentiated neuroanatomically and functionally.

The *neural chassis*, the foundation for the three brains, is the oldest part. It is composed of the spinal cord, medulla, and pons (hindbrain), and the midbrain. Basic neural mechanisms for reproduction and self-preservation, including regulation of the heart, circulation, and respiration, are contained here. The neural chassis represents almost all of the brain in a fish or amphibian.

According to McLean, this neural chassis has three drivers:

R-Complex: This is composed of the olfactostriatum, corpus striatum, and globus pallidus. It is important in aggressive behavior, territoriality, ritual, and in the establishment of social hierarchies.

Limbic System: This includes the olfactory cortex, thalamus, hypothalamus, amygdala, pituitary gland, and hippocampus. It is involved in generating strong emotions (as opposed to the reptilian mind). Rage, fear, or sentimentality have been observed in malfunctions of the limbic system. The beginnings of altruistic behavior may be here. Emotional aspects of smell (olfactory cortex), remembering and recall (hippocampus), oral and gustatory functions, and sexual functions are also related to the limbic system.

Bhatnagar (2008) has noted that the major structures of the limbic system are the amygdale, the hippocampus, the septal nuclei, and the cingulated gyrus. The only structure not involved in memory and learning is the cingulated gyrus. The limbic system regulates emotion, motivation, learning, and memory. Limbic projections to the forebrain contribute to emotions and provide motivation for behaviors that are fundamental to survival (feeding,

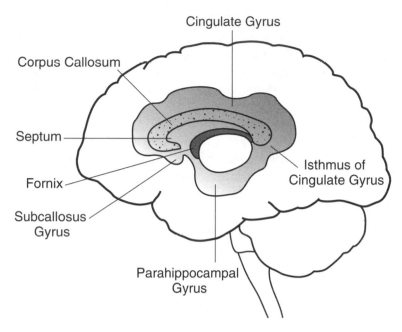

FIGURE 2.15 Midsaggital view showing the limbic structures.

mating, aggression, and flight). With connections into the prefrontal lobe and hippocampus, the limbic structures also participate in memory and learning (see **Figures 2.15** and **2.16**).

Neocortex: This includes the frontal, parietal, temporal, and occipital lobes. It mediates characteristically human cognitive functions. The various subdivisions may have different functions and some may share functions.

    a. *Frontal lobes*: deliberation and regulation of action.
    b. *Parietal lobes*: spatial perception and the exchange of information between the brain and the rest of the body.

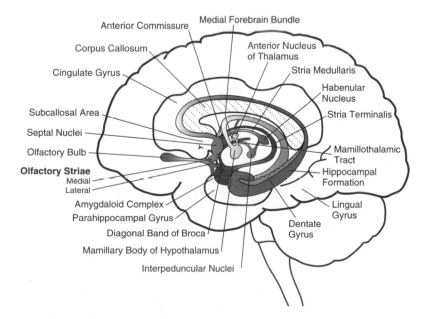

FIGURE 2.16 Medial view of the major limbic structures and their connections.

    c. *Temporal lobes*: complex perceptual tasks.

    d. *Occipital lobes*: vision, the dominant sense in humans and other primates. Frontal lobes may have been responsible for the human bipedal posture, which, in turn, freed our hands and mouths. Sections of the frontal lobes and the temporoparietal region in conjunction with various thalamic nuclei are responsible for spoken language.

Integration–Elaboration Concept

The triune brain model suggests the progressive incorporation of lower brains by higher ones and the subsequent control, modification, and elaboration of all behaviors associated with earlier or lower brains by the highest or latest-to-evolve brain.

Reflexization of Movement

Reflexes form the basis of voluntary movements. Basic respiratory activities of coughing, sobbing, sighing, and yawning; the laryngeal or glottic closing reflex; the rooting reflex; the lip reflex; the mouth-opening reflex; basic biting, suckling, chewing patterns; and suckling, swallowing, pharyngeal, palatal, and yawn reflexes may all be viewed as precursory patterns to prelinguistic phonatory and articulatory patterns, and, finally, to skilled speech movements.

That is, from these basic reflexive movements emerge, respectively, skilled movements necessary for speech breathing; speech voicing; speaker-listener postural attitudes; labial sounds; mandibular sounds; linguadental, lingua-aleolar, linguapalatal, and linguavelar sounds; and for producing nasal/non-nasal sound distinctions.

Phylogenesis of Humans and Speech

Speech phylogenesis is related to the development of the bipedal posture, manual dexterity, the liberation of the mouth from use in crude grasping and manipulative activities, and the development of the communisphere. The ontogenetic reflection of this phyletic heritage is noted when observing the development of true speech in the infant. True speech development in the infant approximately co-occurs with the development of bipedal head, neck, and trunk balance; the use of a preferred hand; the integration of various cranio-oropharyngeal reflexes such as protective, feeding, and emotional reflexes; and the growing need to communicate.

Advanced Study

Translational research refers to original investigations in the broad fields of laboratory, clinical, and public health research, and is interdisciplinary and cross disciplinary in scope. The goal is to expedite the translation of scientific discovery into new or improved standards of care. Some medical journals devoted to translational research began publishing articles in this field more than 10 years ago.

Our profession is somewhat behind the curve with regard to translational research, although there certainly have been efforts in this direction by individuals. The term "aphasiologist" may refer to a physician (usually a neurologist), neurolinguist, neuropsychologist, speech-language pathologist, or other professional. They may have different perspectives on aphasia, but may work together to test hypotheses. For example, localizing brain functions has been typically supported by evidence of shared areas of brain damage in individuals with a similar language deficit, and is sometimes called the "lesion overlap" approach. That is, if there is a functional deficit, then the area of the brain damaged in most of these individuals must have been responsible for that function. When the reciprocal association (the probability that the lesion caused the deficit) is evaluated, then the relationship may not be supported.

Hypoperfusion (reduced blood flow) does not necessarily specify the area of infarct. For example, structural damage or low blood flow in the left posterior inferior frontal gyrus may result in poor drainage into the anterior insula. Reperfusion of the anterior insula will not relieve symptoms of apraxia of speech, a motor programming speech disorder associated with left frontal lobe damage (Hillis et al., 2004).

A recent paper (Goldfarb & Davis, 2010) proposes oceanographic models for measuring regional cerebral blood flow (rCBF). It may be possible to measure blood flow in the middle cerebral artery by applying the acoustic Doppler profiler technique used to measure ocean currents. Accommodations for dune troughs that complicate measurement of ocean currents may provide a model for measuring arterial blood flow, complicated by arteriosclerotic disease.

CLINICAL DESCRIPTION

One of the authors established a stroke club at a Veterans Administration Extended Care Center. The purpose of the club was to provide communication and recreational opportunities for a group of people with aphasia and dysarthria who were no longer eligible for traditional speech-language therapy. About 20–30 men (very few women were patients in the facility) attended a 2-hour meeting each week, while their caretakers were invited to attend a support group led by an SLP and a clinical psychologist.

Accommodating a large group of wheelchair-borne individuals threatened to become a demolition derby. Even though all furniture was cleared out of the waiting room, the men with left-hemisphere CVA (and right-homonymous hemianopsia) often bumped their wheelchairs into those of the men with right-hemisphere CVA (and left visual field neglect). Seating was arranged in several small circles, with chairs set at about 45-degree angles from each other. (See the following chapter for a transcript and analysis of a conversation between one stroke club member with fluent aphasia and another with nonfluent aphasia.)

Food and drinks had to be sugar-free (for those with Type II diabetes) and salt-free (for those with hypertension), and closely monitored for those individuals with dysphagia. Many of the individuals with difficulty or pain/discomfort when swallowing did not cough when fluids escaped into the trachea, nor did they exhibit a gurgly voice when food or fluids escaped into the valleculae. These "silent aspirators" in particular needed supervision for each swallow.

Among the humbling experiences the authors can report in their many years of clinical intervention, one remains crystal clear. The wife of one of the veterans asked to speak to the author privately, as she did not want to raise this issue in the communication support group for caretakers. The conversation went something like this (W is the wife and A is the author):

W: This is uncomfortable for me to say, but I'm having problems with marital relations with my husband.

A: That's not at all unusual. Let me refer you to the urologist in the hospital.

W: No, no, he's functioning fine.

A: It's not at all unusual for there to be anxiety. Would you like to talk to Dr. P., the psychologist in our support group?

W: No, no, it's about communication.

A: (Realizing there is no longer any way he can pass this along) OK, I'm listening.

W: When we had relations before, he always used to say the most wonderful things to me, but now that he can't talk, it feels so different.

A: There are many ways to communicate. Sometimes a gesture or a facial expression can be as meaningful as a word.

W: But I can't see any of that when it's completely dark in the room.

Sometimes the job of the SLP is to help the patient and communicative partner turn on the light of communication, either figuratively or, as in the present example, literally.

Discussion Questions: Theory

1. What is involved in responding to auditory feedback from oneself or from others?

2. How is information transmitted to and away from a brain cell body?

3. What are some multipotential functions of glial cells?

4. How does the anatomy of the vagus nerve (CN X) falsify the neurochronaxic theory of phonation?

5. Use the triune brain model to explain how an infantile suckle reflex may be integrated and elaborated to become /w/ and /u/ sounds in healthy speakers, but released following brain trauma.

Discussion Questions: Therapy

1. How does language improvement in spontaneous recovery from stroke occur?

2. How does language therapy for aphasia facilitate rewiring of brain connections which have been "stunned" following a stroke?

3. A major goal of Lee Silverman Voice Therapy (LSVT) is to have the individual with Parkinson disease think about speaking loudly. How is the brain involved in achieving this goal?

4. Speech therapy for individuals with dysarthria often focuses on improving precision of articulation by developing procedural or muscle memory. What is the neural mechanism underlying this therapy?

5. Augmentative/alternative communication devices using eye tracking may be effective when used with an individual with "locked-in syndrome" following a brainstem stroke. These devices may have been helpful for the late Jean-Dominique Bauby, whose case of locked-in syndrome was described in *The Diving Bell and the Butterfly*. Explain how cranial nerves involved in moving the eyeballs may still function following brainstem stroke.

Assignment: Write a multiple-choice question with five options. Explain why the key option is correct, and why the distractors or decoys are incorrect. Avoid using forms such as, "All of the following are (in)correct *except*" in the stem, and "All (or none) of the above" in the options.

Example: After a CVA (stroke), some cells, not seriously damaged, may respond to natural recovery processes and survive: organelles resume their normal appearance (swelling recedes), and the nucleus assumes a central location. This process follows:

a. Wallerian degeneration

b. Neuroglial responses

c. Stenosis

d. Stunning

e. Axonal reaction

The correct answer is *d*: stunning is associated with spontaneous recovery; *a* is incorrect because, in a Wallerian reaction, there is degeneration of the axonal part that is separate from its cell body; *b* is incorrect because glial cells displace presynaptic and postsynaptic terminals and cell bodies, impairing transmission between neurons; *c* is incorrect because stenosis relates to narrowing of arteries; *e* is incorrect because damaged neurons do not reconnect to the distal axonal segments to reinnervate their target structures.

References

Arroyo, C., Goldfarb, R., Cahill, D., & Schoepflin, J. (2010). AAC interventions: Case study of in-utero stroke. *Journal of Speech-Language Pathology and Applied Behavior Analysis, 5*, 32–47.

Bhatnagar, S. C. (2008). *Neuroscience for the study of communicative disorders* (3rd ed.). Philadelphia, PA: Lippincott Williams & Wilkins.

Damasio, A. (1994). *Descartes' error*. New York, NY: G.P. Putnam's Sons.

Duffy, J. R. (2005). *Motor speech disorders: Substrates, differentiald diagnosis and management* (2nd ed.). St. Louis, MO: Elsevier Mosby.

Goldfarb, R., & Davis, R. (2010). Oceans of the brain. *Journal of Experimental Stroke and Translational Medicine, 3*, 22–26.

Hillis, A. E., Work, M., Barker, P. B., Jacobs, M. A., Breese, E. L., & Maurer, K. (2004). Re-examining the brain regions crucial for orchestrating speech articulation. *Brain, 127*, 1479–1487.

Kent, R. (1997). *The speech sciences*. San Diego, CA: Singular.

McLean, P. D. (1978). A mind of three minds: Educating the triune brain. In J. S. Chall & A. F. Mirsky (Eds.), *Education and the brain: The seventy-seventh yearbook of the National Society for the Study of Education* (pp. 308–342). Chicago, IL: University of Chicago Press.

Webb, W. G., & Adler, R. K. (2008). *Neurology for the speech-language pathologist* (5th ed.). St. Louis, MO: Mosby Elsevier.

Webster, D. (1999). *Neuroscience of communication*. San Diego, CA: Singular.

Weiss, D. (1959). Discussion of the neurochronaxic theory (Husson). *AMA Archives of Otolaryngology, 70*, 607–618.

Zemlin, W. (1998). *Speech and hearing science: Anatomy and physiology*. Needham Heights, MA: Allyn & Bacon.

Aphasia

Definition

Aphasia can be defined as a multi-modality language disturbance (of the person's regular language of communication) due to brain damage. The language modalities involved are auditory comprehension, reading comprehension, oral expression, and written expression. Typically, the language components that are disturbed are the phonologic (sound system), the morphologic and syntactic (grammar), and the semantic (meaning).

The language component most preserved in aphasia is the pragmatic (social use). The wife of a severely impaired adult with aphasia who was wheelchair-borne once told the authors that the grandchildren didn't think anything was wrong with Grandpa. At first glance, the grandchildren noticed the wheelchair and that Grandpa wasn't talking very much. In a split second, Grandpa beckoned the kids with his left hand, his facial expressions, and his general warmth. In no time, the kids were on his lap, and he was hugging and kissing and communicating with them as he usually did.

Aphasia is not caused by a motor problem affecting the person's ability to speak (e.g., paralysis of the lips), by a sensory problem affecting the ability to hear (e.g., hearing loss), or by a thought disorder affecting the ability to speak or listen (e.g., dementia). To be diagnosed as having aphasia, the person's language disturbance has to stand out in relation to the other problems. For instance, the patient with schizophrenia may have language symptoms in common with those of aphasia (see, for example, DiSimoni, Darley, & Aronson, 1977; Halpern & McCartin-Clark, 1984). However, this patient is not identified as having aphasia because of the other apparent behavioral, thought-related, social, and communicative problems caused by schizophrenia.

Is aphasia language without thought or thought without language? This question, raised more than 30 years ago by Wepman (1976), follows the concept of brain function relating to thought as being nonverbal as well as verbal, the former preceding the latter in development and use. The interdependence of aphasia and various aspects of intelligence are seen as playing a prominent role. Treatment should involve thought-provoking therapy rather than the usual sole concern with direct use of language. This opens the way to treatment of the whole person in recovery from aphasia.

We have noted aphasia to be an impairment of the acquired capacity to comprehend and use verbal symbols for interpersonal communication. We may consider intelligence to be an innate capacity to use one's thought processes. This innate capacity includes the ability to adapt to life situations; to symbolize both verbally and nonverbally at levels of both concrete and abstract operations; to preplan actions; to comprehend both verbal and nonverbal stimuli; and to integrate feelings, attitudes, and emotional states into thoughts.

The literature in both areas, aphasia and intelligence, has addressed the two extremes that language is identical to thought, or that language and thought are independent characteristics of human behavior. Some investigators have held that intelligence suffers because language is impaired, while others claim that language is disturbed because of the intellectual disorder. The middle ground position is that language use is inextricably related to thought, but is not identical with it. Language is the product of thought; thought is our highest mental process, and language is its servant. The ability to think is innate in humans, but language is acquired. According to Wepman (1976), and Piaget before him (1966), language is not the source of logic, but is structured by logic. Without thought there would be no meaningful language. Language without thought would be the kind of repetition observed in some types of birds whose utterances, regardless of their content, mean only, "Give me food."

Is aphasia a reduction of efficiency or a loss of language? According to a classic text on aphasia (Schuell, Jenkins, & Jimenez-Pabon, 1964), all aphasias are part of a general hierarchy of language deficit. Conditions such as "pure word deafness," "pure word blindness," "expressive aphasia," and "receptive aphasia" do not exist independently of a general language deficit. The polytypic nature of aphasia (Schwartz, 1984) highlights the limitations of classifications that require separate groupings and imply independence of individual language functions. Virtually all aphasias involve reduction of available vocabulary, linguistic rules, and verbal retention span, as well as impaired comprehension and production of messages.

Language is the result of the dynamic interaction of complex cerebral and subcortical organizations. It may not be possible to separate the various elements of language neuropsychologically. Indeed, attempts to correlate the aphasias to lesions viewed through computerized tomography (CT) failed about one-sixth of the time (Basso, Lecours, Moraschini, & Vanier, 1985).

Communication problems of adults with aphasia seem to be more related to linguistic performance (actual acts of speaking and hearing, with temporal limitations, subject to a variety of distractions) than to linguistic competence (underlying set of rules for syntax, meaning, and sound that makes performance possible). Auditory processes are the most important of the interacting systems that aid in the acquisition, processing, and control of language. After all, humans learn oral language by listening to it, not by looking at it. Deaf children need special instruction to learn oral language, but blind children often do not.

The adult with aphasia does not, except in the most severe cases, lose the ability to comprehend and use language, but may lose the ability to comprehend and use it in certain ways. It is the speech-language pathologist's task to increase efficiency of residual language abilities.

Symptoms

Auditory Comprehension Deficit

Difficulty in the comprehension of spoken language is generally known as *auditory comprehension deficit*. The deficit is linguistic in nature and is not due to perceptual factors (see Gandour, Holasuit Petty, & Dardarananda, 1988) or attentional factors (see Wiegersma, Post, Veldhuijsen, & DeVries, 1988). Wright and Shisler (2005) provided a review and discussion of working memory theories that have been influential in the aphasia literature, research findings of working memory in aphasia, and assessment measures, and how they relate to language comprehension and production in aphasia.

Neglect, also known as *hemispatial inattention*, is a condition that causes difficulty in receiving sensory stimuli (auditory, visual, tactile) in the field opposite to the involved hemisphere. A major cause of neglect is damage to the parietal lobe or occasionally damage to other cortical or subcortical areas. Neglect problems are far greater after right—rather than left hemisphere damage (Myers & Blake, 2008). Because most cases of aphasia are caused by left hemisphere damage, the chance of neglect is not great. However, further compounding the problem, some measure of neglect (Benson & Ardilla, 1996) and/or attention allocation deficits (King & Hux, 1996; Murray, Holland, & Beeson, 1997; Murray & Holland, 1998; Tseng, McNeil, & Molenkovic, 1993) may exist with some patients who have aphasia. For further discussion of neglect and attention see the sections on communication disorders associated with right hemisphere damage and those associated with traumatic brain injury.

The individual with auditory comprehension deficit may have difficulty in understanding the following:

1. Abstract words as opposed to concrete words (e.g., *The Big Apple* vs. *apple*)
2. Longer words as opposed to shorter words
3. Infrequently used words compared with frequently used words (e.g., *domicile* vs. *house*)
4. Closely associated words (e.g., *banana* and *apple*)
5. Word forms involving tense, pluralization, prefixes, suffixes, possessives, comparatives, and grammatical class
6. Sentences that are long or grammatically complex (word order) or include several ideas

The patient can have a reduced auditory retention span (Halpern, Darley, & Brown, 1973) and a general slowness of comprehension. Brookshire (1974) has noted that some patients have a "slow rise time" where they miss the beginning of a sentence; some have a "noise buildup" where they miss the end of a sentence; some have an "information capacity deficit" where an increase in sentence length brings a decrease in performance; and some have "intermittent auditory imperception" where the patient's understanding of auditory input fluctuates.

Some factors that aid the patient with auditory comprehension deficit are as follows:

1. Pauses and imposed delays in the right spots will help the patient.
2. Stressed words are easier to comprehend, or as Kimelman (1991) noted, the words prior to the stressed word may be the important factor.
3. Vocabulary related to work, family, functional use, and recreation is easier.
4. The speaker's facial expressions, tone of voice, and use of gestures all aid the patient's comprehension. The use of a conversational tone in the form of a question will be better understood than a direct command (e.g., "Can I use your phone?" instead of "Point to the phone," or "What time is it?" instead of "Point to your watch.").
5. Tompkins (1991) has noted that patients with aphasia retain knowledge of emotional meanings, and Reuterskiold (1991) found that participants with aphasia had better auditory comprehension on emotional words than on nonemotional words.

Schulte and Brandt (1989) have reviewed some nonlinguistic factors that play a role in auditory comprehension deficit. They are (1) fatigue—the more tired the patient, the poorer the response, (2) scheduling—earlier in the day is better, (3) medication—side effects come into play, (4) illness—the healthier patient does better, (5) hearing loss and words that sound alike (e.g., *neck* and *leg, hair* and *ear*)—these can interfere with comprehension, and

(6) emotional status and psychological factors—negativity and self-isolation can interfere with comprehension.

Typically, incidence of the syndrome called *clinical depression* is not high in aphasia (Damecour & Caplan, 1991). However, it is not uncommon for the patient to feel depressed under the combined burdens of a communication problem, a physical problem, and loss of status as breadwinner and/or homemaker (Benson & Ardilla, 1996; Mlcoch & Metter, 2008; J. Sarno, 1991; Swindell & Hammons, 1991).

According to Code, Hemsley, and Herrmann (1999), emotional stability involves a continuum whereby at the beginning, neurochemical changes resulting from the brain lesion play a major role. After a period of time when the brain has stabilized, along with the intake of antidepressant medication it may produce another emotional set.

Reading Comprehension Deficit

Alexia refers to an acquired impairment in reading comprehension due to brain damage. Many of the same disturbances that apply to auditory comprehension deficit can be observed in alexia, except that here the difficulty is in reading comprehension. Instead of confusing closely associated words that the patient hears (e.g., *banana* and *apple*), as in auditory comprehension deficit, the adult with aphasia will confuse closely associated words that are in printed or written form.

Reading comprehension is not a person's ability to read out loud. Reading aloud is going from one modality (visual) to another (speaking), with or without comprehension. For example, the authors can read aloud a word, sentence, or paragraph in Spanish or German, with all the proper pronunciations and rhythms of the language; in some cases they will understand what is being read and in other cases they will not.

Benson (1979), Benson and Ardila (1996), and Brookshire (2007) have described three types of alexia that are based upon the neuroanatomical site of the lesion. One type called *parietal-temporal alexia* (alexia with agraphia) is associated with the fluent aphasias. The chief characteristics are the almost total loss of reading comprehension and written expression. A second type called *frontal alexia* is associated with the nonfluent aphasias. The chief characteristic is the ability to understand single words more easily than sentences. A third type called *occipital alexia* is not associated with other language problems. The major characteristic is the inability to comprehend through reading, while other language modalities are normal. Written expression is preserved, but the patient cannot understand through reading what was just written correctly.

Oral Expression Deficit

Difficulty in the formulation of spoken language is called an *oral expression deficit*. The problem is most likely influenced by the same factors cited under auditory comprehension deficit, and manifests itself as the following:

1. A reduced vocabulary with infrequent words mostly gone.
2. Jargon, which can be unintelligible words that usually follow the phonological rules of our language (e.g., "freach") or unintelligible words that bear no relationship to the stimulus.

    If consistent sound combinations occur that do not follow our phonemic rules, another language may be in the background of the patient. If one listens closely to jargon, one may detect whether some amount of auditory or reading comprehension is taking place. For example, when one patient was asked, "Where is your wife?" he responded with "she" in the middle of a good deal of jargon. Another, when asked, "How's the weather?" responded with jargon and "outside." Another, when asked if he was going outside, responded with jargon and "car" and "walking." Another, when asked if he would be eating soon, responded with jargon and "lunch."

3. Reduced fluency (nonfluent) or excessive fluency (fluent), determined by the number of words spoken, although the number of different words divided by the total number of words spoken (type–token ratio) may be a small fraction in both cases.

4. Circumlocutions, which can be empty speech (e.g., "The thing that's on the thing with the thing there"), a description of the use or function of the item to be named (e.g., "You carry it" or "It has handles" for *bag*), or using a word that is correct semantically and syntactically but is not in common usage (e.g., in response to, "We sleep in a _____," one patient said "tent" and another said "building"; in response to "There is someone at the _____," a patient replied, "window").

5. Neologisms, which are made up of new words, expressions, or usages that are understandable (e.g., "skymobile" for *airplane*, "windglass" for *window*, "chead" for *chin*, "inkpencil" for *pen*).

6. A semantic error or a verbal paraphasia, which represent confusion with closely associated words (e.g., "driving range" for *parking lot*); there are also literal or phonemic paraphasias, described in #7, below.

   The confusion can occur with words in the same category (e.g., "chair" for *table*), through description of use (e.g., "it sleep" for *bed*), with opposites (e.g., "no" for *yes*), through visual spatial contiguity (saying the name of an object or picture that is visually adjacent to the intended stimulus, e.g., in response to a picture of a train passing through fields, with a cow in sight, the patient says, "cow" for *train*), or through visual perception confusion (e.g., "fan" for *windmill*).

7. Articulation errors.

   The misarticulation can be a substitution, omission, distortion, or addition of a sound. A substitution error is the production of a different standard sound in our language for the target (correct) sound (e.g., "thing" for *sing*). An omission error is leaving out the target sound completely (e.g., "ing" for *sing*). A distortion error is producing a nonstandard sound in our language for the target sound (e.g., a lateral emission /s/ for sing). An addition error is the production of an extra sound to the target sound (e.g., "suhing" for *sing*).

   The articulation error can be at the *phonetic level,* where the sound as part of the word has been retrieved but there is a mechanical problem in producing it. This type of error typically can be found in patients with Broca's aphasia, apraxia of speech, dysarthria, or any combination of those disorders. The articulation error can be at the *phonemic* level, where the sound as part of the word is still in the process of being retrieved. This type of error, also called a *literal* or *phonemic paraphasia* (e.g., saying *corned beef and garbage,* or saying *fable, sable,* or *cable* for *table*), typically can be found in patients with conduction or Wernicke's aphasia (for further elaboration, see the rest of this section and the sections on dysarthria and apraxia of speech). Finally, there are patients with aphasia who produce few or no phonetic or phonemic articulation errors (see Darley, 1982; Halpern, Keith, & Darley, 1976).

8. Grammatical errors.

   Grammar represents the form and structure of language and is composed of the phonologic, morphologic, and syntactic aspects of language. The phonologic aspect has been noted previously, under "articulation errors." *Morphology* is the system that governs the structure of words and the construction of word forms. *Syntax* is the system that governs the combination of words to form sentences, and the relationship among the elements within a sentence in order to convey meaning. Errors at the morphologic level can involve confusion with tense, pluralization, prefixes, suffixes, possessives, comparatives, and grammatical class. Errors at the syntactic level can involve confusion with word order in producing phrases and sentences.

In the language of aphasia, the words *agrammatism* and *syntactic error* have been used interchangeably to describe morphologic (word) and syntactic (sentence) errors, and the word *paragrammatism* has been used to describe syntactic errors. Agrammatism, associated with nonfluent or Broca's aphasia, is characterized by omission of function words, while paragrammatism, associated with fluent or Wernicke's aphasia, is characterized by substitution of functors. Following are descriptions and examples of agrammatism and paragrammatism at the sentence level.

Agrammatism is a nonfluent output that is rich in substantive words (e.g., verbs, nouns, adjectives) but sparse in function words (e.g., prepositions, pronouns, articles). Although sentences are short and constructed in a primitive manner, they frequently provide a good deal of information. A nonfluent output containing agrammatisms is also described as telegraphic or condensed speech (e.g., "Water in mouth" for *I am thirsty and would like a drink of water*).

Paragrammatism is a fluent output lacking substantive words and overusing function words. The sentences are long and without defining limits, contain verbal paraphasias and neologisms, show facile articulation, and tend toward logorrhea (pressure to speak). The sentences are lacking in semantic content and often provide little information. (One patient with aphasia, when asked to *point* to the tape recorder, *spoke* without being asked to do so, and without a pause said, "I've tried to all I had on my own but it doesn't make it I tried to make it but it doesn't work right why I have the recording but it was very, very good but the whole part of the radio itself I've tried to do it myself I can even show it to you I haven't but what I want to say about it that is why I tried to do it by myself but I could stay and pay I would like to do it just one more minute that I would try some place to have it done." The patient was probably trying to say that his own tape recorder or radio or stereo set was in need of repair, and that he tried unsuccessfully to fix it and would now have to send it out to be repaired.)

9. Word-finding difficulty.

   This is present in all types of aphasia as well as in other neurogenic language disorders. Because word-finding difficulty is so prevalent in neurogenically caused language disorders, it might be unreliable as a differential diagnostic indicator of a specific condition.

10. Perseveration, which is the repetition of a response that is no longer appropriate.

   Perseveration can occur on the level of sound (<u>s</u>oap—<u>s</u>chair), syllable (<u>baby</u>—<u>bay</u>nana), prefix (<u>un</u>happy—<u>un</u>hat), suffix (wonder<u>ful</u>—children<u>ful</u>), word (<u>boy</u>—<u>boy</u>), phrase (<u>a lovely person</u>—<u>a lovely person</u>), sentence (<u>I can't say it</u>—<u>I can't say it</u>), or incomplete sentence (<u>The boy is going</u> to the store—<u>The boy is going</u> bread).

11. Automatic speech, which can be best described as verbal stereotypes.

   Typically, automatic speech is language that is overlearned, such as counting, reciting the days of the week, or saying the alphabet, jingles, parts of songs, parts of prayers, curse words, and so forth. It is a sort of sublanguage that can appear at any time. When words are taken out of their automatic mold and put into a more formulative framework, this can cause problems for the patient (the patient is able to correctly rattle off 1, 2, 3, 4, 5, 6, 7, 8, 9, 10, but has difficulty when asked what comes after the number 3).

12. Failure to respond at all, or the use of only a single word (e.g., "no no no") or part of a sentence (e.g., "I know it but I can't, I know it but I can't" or "You know it and I know it, You know it and I know it") in response to most stimuli.

   Many times, the response will take on the prosodic changes that reflect the mood of the patient. The patient who responded with "You know it and I know it" said it in the manner of Robert De Niro, James Cagney, or James Gandolfini in their best tough-guy roles.

13. Responses that do not fit into any of the other categories mentioned (spelling a word out loud when asked to name it or making the sound of an object when asked to name it, e.g., "vooooom" for *car* or *airplane*, or "mmmmm" for *motor*).

Written Expression Deficit

An acquired impairment in the formulation of written language due to brain damage is called *written expression deficit*, or agraphia. Many of the problems and influencing factors cited in the other symptom categories would apply here. For example, if shown a picture of a pen, the patient responds by writing closely associated words such as *paper, ink*, or *pencil* (semantic error). The patient may write *pens* for *pen* (grammatical error), keep writing the same word over and over again inappropriately (perseveration), and so on.

It doesn't matter what sort of handwriting the patient has. The letters can be wiggly, out of line, or written in a slow, groping manner; if the language is correct, it is not agraphia. On the other hand, the letters and words can be written perfectly in a fluent and easy manner; if the language is incorrect, it is agraphia.

Benson (1979) and Brookshire (2007) have described two types of aphasic agraphia (see Benson & Ardila, 1996, for additional types of aphasic agraphia) that are based upon the neuroanatomical site of lesion. One type is called *dominant frontal (anterior) agraphia* and is often associated with the nonfluent aphasias and hemiplegia. Output is limited to single, substantive words with spelling errors, and if sentences are required, many short grammatical words are omitted. The mechanics of writing are large and messy.

A second type is called *dominant parietal-temporal (posterior) agraphia* and is often associated with the fluent aphasias. Output contains many spelling errors and verbal paragraphia (semantic), and if sentences are required, many patients will offer wordy, empty sentences. The mechanics of writing are normal or nearly so, and usually these patients will have no hemiplegia.

Classification

Through the years, patients with aphasia have been classified in many ways. It is beyond the realm of this text to go into all of the classification systems and the controversies surrounding them (see Benson & Ardila, 1996). Several of the more popular ones are noted here. Wernicke (1874) suggested a motor and sensory division. The *motor classification* involved a lesion in the anterior cortex and included motor speech activities, whereas the *sensory classification* involved a lesion in the posterior cortex and included auditory reception activities.

Weisenburg and McBride (1935) gave us *expressive, receptive*, and *mixed expressive and receptive* classifications. With this classification system, expressive aphasia was linked with anterior lesions, and receptive aphasia was linked with posterior lesions. Because almost all patients with aphasia show deficits in the four language modalities (auditory comprehension, reading comprehension, oral expression, and written expression), the Wernicke and Weisenburg and McBride classifications appeared too vague and thus lost their momentum as tools for diagnosis. However, their classification systems led to a division based on *anterior* or *posterior* site of lesion; most aphasiologists associate an anterior lesion with the motor and expressive classification, and a posterior lesion with the sensory and receptive classification.

Currently, there are three popular ways to classify patients with aphasia. One method is assessing patients as having a mild, moderate, or severe impairment. In this approach, the symptoms appearing in the various modalities are described and given a ranking of impairment within each modality and/or across all the modalities.

Aphasia can also be classified into *nonfluent aphasia*, usually caused by damage to anterior portions of the language-dominant side of the brain, and *fluent aphasia*, usually caused by damage to posterior portions of the language-dominant side of the brain. Authors such as Benson (1979), Benson and Ardila (1996), Brookshire (2007), and Goodglass and Kaplan (1983) have reviewed both types as follows. Nonfluent aphasia is characterized by:

1. Decreased output (50 words or less per minute, and often fewer than 10 words per minute)
2. Increased effort in producing speech
3. Defective articulation (because of the last two characteristics, prosody may be abnormal)
4. Decreased phrase length (fewer than four words, and often only single words per phrase)
5. Primitive syntax but a lot of information conveyed
6. Fewer paraphasias of the phonemic (literal), verbal (semantic), neologistic, and jargon types
7. Awareness of impairment and, as a result, frustration

Fluent aphasia is characterized by:

1. Increased output (mostly within the normal range of 100–150 words per minute, and sometimes as high as 200 words per minute)
2. Effortless production of speech
3. Relatively normal articulation (because of the previous two characteristics, prosody may be normal)
4. Normal phrase length (about five or more words per phrase);
5. Long sentences without defining limits, a lot of meaningless, empty talk characterized by a lack of substantive words, and a tendency toward logorrhea (a pressure to speak)
6. Many paraphasias of the phonemic (literal), verbal (semantic), neologistic, and jargon types
7. Frequent lack of awareness of the impairment and, as a result, no frustration over the condition

A third way of categorizing aphasia is by site of lesion. The *perisylvian* area (Benson, 1979; Benson & Ardila, 1996; Damasio, 2008) is located around the lateral fissure in the dominant hemisphere and contains the major language areas used for comprehension and expression (**Figure 3.1**). The aphasias caused by lesions in the perisylvian area would include Broca's, Wernicke's, and conduction. The *borderzone* area (Benson, 1979) or *extrasylvian* area (Benson & Ardila, 1996) or *watershed* area (Damasio, 2008) of the dominant hemisphere is located outside the perisylvian area, in the vascular borderzone between the territory of the middle cerebral artery and the territory of the anterior or posterior cerebral artery (Figure 3.1). The aphasias caused by lesions in the borderzone area would include transcortical motor aphasia, transcortical sensory aphasia, and mixed transcortical aphasia (isolation of the speech area). The aphasias caused by a nonlocalizing lesion would include anomic and global.

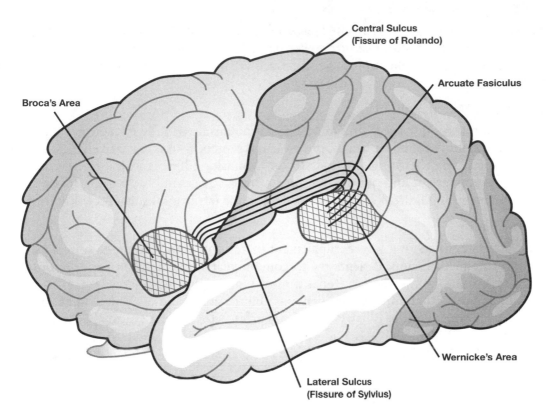

FIGURE 3.1 Lateral view of the left hemisphere (language dominant), showing the location of the borderzone or extrasylvian area and the perisylvian area.

Nonfluent Aphasia Syndromes

The nonfluent aphasias typically include Broca's aphasia, transcortical motor aphasia, global aphasia, and mixed transcortical aphasia or isolation syndrome.

Broca's Aphasia

Broca's aphasia is characterized by a sparse output of words and sentences, misarticulations, and agrammatisms. Speech is laborious, filled with many pauses, and is telegraphic. Auditory and reading comprehension are better than oral expression, and written expression tends to mirror oral expression. Repetition of words, phrases, and sentences is poor. The right side of the body is often paralyzed, and patients are aware of their difficulties, which can lead to frustration or catastrophic reaction (extreme emotional behavior such as complete withdrawal, prolonged crying, and intense hostility when the patient is unable to cope with demands made upon him or her).

Typically, the lesion (Benson & Ardila, 1996; Damasio, 2008) is in the posterior portion of the frontal lobe of the dominant hemisphere. It is in the perisylvian zone and may involve not only Broca's area but also premotor and motor regions immediately behind and above (Figure 3.1). In addition, the lesion may involve the underlying white matter and basal ganglia, as well as the insula, which is in the paralimbic area and may be seen by pulling apart the two borders of the lateral fissure (or the fissure of Sylvius).

Curiously, the patient Broca (1861, as cited in Damasio, 2008) described, called "Tan" because that was his stereotypic utterance, had a severe oral expressive deficit along with a severe auditory comprehension deficit. Currently, that combination of symptoms would probably be indicative of a global aphasia.

Transcortical Motor Aphasia

Transcortical motor aphasia is similar to Broca's aphasia, with the exception that these patients have the ability to repeat words, phrases, and sentences. It is a relatively rare syndrome. Generally, the lesion (Benson & Ardila, 1996; Damasio, 2008) is in the frontal lobe of the dominant hemisphere, is anterior or superior to Broca's area, and lies within the extrasylvian or watershed region (Figure 3.1). It is either deep in the left frontal substance or in the cortex.

Global Aphasia

Global aphasia consists of a severe impairment in auditory and reading comprehension, and oral and written expression. Patients try to communicate but often can produce only verbal stereotypes and automatic speech. Repetition of words, phrases, and sentences is defective. Nonlanguage perceptual and problem-solving abilities may be impaired (nonlanguage abilities are mostly intact in the other types of aphasia). Mostly, the lesion (Benson & Ardila, 1996; Damasio, 2008) involves a widespread area of the perisylvian zone of the dominant hemisphere, affecting all areas whose damage correlates with the aphasias (Figure 3.1).

Mixed Transcortical Aphasia

Mixed transcortical aphasia, or isolation syndrome, is similar to global aphasia, except that these patients can repeat and show echolalia of words, phrases, and sentences. It is a relatively rare syndrome. Mostly, the lesion (Benson & Ardila, 1996) involves a widespread area of the anterior and posterior extrasylvian regions or watershed areas (Damasio, 2008) of the dominant hemisphere (Figure 3.1).

Fluent Aphasia Syndromes

The fluent aphasias typically include Wernicke's aphasia, transcortical sensory aphasia, conduction aphasia, and anomic aphasia.

Wernicke's Aphasia

Wernicke's aphasia is characterized by fluent, verbal paraphasic, and generally well-articulated speech. Jargon, neologisms, and empty speech are common features. Auditory and reading comprehension and written expression are impaired. Repetition of words, phrases, and sentences is poor. Patients show few or no other neurologic signs and are often unaware of their errors, which leads to less incidence of frustration. On the other hand, some of these patients can become suspicious or even paranoid about their circumstances.

Generally, the lesion (Benson & Ardila, 1996; Damasio, 2008) is in the posterior portion of the temporal lobe of the dominant hemisphere. The lesion is near Heschl's gyrus (Brodmann's area 41), which is the primary auditory cortex. It is in the perisylvian zone involving Wernicke's (left superior temporal gyrus) and surrounding areas (Figure 3.1).

Transcortical Sensory Aphasia

Transcortical sensory aphasia is similar to Wernicke's aphasia, except that these patients have the ability to repeat and show echolalia of words, phrases, and sentences. It is a relatively rare syndrome.

Mostly, the lesion (Benson & Ardila, 1996; Damasio, 2008) is in the posterior portion of the temporal or parietal lobes; in the middle temporal gyrus or occasionally in the angular gyrus, in the white matter underlying these cortices, or a combination of both. The lesion is in the watershed area in the dominant hemisphere (Figure 3.1).

Conduction Aphasia

Conduction aphasia consists of fluent, verbal, and phonemic paraphasic speech, although usually less severe than that in Wernicke's aphasia. Auditory and reading comprehension are relatively good, whereas written expression is defective. Repetition of words, phrases, and sentences is disproportionately severely impaired in relation to the level of fluency in spontaneous speech, and the near normal level of auditory comprehension. Other motor signs may be present, and because of the patient's awareness of errors, speech can be filled with unsuccessful attempts at self-correction.

Typically, the lesion (Benson & Ardila, 1996; Damasio, 2008) can be in the arcuate fasciculus (the fibers that connect Wernicke's area with Broca's area) or deep in the supramarginal gyrus. The lesion can also be in a subsylvian involvement of Wernicke's area, in the primary auditory cortex, or to a variable degree, the insula and its subcortical white matter. The lesion is in the perisylvian area in the dominant hemisphere (Figure 3.1).

Anomic Aphasia

Anomic aphasia is characterized by fluent, well-articulated, mildly paraphasic, grammatically intact, and somewhat empty speech. The outstanding symptom is a naming or word-finding problem that can affect any of the modalities. Generally, if other symptoms appear, they do so mildly in the various modalities. These patients have no difficulty with repetition of words, phrases, and sentences. They know when they make errors, and because of unsuccessful attempts at self-correction, they often become frustrated. As mentioned previously, word-finding difficulty is probably the most common symptom found in aphasia and other neurogenically caused language disorders. Many times, word-finding difficulty is the only residual symptom as the patient gets better.

Generally, the site of lesion (Benson & Ardila, 1996; Damasio, 2008) is variable, but damage to the left anterior temporal cortex is an essential element.

Communication Between Two Individuals with Aphasia

Following is a transcription of a videotaped recording from an anniversary party for members of the stroke club at the Veterans Administration Extended Care Center in St. Albans, New York (see Goldfarb & Amsel, 1982, for more information about the club). There are many clues in the transcription regarding type of aphasia and symptomatology. Try doing some detective work on your own, before reading the comments at the end.

Isadore (holding the microphone in his right hand and looking straight ahead at the camera): My name is Isadore, and I'm having a very nice time. Gee, what else?

Bob (seated to the left of Isadore and turning right to face him. Bob is making the letter "U" with his left thumb and index finger, and stroking his chin): What's happening over here? Looks like two months ago. What's happening?

Isadore (now turning his head left so he can see Bob): Yeah. I have the apartment.

Bob (repeating the pantomime of stroking a beard): No, about this.

Isadore: Oh, the whiskers.

Bob: Yeah, what happened?

Isadore: Tomorrow.

Bob: What, 14 days.

Isadore (laughs): Yeah.

Bob: I think it looks nice for a while.
Isadore laughs.
Bob (repeating the pantomime of stroking a beard): In May.
Isadore laughs and uses his right hand to offer the microphone to Leon, who is seated on his right. Leon, who has already had a turn to introduce himself, uses his left hand to point to Bob. Isadore passes the microphone to the left to Bob, who takes it with his left hand.

Comments

Notice the references to left and right hands. Both Bob and Leon hold the microphone in their left hands. For Leon, this is because of right hemiplegia. He is wheelchair-borne, and cannot move his right arm or hand. For Bob, this is because of a contracture of the right hand, which causes his fingers to curl up and maintain a loose fist. Bob also walks with a distinct limp, with weakness in his right leg. For both Bob and Leon, anterior left hemisphere damage is implicated, as opposed to Isadore, who has fluent aphasia, is ambulatory, and has posterior left hemisphere damage. Both men also have nonfluent aphasia, Leon's being a severe form of Broca's aphasia, and Bob's a mild–moderate form. Isadore holds the microphone in his right hand, suggesting the motor area of his left hemisphere is not damaged. Of course, based only on this observation, we do not know if Isadore has weakness or paralysis on his left side. He might still have nonfluent (Broca's) aphasia if his left side was affected and he was left-handed or had a crossed aphasia (where the language center and the center for handedness are in different brain hemispheres). In fact, Isadore had a stroke in posterior portions of his left hemisphere, resulting in fluent (mild Wernicke's) aphasia, with no effect on his limbs or ambulatory ability.

Both Bob and Leon use the adaptive behaviors of gesture and pantomime to substitute for and supplement vocal language efforts. Bob pantomimes stroking a beard, and Leon points to where Isadore should pass the microphone. These adaptive behaviors may indicate that both men are using self-monitoring strategies (prerequisite for self-correction), and that they have employed adaptive behaviors to compensate for word-retrieval difficulties. Isadore gestures only to pass the microphone in the wrong direction. That he does not use adaptive behaviors is consistent with the poor auditory comprehension, poor self-monitoring, and lack of self-correction associated with Wernicke's aphasia.

In the first interaction, the message Bob sends is obviously not received by Isadore. Bob tells Isadore to get a shave, and Isadore says he has the apartment. Bob also uses a semantic paraphasia, selecting *months* to represent *weeks*. We know this is so, because he later modifies "*2 months ago*" to "*14 days.*"

When Isadore is looking directly at the camera, he is limited to auditory comprehension to receive and decode Bob's message. After Isadore turns to face Bob, the information from the beard-stroking pantomime is readily understood, and Isadore replies, "Oh, the whiskers."

Isadore's fluency is evident in his grammatically well-formed sentences and absence of struggle behavior in producing them. Bob's impaired fluency is characterized by omission of functors (pronoun, article, auxiliary verb), with preservation of grammatical morphemes (plural, gerund form of verbs). While there is no need to modify the syntax in Isadore's sentences "I'm having a very nice time" or "I have the apartment," Bob's sentences require the following syntactic modifications, shown in parentheses: "(It) looks like (it was) two months ago (. . . *that you last shaved* is understood by Bob's pantomime)." "(It should grow in) in May."

Both speakers give evidence that they communicate better than they speak (the opposite of which is said to occur in traumatic brain injury). When Isadore says, "Tomorrow," Bob understands that to mean Isadore has scheduled a shave. When Bob says, "In May," Isadore shows he gets the joke by laughing.

Aphasia in Bilingual or Multilingual Individuals

In their review, Benson and Ardila (1996) looked at whether patients with aphasia who are bilingual or polyglot (multilingual) show equal impairment in the different languages, or better recovery in just one of them. Those who observe that one language recovers better than the others cite such factors as the language learned early in life, the language most consistently used at the onset of aphasia, and the language milieu during recovery. Benson and Ardila have concluded that no set pattern exists for the recovery of language in the bilingual or polyglot patient.

Roberts (2008) noted that bilingualism is a continuum, with different levels of ability for varied linguistic tasks and assorted domains of use. Out of five types of impairment and five types of recovery in bilingualism, she states that clinical experience suggests that parallel impairment and parallel recovery are overwhelmingly the most frequent patterns, especially after the first couple of weeks. Parallel impairment is where the two languages are impaired in the same manner and to the same degree, relative to premorbid abilities.

Kohnert (2005) talks about two intervention approaches that can be used in bilingual aphasia. One is the bilingual approach, which is aimed at those cognitive-linguistic skills that are common to both languages. The second is the cross-linguistic approach, which is directed at the linguistic features or social uses of language that are unique to each language.

Lorenzen and Murray (2008), in their theoretical and clinical review, stated that despite a growing understanding of bilingualism and the various recovery patterns identified with bilingual aphasia, there remains a dire need for empirically validated management techniques, particularly in terms of determining which language to treat, identifying which aspects of various languages are most vulnerable to insult as well as most responsive to treatment, and establishing how to exploit language similarities to maximize treatment efficiency.

Primary Progressive Aphasia

Occasionally, an ongoing cerebral atrophy in a language area of the brain can result in progressive language deterioration. If the person's nonverbal memory and intellect remain intact, the language deterioration is known as a *primary progressive aphasia (PPA)*.

Duffy and McNeil (2008), in their review of 147 cases with PPA, note the following key points of the condition:

1. PPA is of insidious onset, gradual progression, and prolonged course, without evidence of nonlanguage computational impairments; is due to a degenerative condition; and presumably and predominantly involves the perisylvian area of the language-dominant hemisphere.
2. Criteria for the diagnosis of PPA include a minimum of a two-year history of language decline.
3. PPA can be very different from Alzheimer disease (AD) or other degenerative diseases that bring diffuse cognitive impairment. It can be strikingly similar to the static etiologies of aphasia (CVA, etc.).
4. More males than females have PPA; age of onset averages about 60 years old.
5. Apraxia of speech (AOS), nonverbal oral apraxia, dysarthria, dysphagia, other neurologic symptoms, and depression can be present in cases with PPA.
6. Magnetic Resonance Imaging (MRI) and Single Photon Emission Computed Tomography (SPECT) are typically used for the neuroradiologic evaluation. When abnormal, they show predominance of left hemisphere damage.
7. Although some cases of PPA can be associated with a variety of histopathologic diagnoses, most will not be associated with AD.

8. Distinguishing between a progressive AOS and PPA may be relevant to prognosis, management, and may be the underlying pathology.
9. Under the right circumstances, language and communication treatment for PPA can be effective.

Recently, Henry and Beeson (2006) in their review have mentioned that treatment for the communication problems found in PPA can work.

Additional Sources

For a further review of the various symptoms and classifications of aphasia, and site of lesion, the reader is referred to Benson (1979), Benson and Ardila (1996), Brookshire (2007), Goodglass, Kaplan, and Barresi (2001), and Webb and Adler (2008).

Etiology

As was stated in the definition, aphasia is caused by brain damage, most likely in the cortical language areas of the left hemisphere. In some cases, aphasia can occur because of lesions in subcortical areas, mostly in the thalamus or basal ganglia. In some cases, a lesion in the right hemisphere of a right-handed person will cause a crossed aphasia. Sheehy (2006) in her review has noted that crossed aphasia was first described in the literature in 1899 and that it occurs in less than 3% of reported aphasia cases.

A major cause of aphasia in middle and old age is the *cerebrovascular accident (CVA)*. Cerebrovascular accidents consist of ischemic strokes (83%) in the form of *thromboses* and *emboli*, or hemorrhagic strokes (17%), usually *aneurysms* or *hemorrhages*, as well as CVA-like syndromes. Ischemia refers to deficient circulation in the brain. A cerebral thrombosis is an occlusion of an artery to the brain by a clot. A cerebral embolus is a clot formed elsewhere that finally lodges in the brain. An aneurysm is a swelling or ballooning of a cranial artery. A cerebral hemorrhage is the rupture of a blood vessel with subsequent bleeding into the brain. All cerebrovascular accidents have one thing in common: they deprive the brain of oxygen and circulation, thus causing brain damage.

Trauma to the brain is another major cause of aphasia. Gunshot wounds, automobile accidents, and falls are the most likely causes of physical trauma to the brain. Brain tumors, both malignant and nonmalignant, are associated with aphasia. Quite often, the extirpation of a brain tumor will cause aphasia. The authors remember one young man in his early 20s who suffered symptoms of brain damage (spasms, blackouts, etc., but no aphasia). A diagnostic workup determined that a brain tumor was present in his left frontal lobe. Although the tumor was benign, the surgery left him with aphasia and a right-sided paralysis. Abscesses, infectious diseases, and degenerative disease of the brain can also result in aphasia.

Ischemic Thrombosis/Embolism. This is the most common cause of CVA. A thrombus is a blood clot forming within and occluding an artery. It is usually the result of an atherosclerotic plaque (a collection of cholesterol and calcium deposited within the arterial wall). The condition is exacerbated by smoking, which may cause *stenosis*, or narrowing of the artery. Finally, the white blood cells, which attack the cholesterol and calcium "invaders," release a growth factor, which may further occlude the artery.

Common sites of thromboses are in the internal carotid artery at its origin in the neck, in the middle cerebral artery (a branch of the internal carotid), and its more distal branches. The pulse of the internal carotid is felt by palpating just in front of and below the ear, near the angle of the mandible. Surgical treatment of accumulated plaque in the carotid is via a procedure called *endarterectomy*. This neurosurgical equivalent of a Roto-Rooter repair of a sewage system uses a cutting tool to remove the plaque and a vacuum pump to remove the debris. However, there is a danger of bits of debris escaping into the circulatory system and occluding a more distal branch of the artery. Thus, a treatment to prevent a stroke entails the risk of a stroke. Recent use of stents (cages to keep the artery open) in the middle cerebral artery have not met with much success.

A low-tech alternative to endarterectomy was introduced in 1999. Called the Merci Retriever, this corkscrew-shaped device permits removal of clots in patients who are not treated within the first three hours of stroke onset by tPA (tissue plasminogen activators, or "clot-busting" drugs). The Retriever is used in conjunction with a balloon catheter, which is inserted through a small incision in the femoral artery in the groin. Under x-ray guidance, the catheter is maneuvered up to the carotid artery in the neck, just beyond the clot. The physician then inserts the Retriever device to ensnare the clot. Inflation of the balloon catheter temporarily stops forward blood flow while the clot is being withdrawn through a wider portion of the artery and then completely out of the body. When the balloon is then deflated, blood flow is restored.

In a cerebral *embolism*, the artery is occluded by a fragment of blood clot or foreign substance carried in the bloodstream. A blood clot often breaks off from the heart. Blood tends to clot when it stops circulating, which is why it is not uncommon to "throw an embolus" when rising after a long airplane flight where one has sat for many hours without exercising the legs. Atherosclerotic plaques on the internal carotid may ulcerate, and calcium and cholesterol may be carried to the brain. Emboli of fat, tumor cells, and even air occur rarely.

Anoxia from drowning, asphyxia, shock, or cardiac arrest may result in an ischemic CVA (especially if the cerebral arteries are stenotic).

Hemorrhagic. In intracerebral hemorrhage, bleeding occurs from an artery within the substance of the brain. The artery usually has been weakened by hypertension, inflammation, injury, or congenital defect. Failure of blood to clot may contribute to hemorrhage. There is a "catch-22" situation between thromboembolic and hemorrhagic CVAs. Within the first three hours of an ischemic CVA, use of tPA (tissue plasminogen activators), or clot-busting drugs, can reverse the effects of the blood clot and save the patient from a devastating stroke. These same drugs, given in error to treat a hemorrhagic stroke, exacerbate the bleeding and may have fatal consequences.

Bleeding within the subarachnoid space that surrounds the brain is usually the result of cerebral aneurysm, which is a dilated, very thin-walled portion of the cerebral artery. Aneurysms are formed by gradual deterioration of the arterial wall at sites where there are irregularities in cerebral blood flow and congenital (present at birth) deficiencies in the vessel walls. Rupture of a cerebral aneurysm causes a hemorrhage.

Arteriovenous malformations (AVMs) are congenital communications between arteries and veins, which tend to bleed and cause subarachnoid hemorrhage. Other causes of subarachnoid hemorrhage are brain tumors, hypertension, and blood-clotting abnormalities.

A pair of internal carotids and two vertebral arteries supply the brain with blood. As both sets of vessels enter the intracranial cavity, they give off a series of branches that spread throughout the brain. Usually there is little mingling of blood from the two carotids by way of the Circle of Willis, located at the base of the brain. In disease, however, the Circle of Willis may become a source of collateral circulation for either hemisphere. Collateral circulation is far from perfect, and seems to compensate for occluded arteries better in males than in females.

CVA-Like Syndromes. Brain tumor, unrecognized head injury with chronic subdural hematoma, multiple sclerosis, and inflammatory diseases may resemble CVAs clinically. They require different medical treatment from that of CVAs.

Additional Sources

Reviews of etiology of aphasia can be found in Benson (1979), Benson & Ardila (1996), Brookshire (2007), and Mlcoch and Metter (2008).

Neuronal Responses to Brain Injuries (see Bhatnagar, 2008)

Nerve cells cannot divide or regenerate. Neural degeneration occurs if either the presynaptic or postsynaptic terminal degenerates. Cells conduct impulses, but they also transmit nutritive (trophic) substances between neurons, which maintain cells on both sides of the synapse. The two types of degenerative changes—axonal (retrograde) reaction and wallerian (anterograde) degeneration—serve as models for understanding physiological events that cells undergo following CVA, and also help us to understand spontaneous recovery.

After an injury to the brain, astroglial cells are important to recovery. Glial (meaning "glue") cells support and protect the nerve cells. Found in the gray and white matter of the brain, there are 40 to 50 times as many glial cells as nerve cells. Glial cells do not generate or transmit nerve impulses. Astrocytes function as connective tissue, providing skeletal support for the brain cells and their processes. They contribute to the *blood–brain barrier* by contacting capillary surfaces with their end feet and using tight junctions. This restricts the movement of certain substances from the blood to the brain through selective permeability. Microglial cells are multipotential, because they sometimes act as phagocytes (which remove dead neural tissue debris), and at other times as astrocytes or oligodendrocytes (which help form and maintain the myelin sheath).

In CVAs, the astrocytes and microglial cells proliferate and migrate to the lesion site. Microglia phagocytose (engulf) cellular debris, leaving a cavity. For large lesions, astrocytes seal the cavity, which is called a *cyst*. In smaller lesions, astrocytes fill the space with a glial scar that is called *replacement gliosis*.

Axonal Reaction. A day or two after suffering a CVA, the microscopic organelles in the cell body (or soma) begin swelling. The coarse clumps of Nissl substance dissolves into fine granules. Cellular edema occurs when the blood–brain barrier is violated or altered, changing the relationship of the gray and white matter, and triggering shrinking (pyknosis) of the cell nuclei. This process is maximal after about 4 days, and completed after 10 to 18 days.

In a process called *stunning*, some cells that are not seriously damaged may respond to the natural recovery process and survive. Organelles resume their normal appearance, swelling recedes, and the nucleus assumes a central location. Following a CVA, this process takes some six months to one year; following head trauma, it may be even longer. Of course, cells that are severely injured do not survive, shrinking and assuming irregular shapes because of the degenerated organelles. Then microglial cells take over for cleanup.

What happens when brain cells die? The cause of death may be direct (as in the area of infarct following a CVA) or indirect (as in increased intracranial pressure). New capillaries (hyperplasia) and macrophages (astrocytes and microglia) invade necrotic tissue (*necrosis* refers to an island of dead tissue surrounded by normal tissue). After a week during which cellular swelling begins to go down, there is liquefaction of necrotic tissue and *phagocytosis*, a process in which lipid-laden microphagic microglia cells engulf and remove the dead tissue.

Wallerian Degeneration. In a wallerian reaction, there is degeneration of the axonal part that is separate from its cell body. Beginning with the distal portion of the sectioned axon, swelling and degeneration begins within 12 to 20 hours; the myelin sheath degenerates later (within 7 days). Within 2 to 3 days the connected muscles become denervated. Microphagy (action of microglial cells) begins in 7 days and is complete in 3 to 6 months.

Neuroglial Responses. We have discussed how neuroglial cells react to cellular injuries and brain tissue necrosis by multiplying in number (hyperplasia) and by increasing their size (hypertrophy). Also of interest when studying the effects of CVAs is the action of infection-fighting *neurotrophils*, the scavenger white blood cells, and the growth factor they release (see "Ischemic Thrombosis/Embolism," above).

Post-CVA, some neurons will become axotomized. Glial cells displace presynaptic and postsynaptic terminals and cell bodies, impairing transmission between neurons. After normal input to the cell body is removed, new synaptic trigger zones develop on its dendritic tree and begin to excite the cell. This is part of the process of spontaneous recovery, and it is crucial for therapeutic intervention to assist in this rewiring process of the injured brain.

Axonal Regeneration in the Peripheral Nervous System. Proliferating Schwann cells fill the interval between opposing ends of the nerve fiber. The sheath of Schwann (similar to the myelin sheath in the central nervous system) and the endoneurial connective tissue form a tube from the proximal fiber end to the distal end. As the proximal end regenerates, processes of axons, or sprouts, form. Some sprouts grow along the tube at a rate of 4 millimeters per day if they pass through the cleft, or astrocytic scar. Problems occur when a regenerated axon attaches to a different sensory or motor fiber (e.g., a pain-mediating fiber connects to a touch receptor, resulting in a sensation of pain from touch). Such incorrectly connected nerve fibers usually atrophy. This process may explain why some patients with aphasia and right hemiparesis (weakness on one side of the body) or right hemiplegia (paralysis on one side of the body) report excruciating pain on the weakened or paralyzed side.

Diagnosis

Procedures for diagnosing aphasia can involve (1) establishing background information, (2) giving a neurologic evaluation, (3) employing four-modality tests, (4) employing functional language tests, (5) employing single-modality tests, and (6) evaluating connected speech.

Establishing Background Information

Establishing background information about the neurogenic patient with a communication disorder can involve obtaining *basic*, *medical*, and *related area information* through questioning the patient and/or the caretaker, and through access to medical and other reports. Procedures for establishing background information are applicable to the other language and motor speech disorders discussed in this text.

Basic information can include the patient's name; age; educational level; occupation; marital and family status; previous speech, language, and cognitive problems; family history of speech, language, and cognitive problems; native language; and communicating language.

Medical information can include the onset and course of the disorder, diagnosis of the disorder, past illnesses, any injuries, general physical condition, past cerebrovascular disorders, previous central or peripheral nervous system damage, disorientation, confusion, paralysis, seizures, loss of consciousness, chronic conditions, and instrumentation findings (CT scan, etc.).

Related area information can include visual deficits; hearing deficits; preonset personality; postonset personality; mood changes; memory functioning; swallowing; drooling; medications that may have affected speech, language, and cognition; substance abuse (alcohol, etc.); and the patient's awareness and perception of the problem.

The Neurologic Evaluation

The neurologic evaluation includes those procedures used in determining the type of pathology and the location of the brain lesion. These neurodiagnostic procedures are applicable to the other language and motor speech disorders discussed in this text.

Benson and Ardila (1996) and Mlcoch and Metter (2008) have reviewed the localization techniques used in determining the neuroanatomical site of brain damage in cases of aphasia. The localization techniques include neuropathology, neurosurgery, posttrauma skull defects, the neurologic examination, and brain-imaging studies.

Neuropathology relies upon direct postmortem anatomical observation of patients who had suffered language impairment. *Neurosurgery* correlates the site of surgical incision and the subsequent aphasia, and prior to surgery the focal stimulation of brain areas (with the patient awake and responding to questions) and its correlation to the elicited language symptoms. *Posttrauma skull defects* correlate the site of skull damage and the aphasic symptoms.

The *neurologic examination* involves a visual sensory examination that checks for visual-field defects, a motor examination that checks for paralysis, a sensory examination that checks for pain and/or temperature loss, and a motor praxis examination that checks for apraxia. The defects in these areas are then correlated to the neural system responsible for their functioning.

Brain-imaging studies include *isotope brain scans, cerebral blood flow and metabolism studies, computed tomography (CT)*, and *magnetic resonance imaging (MRI)*. An isotope brain scan involves an injection of an isotope followed by counts of radioactivity over brain areas. Cerebral blood flow and metabolism studies involve the use of positron isotopes, as in positron emission tomography (PET) studies, which provide relatively precise neuroanatomical delineation based on variations in glucose metabolism. Dynamic isotope studies reveal brain areas with increased blood flow or alterations of metabolic rate when the participant performs certain activities. Single-photon emission-computed tomography (SPECT) uses relatively stable isotope products to demonstrate cerebral blood flow and, to a lesser degree, perfusion of metabolites.

Computed tomography relies on the penetration of x-ray beams processed through computerized mathematics, which provides a tomographic (pictures of body section) image of the brain without physical invasion of the body. Magnetic resonance imaging uses a powerful magnetic field to alter electrical fields in the brain, which can then be monitored electronically to produce computerized images (slices) of brain tissues. MRI does not use x-ray and does not introduce radioactive material into the patient's body.

In addition to the above, Mlcoch and Metter (2008) describe the use of *x-rays* (for observing the skull and/or spine), *cerebral angiography* (for observing the veins and arteries of the brain and brainstem), *myelography* (for observing the spinal cord and spinal nerves), *B-mode carotid imaging* (for observing extracranial blood vessels with ultrasound), *electroencephalograms* (EEG) (for obtaining a graphic record of the electrical activity of the cerebral cortex), *electromyography* (for recording the electrical activities of muscles), *nerve conduction studies* (for measuring stimulation and response points along the nerve fiber), *lumbar punctures* (for analyzing a sample of cerebrospinal fluid), and *biopsies* (for analyzing samples of tissue).

Mayer (2003) presented a review on the uses of MRI in aphasia, and Shuster (2007) has provided an overview of brain-scanning procedures involving MRI, functional MRI (fMRI), and a combination of PET/CT. Abou-Khalil and Abou-Khalil (2003) show how cortical stimulation following cerebral injury provides greater accuracy in mapping brain functions.

Four-Modality Tests

Most of the tests used for aphasia evaluate all four modalities of speaking, listening, reading, and writing. Each modality is tested individually, with stimulus items generally ranging from simple to more complex. For example, auditory comprehension might be tested by the examiner's saying single words, multiple words, sentences, and paragraphs (e.g., "Point to the window") and having the patient respond by pointing, nodding, or gesturing in response to the auditory stimuli. Reading comprehension might be tested by the examiner's presenting printed words, sentences, and paragraphs (e.g., *Do cows fly?*) and having the patient respond by pointing to, circling, or underlining the printed words *yes* or *no,* or by nodding or gesturing.

Oral expression might be tested by having the patient produce sublanguage items such as serial speech (e.g., reciting the alphabet or days of the week) and repeating words after the examiner, and language items such as sentence completion (e.g., "We sleep in a __"), naming pictures or objects, defining words and sentences, and talking spontaneously about everyday activities. Written expression might be tested by having the patient produce sublanguage items such as copying letters and words and writing words to dictation, and language items such as writing the name of an object or item shown in a picture and writing a narrative from an action picture.

Tests that evaluate the four modalities in the manner described include the following: *Acute Aphasia Screening Protocol* (AASP) (Crary, Haak, & Malinsky, 1989); *Aphasia Language Performance Scales* (ALPS) (Keenan & Brassell, 1975); *Bedside Evaluation Screening Test* (BEST) (Fitch-West, Sands, & Ross-Swain, 1998); *Bilingual Aphasia Test* (BAT) (Paradis, 1987); *Boston Assessment of Severe Aphasia* (BASA) (Helm-Estabrooks, Ramsberger, Morgan, & Nicholas, 1989); *Boston Diagnostic Aphasia Examination-3* (BDAE) (Goodglass, Kaplan, & Barresi, 2001); *Examining for Aphasia-4* (EFA-4) (LaPointe & Eisenson, 2008); *Language Modalities Test for Aphasia* (LMTA) (Wepman & Jones, 1961); *Minnesota Test for Differential Diagnosis of Aphasia* (MTDDA) (Schuell, 1972); *Multilingual Aphasia Examination* (MAE) (Benton & Hamsher, 1978); *Neurosensory Center Comprehensive Examination for Aphasia* (NCCEA) (Spreen & Benton, 1969); *Porch Index of Communicative Ability* (PICA) (Porch, 1981); *Sklar Aphasia Scale* (SAS) (Sklar, 1973); and *Western Aphasia Battery-Enhanced* (WAB) (Kertesz, 2006). Of the above tests, the AASP omits evaluating reading comprehension, and the BEST omits evaluating written expression.

Currently, the most popular tests are the BDAE, MTDDA, and WAB. The formerly popular PICA is out of print. The BDAE and the WAB are the only tests among those cited above that place patients in the classic aphasia categories of Broca's, transcortical motor, global, mixed transcortical, Wernicke's, transcortical sensory, conduction, and anomic. The MTDDA contains the categories of simple aphasia, aphasia with visual involvement, aphasia with sensorimotor involvement, aphasia with scattered findings compatible with generalized brain damage, and irreversible aphasic syndrome. Two minor syndromes are aphasia with partial auditory imperception and aphasia with persisting dysarthria.

Hegde (1998) and Patterson and Chapey (2008) have provided details about the purposes and descriptions of the standardized diagnostic tests for aphasia. The BDAE uses a 5-point severity rating scale and a profile of speech characteristics to help assign severity and type of aphasia. However, the test fails to classify about half of the individuals with aphasia who are tested with the instrument. In addition, its length (about 1–4 hours to administer) may make it impractical for clinical aphasiologists. The WAB was based on the BDAE, and the two tests correlate well, but they classify only about 1/4 of the individuals with aphasia into the same types. That is, an individual classified as having Wernicke's aphasia on one test may be diagnosed with anomic aphasia on the other.

Desirable features of the WAB include the *Aphasia Quotient* (AQ), which is a functional measurement of severity of language impairment, based on oral language subtests; and the *Cortical Quotient* (CQ), which measures cognitive functioning. The MTDDA takes the longest to administer in full (4–6 hours). The five sections assess the primary areas of language and symbolic disturbance. Items increase in difficulty within each group of subtests. The PICA uses a 15- or 16-point multidimensional scoring system (depending on the edition of the test) rather than correct/incorrect scoring. It has the greatest psychometric strength, but provides limited measurements of speech and language, and requires a 40-hour training course for administrative competence.

Molrine and Pierce (2002) found no statistically significant differences between 24 non-brain-damaged black adults and 24 non-brain-damaged white adults in expressive language performance from three popular tests of aphasia (*Boston Diagnostic Aphasia Examination*; *Minnesota Test for Differential Diagnosis of Aphasia*; *Western Aphasia Battery*). All participants were equally represented in the middle and upper levels of the socioeconomic scale, and across gender.

Ellis (2009) reviewed articles related to adult neurogenic communication disorders in the *American Journal of Speech-Language Pathology* (AJSLP) and the *Journal of Speech, Language, and Hearing Research* (JSLHR) from 1997 through 2007 and reported the race/ethnicity of the participants. He concluded that because few studies report race/ethnicity or consider how race/ethnicity has the potential to confound the results and conclusions drawn, the generalization of the reported findings may be limited. He further stated that reporting race/ethnicity is likely critical to the external validity of studies in adult neurogenic communication disorders, and when available can enhance the relevance of the findings reported.

Functional Language Tests

Some tests evaluate functional language through the various modalities. Many times these tests are used as adjuncts to the more traditional tests used for aphasia. They include the following: *ASHA Functional Assessment of Communication Skills for Adults* (ASHA FACS) (American Speech-Language-Hearing Association, 1994); *Assessment Protocol of Pragmatic-Linguistic Skills* (APPLS) (Gerber & Gurland, 1989); *Communicative Effectiveness Index* (CETI) (Lomas et al., 1989); *Communicative Abilities in Daily Living* (CADL-2) (Holland, Frattali, & Fromm, 1999); *Functional Communication Profile* (FCP) (Sarno, 1969); and *The Stocker Probe for Fluency and Language* (Stocker & Goldfarb, 1995). Items in these tests elicit language related to everyday activities (greetings, shopping, family matters, etc.), and the tests are administered in a relatively informal manner. The authors of these tests feel that because of the emphasis on functional language or social-communicative interaction and the informal setting, the psychological barriers of tension and anxiety that accompany formal test taking would be ameliorated.

Single-Modality Tests

Other tests evaluate the patient's language abilities through only one modality. Usually, these tests evaluate in-depth and are quite sensitive, thus enabling the detection of even the mildest language impairment. These tests are used mostly as adjuncts to the more traditional ones and include the following: *Auditory Comprehension Test for Sentences* (ACTS) (Shewan, 1980); *Boston Naming Test* (BNT) (Kaplan, Goodglass, & Weintraub, 1983); as well as a short version of the BNT, which del Toro et al. (2011) developed for individuals with aphasia and compared with two existing short forms originally analyzed with responses from people with dementia and neurologically healthy adults. The authors concluded that their new short form demonstrates good psychometric properties when used with individuals with aphasia. However, the Mack et al. (1992) form (as cited by del Toro et al., 2011) was as psychometrically sound as the BNT-aphasia short form, and is also appropriate for individuals with aphasia. In addition, there is the *Reading Comprehension Battery for Aphasia* (RCBA) (LaPointe & Horner, 1980); *The Reporters Test* (DeRenzi & Ferrari, 1978), which evaluates oral expression; *The Token Test* (DeRenzi & Vignolo, 1962), which evaluates auditory comprehension; *Revised Token Test* (RTT) (McNeil & Prescott, 1978); and *Word Fluency Measure* (Borkowski, Benton, & Spreen, 1967), which evaluates oral expression.

Odekar and Hallowell (2005) used the *Revised Token Test* (RTT) (McNeil & Prescott, 1978) to compare traditional multidimensional scoring with three alternate scoring forms that would require less time in administration: one simpler form of multidimensional scoring and two forms of correct/incorrect scoring. The findings of the study suggest that simpler, less time-intensive scoring systems might yield equivalent data to the traditional multidimensional scoring.

Thompson and Shapiro (2007), in reference to the treatment of syntactic deficits in individuals with aphasia, summarized the benefits of training complex, rather than simple, sentence structure.

Evaluating Connected Speech

As an adjunct to the aphasia tests mentioned previously, several studies have looked at the connected speech of adults with aphasia as a means for evaluation. Nicholas and Brookshire (1995b) noted that various measures have been used to compare the connected speech of adults with aphasia to that of typical, non-brain-damaged adults, and to evaluate changes in connected speech over time. Such measures range from those used to assess adherence to standard language rules and patterns of use to those used to evaluate the informativeness and efficiency of connected speech.

Measures of adherence to standard language rules and patterns of use include counts of syntactic errors (Shewan, 1988; Wagenaar, Snow, & Prins, 1975); ratio of clauses to terminal units (Hunt, 1965); and type-token ratio, mean length of utterance, and number and types of cohesive ties (Halliday & Hasan, 1976). Measures of communicative informativeness and efficiency include content units per minute (Yorkston & Beukelman, 1980); percent of words that are correct information units (Nicholas & Brookshire, 1993); presence, completeness, and accuracy of main concept production (Nicholas & Brookshire, 1995a,b); and subjective ratings of coherence (Ulatowska, Freedman-Stern, Doyel, & Macaluso-Haynes, 1983). Ulatowska, et al. (2001) held that fable and proverb discourse tasks may be valuable supplemental measures for characterizing competence in African American adults who have aphasia. Brodsky et al. (2003) found that persons with aphasia recall discourse length information using similar memory functions as the nonimpaired subjects though at a reduced level of efficiency or quantity.

The *Discourse Comprehension Test* (Brookshire & Nicholas, 1997) was designed to assess listening and reading comprehension, and retention of stated and implied main ideas and details from narrative discourse. The authors maintain that the test is appropriate for adults with aphasia, right hemisphere brain damage, or traumatic brain injury. Main idea questions test central information that is repeated or elaborated on by other information in the story. Detail questions test peripheral information that is mentioned only once and not elaborated on by other information in the story. Stated questions test information that appears in a story in essentially the same form in which it is subsequently tested. Implied questions test information that is not directly stated but has to be inferred from other information in the story; answering these questions requires the listener to form bridging assumptions and draw inferences.

Nicholas and Brookshire (1995a), using an earlier version of the *Discourse Comprehension Test*, found that the performance of groups of patients with brain damage (20 patients had left hemisphere brain damage and aphasia, 20 had right hemisphere brain damage, and 20 had traumatic brain injury) was qualitatively similar to that of the group with no brain damage (40 subjects), but quantitatively inferior. The performance of the groups with brain damage was qualitatively and quantitatively similar. The performance of all groups was strongly affected by the salience of information in the stories. All 100 participants responded correctly to main idea questions more often than to detail questions. The effect of directness was less strong than that of salience, but all groups produced more correct responses when questions assessed stated information than when they assessed implied information. The effect of directness was greater for detail questions than for main idea questions.

Pak-Hin Kong (2011) evaluated 16 participants with aphasia on the main concept (MC) analysis, the Cantonese version of the *Western Aphasia Battery* (CAB), and the Cantonese linguistic communication measure (CLCM). He found significant associations between the MC measures and the corresponding CLCM indices and CAB performance scores that were relevant to the presence, accuracy, and completeness of content in oral narratives, and concluded that the present study has further established the external validity of MC analysis in Cantonese.

Additional Sources

For all of the tests mentioned, if a complete evaluation is not made during the initial diagnostic session, additional sessions may be required to ascertain the full picture of the patient's abilities. On the other hand, Marshall and Wright (2007) are developing the *Kentucky Aphasia Test* (KAT) which, according to the authors, is an objective measure of language functioning for persons with aphasia. The authors claim that the test is "clinician-friendly" in that it offers a rapid, convenient means of determining changes in language functioning during the early postonset period. They state that clinicians have less time for assessment, now that we're in the managed care era, and thus the KAT would be beneficial in this environment.

Ross and Wertz (2003) administered two general language measures (the PICA and the WAB) and two functional communication measures (the CADL and the ASHA FACS) to 18 persons with mild aphasia, and 18 typical elderly persons. Results showed that expressive language ability and efficiency of performance best differentiated the two groups. However, group performance ranges overlapped at least 10% on each measure. To enhance the differential diagnosis of aphasia, the authors recommend adding subjective and objective evidence to formal test results.

Milman et al. (2008) found that the scales of cognitive and communicative ability for neurorehabilitation (SCAN) accurately classified 95% of neurologically healthy control participants and 90% of the participants diagnosed with neurological disorders. Results indicated that the test also differentiated the performance profile of the three clinical populations (left-hemisphere pathology, right-hemisphere pathology, or probable Alzheimer disease). The test was designed to provide an overview of impairment and activity limitation across 8 cognitive scales (speech comprehension, oral expression, reading, writing, orientation, attention, memory, and problem solving).

Reviews of testing procedures for aphasia and other adult neurogenic communication disorders can be found in Benson and Ardila (1996), Brookshire (2007), and Patterson and Chapey (2008). Kennedy and Chiou (2005) offer a review of 33 assessment tools that are available in languages other than English, some of which might be used with the patient with aphasia.

Finally, *Time-Altered Word Association Tests* (TAWAT) (first reported in Goldfarb & Halpern, 1981; see the appendices at the end of the text) can help in differential diagnosis among typical young adults, typical older adults, older adults with aphasia, institutionalized elderly with and without dementia, and adults with the language of chronic undifferentiated schizophrenia.

Therapy

A Model for Aphasia Therapy

Following is a model based on set theory, used in describing assessment and treatment of aphasia in adults (Santo Pietro & Goldfarb, 1995), Alzheimer dementia (Ostuni & Santo Pietro, 1991), and stuttering (Goldfarb, 2006a). In mathematics, the intersection of two sets consists of the elements the sets have in common. For example, if the patient's communicative goals are to improve recitation of prayers and hymns, saying the names of family members, and ordering in a restaurant, and the clinician's goals for the patient are reading the newspaper, writing with the nondominant hand, and saying the names of family members, then there is only one targeted goal that intersects both clinician and patient. Mathematically, the intersection of patient's goal set A and clinician's goal set B becomes set C, or A ∩ B = C. What looks like an upside-down capital "U" is pronounced *cap*.

Intersections of sets are depicted graphically as interlocking circles (think of the logo for the Olympic games) called a Venn diagram. Areas of assessing and treating a person with aphasia are grouped according to the intersections in the drawing, or Venn diagram, in **Figure 3.2**.

The diagram portrays a person with an acquired language impairment communicating with a communication partner within an environment. None of the component sets should be assessed or treated independently of the others. Furthermore, the approach is best conceived in terms of the intersection it targets. For example, the clinician focusing on the syntactic and semantic deficits caused by the individual's aphasia is working on impairment [I]. However, [I] is contained completely within the set of the person [P], who is contained completely within an environment [E]. It also intersects the communication [C] between the person with aphasia and the communication partner [CP], as well as the communication partner as an individual, as seen in **Figure 3.3**.

Assessing and treating aphasia will have a direct effect on the total person [P], the communication partner [CP], the level of communication between them [C], and their shared environment [E]. Conversely, [P], [CP], [C], and [E] will have a direct effect on the level of impairment as therapy proceeds. Therapy and assessment must not be confined to circle [I], which may be considered *treating to deficit*. To be effective, treatment should address all the

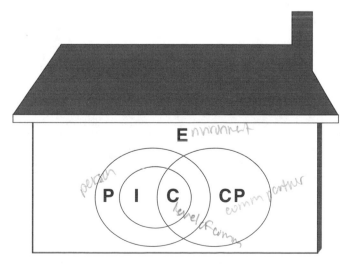

FIGURE 3.2 The intersection of sets.

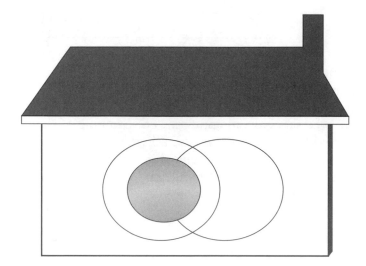

FIGURE 3.3 Treating to deficit.

other intersections in the diagram to maximize the person's unimpaired communication skills (*treating to strength*) (**Figure 3.4**), repair communication acts between adults with aphasia and their communication partners (**Figure 3.5**), educate and support communication partners (**Figure 3.6**), repair the communication-impaired environment and provide opportunities for communication (**Figure 3.7**), and treat the whole person to reduce psychosocial handicap (**Figure 3.8**).

There are two major points of applying set theory:

1. Diagnosis of aphasia must be comprehensive. The whole person as well as the communication partners and environment must be treated. Ask questions such as, "Who is your best friend?" and "What is your favorite food?" in addition to those indicated in standardized aphasia batteries.
2. The individual's needs and wishes must be integral components in determining approaches to treatment.

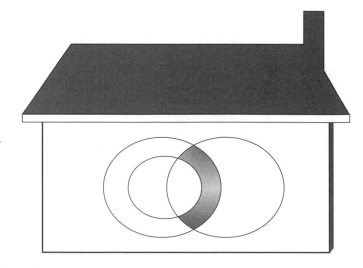

FIGURE 3.4 Treating to strength.

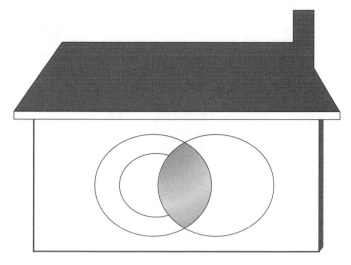

FIGURE 3.5 Repairing communicative acts.

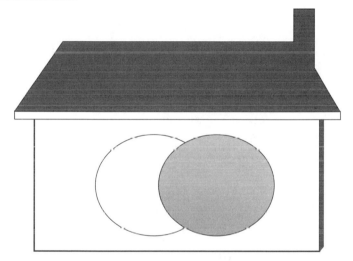

FIGURE 3.6 Educating and supporting communicative partners.

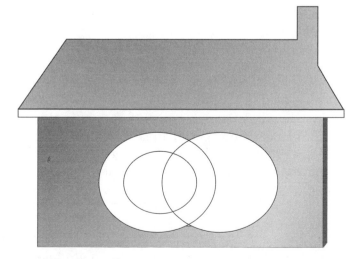

FIGURE 3.7 Repairing the communication environment.

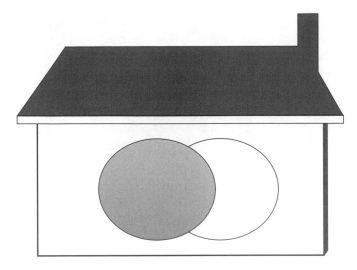

FIGURE 3.8 Treating the whole person, not just the disability.

Goals of Therapy

There are three basic goals of therapy that are applicable to all the communication disorders described in this text.

The first goal is to inform the patient and the caretaker(s) about the nature and consequences of the disorder. This is done to help alleviate any misconceptions about the condition and to provide the proper counseling and psychological support for the patient and the caretaker(s). Information about spontaneous recovery, prognosis, stages of the disorder, and reactions of the patient and/or family may be included in this goal.

The second goal is to provide the appropriate treatment approaches and techniques. This is done to teach the patient how to compensate and use various strategies in his or her efforts to communicate in a functional manner. Information about the efficacy of therapy may be included in this goal.

The third goal is to encourage the patient and the caretaker(s) to continue the rehabilitative process outside of the clinical setting. This would involve practice and environmental changes at home or at the care facility to achieve the carryover or generalization of what occurs in the clinical setting. Information about family and spousal attitudes, and general and specialized home or facility treatment by caretakers, may be included in this goal.

The first goal of therapy is to inform the patient and the caretaker(s) about the nature and consequences of the disorder.

After a language evaluation is completed, usually the speech-language pathologist, and occasionally another professional, will relate the findings to the patient and/or caretaker. It makes life a little easier for the patient and caretaker if the one explaining the evaluation can say where needed, "You have a condition called aphasia, and all aphasia means is a language disturbance. Your thinking abilities should be close to normal. Aphasia is very common after strokes [or trauma or tumor]. You have no motor problems of the lips or tongue [or you have a motor problem, or dysarthria or apraxia of speech, and that is why your articulation is disturbed]. Your brain is healing every second and with that can come some restoration of function. Of course, everybody is not the same. Some will heal faster than others."

The above sounds so obvious, but the authors have dealt with a number of patients and caretakers who were still completely in the dark about the condition even after seeing the appropriate professionals. One patient with aphasia came on a bus to the rehabilitation center for his therapy. Using his aphasic language along with gestures, he explained that people on the bus and elsewhere thought that he was either drunk (forming his hand like a cup and making a drinking motion) or crazy (moving his index finger in a circle near his right temple). Uninformed or poorly informed patients and caretakers may feel the same way about the condition called aphasia.

Holland and Fridriksson (2001) and Fridriksson and Holland (2001) proposed some thoughts on how clinicians might maximize patient resources during the acute care stage. Their approach emphasizes patient and family counseling instead of focusing on impairment-based treatment. It stresses social support during this difficult stage, and is not designed specifically on language improvement. It employs the skills of the clinician to abbreviate the burden of the crisis facing both patients and families during the early days following the stroke. The authors feel that structured language treatment is best employed when the aphasia symptoms become more chronic.

On the other hand, Peach (2001) states that treatment for aphasia during the acute stage should be based on the assessment results derived from standardized instruments that have shown validity and reliability and that meet the demands of practice in the present healthcare environment. Peach (1993) as cited in Peach (2001) further notes that although treatment during the acute stage may include attempts to offer an immediate source of basic communication, the great focus should be on remediation of language impairment using multimodality stimulation on these deficits to improve long-term outcome.

Glista (2006) cites a study by Avent et al. (2005) that provides a list of 20 questions that were derived from the experiences of other family members that relate to the onset of aphasia, the beginning of treatment, and the chronic phase of aphasia. Questions may include: "What is a stroke?", "Can we watch or participate in therapy?", and "What support services are available?" The SLP can give the list of questions to the family and let them decide which ones they want answered, or the SLP might discuss some of the issues as they come up.

Spontaneous Recovery

Before getting into the specifics of therapy, there are several factors that influence the language intervention process. One factor is the concept of spontaneous recovery, which is the body healing itself without any therapy. Spontaneous recovery is most likely due to a reduction of edema or swelling in the damaged hemisphere, a return to normal blood flow or circulation in the undamaged hemisphere, and collateral or compensatory blood circulation in the damaged hemisphere.

The greatest amount of spontaneous recovery takes place within the first two months postonset of the brain lesion. More spontaneous recovery will take place from the third through the sixth month postonset, but to a lesser extent than in the first two months. More recovery will take place from the seventh through the twelfth months, but this will not be as much as in the first six months. Reviews of spontaneous recovery can be found in Benson (1979), Benson and Ardila (1996), Cherney and Robey (2008), Kertesz, Lau, and Polk (1993), Mlcoch and Metter (2008), and M. Sarno (1991).

Prognosis

Prognosis is another feature in language rehabilitation. Before deciding who would make a good candidate for therapy or providing information to patients and their families about the prospects for improvement, the clinician could gain insight into these processes through a number of prognostic indicators. These indicators might also predict improvement through spontaneous recovery.

Although the prognostic factors cited are gleaned from the literature in aphasia, many of these indicators might apply to patients with other communicative disorders. The following prognostic indicators have been outlined by Benson and Ardila (1996), Darley (1982), Patterson and Chapey (2008), and M. Sarno (1991).

1. The younger the patient, the better the prognosis.
2. The sooner the patient enters therapy after the onset of aphasia, the better the prognosis.
3. The less extensive the neurological damage, the better the prognosis.
4. Borderzone and subcortical lesions offer a better prognosis than perisylvian lesions.
5. Broca's, transcortical motor, conduction, and anomic aphasia offer a better prognosis than the other types of aphasia.
6. Hemorrhage as a cause of cerebrovascular accident seems to offer a better prognosis than ischemia.
7. If the patient with aphasia has the will to improve and accept limitations, the prognosis is better.
8. If the family of the patient with aphasia has the proper attitude and provides encouragement to the patient, the prognosis is better.
9. The milder the language impairment at the initial evaluation, the better the prognosis.
10. If the patient receives a longer and more intense period of speech and language therapy, the prognosis is better.
11. The better the physical condition with no sensory defects, the better the prognosis.

Darley (1982) cited several studies indicating that when dysarthria accompanies aphasia, the prognosis for recovery in aphasia is poorer. However, other studies he cited differed about prognosis when apraxia of speech or oral apraxia accompanies aphasia. Although there are always exceptions, these prognostic factors might provide insight and guidelines for therapy and help in guidance and counseling procedures for the family.

Patients' Reaction to Illness

Patients with aphasia may react to their illness with depression, anxiety, denial, guilt at being sick, anger, counterproductive coping, fear, frustration, and embarrassment. One was a 75-year-old, wheelchair-confined patient with aphasia, whose nephew built a wooden ramp with handrails leading from the house to the backyard. With the ramp providing easy access, the patient still refused to sit in his own backyard because he was embarrassed to have the neighbors see him sitting in a wheelchair.

Patients may also have emotional lability (emotional incontinence) and catastrophic reactions (Damecour & Caplan, 1991; Mlcoch & Metter, 2008; Sapir & Aronson, 1990; Swindell & Hammons, 1991). These reactions can interfere with the whole rehabilitative process, especially language therapy. As Damecour and Caplan (1991) noted in their study of patients with aphasia, depression was not correlated with lesion site or size of lesion, and there was no difference in the degree of depression between Broca's and Wernicke's subjects.

A particular patient with Broca's aphasia and a right-sided paralysis mentioned that he was in the infantry in World War II and fought in the Battle of the Bulge. The fighting was extremely difficult, but finally the Americans were victorious over the Germans. In spite of those horrendous wartime conditions, he said nothing is as bad as having a stroke and all of its symptoms. In that vein, Ross (2005) has provided a number of articles related to quality of life research, with the hope of helping clinicians to use quality of life issues in diagnosis, intervention, and interpretation of intervention outcomes.

The second goal of therapy is to provide the appropriate treatment approaches and techniques.

Efficacy of Aphasia Therapy

Applying the scientific method, rather than an educational model, to speech-language therapy requires that the clinician prepare a clinical hypothesis, not a lesson plan to guide treatment (see Santo Pietro & Goldfarb, 1995, for a clinical hypothesis template). It makes sense that clinicians should test hypotheses, rather than follow a curriculum. If the hypothesis is falsified as a result of clinical intervention, then it can be abandoned, and another hypothesis tested; if the clinician follows a curriculum which does not seem to work, there are few alternatives based on an educational model.

Evidence-based practice supports the hypothesis-testing model, and individual therapy can model an experiment where N = 1. The cognitive shift that the speech-language pathologist makes when switching from applying curricula to testing hypotheses also serves to shorten, or even eliminate, the distance between the clinician and the researcher. The problem is that single-subject treatment research is not easy to evaluate. Any attempt to generalize findings will necessarily suffer from a lack of statistical power. Even if the patient's responses, which may be quite numerous, are treated as the subjects of the experiment, then the results will apply to characteristics of a sample, rather than characteristics of a population.

Beeson and Robey (2006) reviewed over 600 articles published over the past 50 years on treating aphasia and related disorders (288 articles used group designs to examine effects of treatment, and 332 were single-subject case reports or experimental studies). The authors found it difficult to assess efficacy of various treatments or to synthesize the findings in a meaningful way. While meta-analyses of the outcomes from group studies (see, for example, Robey, 1998) suggest that treatment for aphasia results in improvement in language performance relative to untreated controls, such analyses are not appropriate when applied to research where N = 1. Some suggestions (Beeson & Robey, 2006) for evaluating single-subject research include the following:

1. Studies with large effect size, where the treatment effect diverges from the null state, that is, where the outcome is more or less than zero
2. Studies that present testable hypotheses, either in pretreatment vs. posttreatment or treatment vs. no treatment conditions
3. Studies that can be grouped because they address a common dependent variable, such as lexical retrieval, speech fluency, or auditory comprehension

There are two types of research design used in studies to determine the efficacy of aphasia therapy. There are *group studies*, which measure the effects of aphasia therapy (in its various forms) as opposed to no therapy or deferred therapy, or the effects of therapy administered by speech-language pathologists as opposed to trained volunteers. The findings of each study are generalized to the greater population. Group study research includes that of Basso, Capitani, and Vignolo (1979), Butfield and Zangwill (1946), David, Enderby, and Bainton (1982), Deal and Deal (1978), Elman and Bernstein-Ellis (1999), Hartman and Landau (1987), Lincoln et al. (1984), Marshall et al. (1989), Meikle et al. (1979), Poeck, Huber, and Willmes (1989), Sarno, Silverman, and Sands (1970), Shewan and Kertesz (1984), Vignolo (1964), Wertz (2005), Wertz et al. (1981), and Wertz et al. (1986).

There are also *single-subject experimental studies*, which measure the effectiveness of specific forms of aphasia therapy administered to an individual patient over a period of time and checked at designated intervals. The findings of each study are applicable only to the individual subject, not to the general population. See, for example, the single-subject studies of Boyle and Coelho (1995), Kearns (1985, 2005), McNeil, Small, Masterson, and Fossett (1995), and Thompson, Shapiro, and Roberts (1993).

By almost all accounts (whether the studies are of group or single-subject design), it appears that language therapy for the patient with aphasia is beneficial for language recovery. As Robey (1994) noted in his analysis of 21 efficacy-of-treatment studies, there is a clear superiority in the performance of patients with aphasia who receive treatment from a speech-language pathologist.

In a follow-up meta-analysis of 55 reports of aphasia treatment outcomes, Robey (1998) found the following:

1. Results for treated patients are superior to those for untreated patients in all stages of recovery. Results are greatest when therapy is begun in the acute stage of recovery (during or before the third month postonset of the neuropathology).
2. Therapy length of two hours or more per week brings more gains than does therapy of shorter durations.
3. Of specifically named therapies, the Schuell-Wepman-Darley Multimodality (SWDM), or "stimulation approach," was reported in a relatively large number of primary studies.
4. Large gains are achieved by patients with severe aphasia when they are treated by a speech-language pathologist.
5. There are too few investigations that examine the differential effects of therapies for the different types of aphasia.

Elman and Bernstein-Ellis (1999) found that adults with chronic aphasia receiving group communication treatment (five hours per week) had significantly higher scores on linguistic and communicative measures than adults with chronic aphasia not receiving treatment. In addition, significant increases were revealed after two months of treatment and after four months of treatment.

Holland, Fromm, DeRuyter, and Stein (1996) have noted several representative treatment techniques that appear to be effective with patients who have aphasia. These treatment approaches and techniques include the following (described later in this section): traditional modality-specific stimulus-response treatment (also known as the "stimulation approach"), language oriented therapy (LOT), group therapy, functional communication therapy, PACE therapy, programmed instruction approaches, melodic intonation therapy, and visual action therapy. Holland et al. (1996) wrote, "Talented aphasia clinicians sample from among available approaches for those that augment their patient's strengths and compensate for deficit. . . . Matching aphasic patients to the most effective clinical technique for management is an area ripe for further investigation" (p. 33).

In conclusion, Brookshire (1994) has stated

> The work is not yet over, for several issues remain—issues which are likely to escalate in importance as resources allocated to health care diminish and as accountability becomes more and more important. Aphasiologists need to demonstrate that specific treatment approaches work for specific communicative disabilities. Although single-case studies seem a natural vehicle for this work, it may be that group studies will be needed to convince consumers (patients, families, physicians, and funding agencies) that the approaches are appropriate and effective for some meaningful segment of the aphasic population (p. 12).

The literature on the efficacy of aphasia therapy has been reviewed by Cherney and Robey (2008), Elman and Bernstein-Ellis (1999), Holland et al. (1996), Robey (1994, 1998), Tompkins et al. (2008), and Wertz (1992).

Stimulation Approach

One of the major approaches to aphasia therapy is the stimulation approach and its variations.

Schuell (Schuell, Jenkins, & Jimenez-Pabon, 1964) conceived the simulation approach to aphasia therapy and noted that stimulation is supported by the following: (1) sensory stimulation affects brain activity; (2) repeated sensory stimuli are essential for the organization, storage, and retrieval of language patterns in the brain; (3) the auditory system is of prime importance for language acquisition and for processing information and feedback in ongoing functional language; (4) nearly all patients with aphasia have auditory deficits, and recovery in this modality will help the other modalities; (5) because of its crucial link to language, gains made through the auditory modality will extend to all other input and output language channels.

General Principles of the Stimulation Approach

Schuell (Schuell, Jenkins, & Jimenez-Pabon, 1964) further elaborated the general principles of the stimulation approach. They are presented here along with additional references: (1) intensive auditory stimulation should be used along with the other modalities; (2) the stimulus must be adequate and get into the brain; (3) repetitive sensory stimulation should be used; Hough, Pierce, and Cannito (1989) and Tompkins (1991) found that redundancy of stimulation will help comprehension in aphasia; (4) each stimulus should elicit a response; (5) responses should be elicited and not forced; (6) a maximum number of responses should be elicited; a large number of adequate responses indicates a large number of adequate stimuli; (7) feedback about accuracy of response should be provided when such feedback appears beneficial; (8) work should proceed systematically and intensively; (9) sessions should begin with relatively easy, familiar tasks and proceed to more difficult tasks after the patient experiences success; (10) the examiner should use abundant and varied materials and present them in the proper manner. Bracy and Drummond (1993) found that the use of pictograms (comic strips) was better than a single picture for eliciting word retrieval in participants with fluent and nonfluent aphasia; and (11) new materials and procedures should be extensions of familiar materials and procedures.

Structure of Stimulation

The structure of stimulation listed below follows the Coelho et al. (2008) outline. Many of the research summaries surrounding each factor can be found in Brookshire (2007), Coelho et al. (2008), Darley (1982), and Rosenbek et al. (1989).

Auditory perceptual clarity (volume and noise). Reducing noise or working in quiet facilitates language performance. Increasing volume is not useful except in specific cases.

Nonlinguistic visual–perceptual clarity (dimensionality, size, color, content, ambiguity, operativity). *Operativity* is described as a stimulus that can involve other senses. For example, a picture of a rock will be easier for the patient to name than a picture of a cloud. A rock can be seen and touched, whereas a cloud can only be seen. Operativity may be another term for concreteness. The clinician should be clear, realistic, and redundant. The most potent visual stimuli are characterized by these dimensions: color, lack of ambiguity, operativity, and redundant physical properties.

Quite often, for a confrontation naming task, the authors use very large (8 ½ × 11 inches) and very clear black-and-white pictures from a popular rehabilitation kit. However, one picture is that of an open box of matches, with the matches lined up in the rectangular box. Many patients have perceived a piano from the shape of the box, with the lineup of matches as a line of piano keys.

Towne and Banick (1989) studied the naming performances of adults with nonfluent and fluent aphasia. They found no significant differences in naming ability when participants were presented with black-and-white or colored versions of pictures.

Linguistic visual–perceptual clarity (size and form). Large print seems better; the clinician should be aware of idiosyncratic preferences.

Method of delivery of auditory stimulation. Auditory stimulation that is direct, with live voice, binaural, and in the free field, is best. Moineou, Dronkers, and Bates (2005) studied some factors (e.g., age-related decrements, processing great chunks of information in a short amount of time) that can interfere with the listening climate.

Discriminability (semantic, auditory, visual). The best approach is to select stimuli that offer few response alternatives. In the semantic area, words that are closely associated in meaning (e.g., *knife* and *fork*) should be avoided when the patient is given a number of responses from which to choose. Similarly, closely related choices should be avoided when presenting words auditorily (e.g., *goat* and *coat*) and visually (e.g., *car* and *oar*). The clinician should particularly avoid stimuli that contain two or three of the factors mentioned above (e.g., *ear* and *hair, neck* and *leg*), where they can be confused semantically and auditorily.

Combined sensory modalities. The best method is combined auditory and visual stimulation. This helps the single modalities and is a good starting point. Using the tactile modality also helps. The multimodality stimulus provides redundancy and additional cues for the patient. The patient should not be overloaded with too much multimodality stimulation. It can cause distraction and exceed the capacity of the patient.

Beukelman, Yorkston, and Waugh (1980) found that patients with aphasia are more successful when given combined verbal and pantomimed instructions than when given these instructions separately. Hough (1993) treated a patient with Wernicke's aphasia who had jargon, using a program concentrating on visual and written stimuli instead of auditory comprehension activities. After two months, the patient improved in naming and general conversation, including a reduction of the jargon.

Stimulus repetition. Repetition of stimuli after the incorrect response appears to increase adequate responses (especially after the first or second repetition).

Rate and pause. The clinician should speak slowly with a slow overall rate. One should pause at appropriate intervals to help auditory retention, and reduce rate of phoneme production by prolonging words (see Goldfarb & Halpern, 1981; Schulte & Brandt, 1989).

Length and redundancy (a factor in all modalities). Through the visual modality, short words, sentences, and paragraphs are better; through the auditory modality, short phrases, sentences, and paragraphs are better. Length may not be a factor at the word level. Redundancy can overcome the limitations of length. For example, Halpern (1965a,b) and Silver and Halpern (1992) found that regardless of modality, long words were more difficult for patients with aphasia than were short words.

Cues, prompts, and prestimulation. These are techniques to facilitate word finding in oral and written expression, or in auditory and reading comprehension (e.g., to stimulate the patient to name a picture of a "watch," the SLP shapes own articulators for the /w/ sound; other examples of this are given in this section). Freed and Marshall (1995), Freed, Marshall, and Nippold (1995), and Lowell, Beeson, and Holland (1995) elaborate further on the use of cues, prompts, and prestimulations in aphasia therapy. Ramsberger and Marte (2007) found that self-administered, computer-based, cued naming therapy using a common mixed-cue (phonological and semantic) protocol may be beneficial to a wide range of persons with aphasia regardless of treatment schedule. Treatments such as this may be a low-cost supplement or extension to traditional aphasia therapy.

Frequency and meaningfulness. Frequency refers to how often a word is used in the English language. Meaningfulness refers to language that contains personal relevance and emotion, and whose content conforms to the expected order of things (e.g., *Dog bites man* rather than *Man bites dog*). The higher the frequency of occurrence in the language (see Halpern, 1965b; Silver & Halpern, 1992) and the more meaningful the word stimuli, the greater the chance of a correct response.

Abstractness. Concrete words represent items that are closely related to the senses (e.g., *apple*; one can see, touch, smell, taste, and hear the biting crunch of an apple), whereas abstract words represent concepts that are distant from the senses (e.g., *justice, mercy*). Typically, concrete words would be easier for the patient than abstract words (Halpern, 1965a,b). However, abstractness can be overcome by frequency of occurrence and redundancy. Redundant (semantically supporting) words in a sentence may facilitate comprehension regardless of abstraction level or even length (e.g., "Point to the *furry* cat" would be easier for the patient than "Point to the cat" in an array of pictures placed in front of the patient).

Part of speech and semantic word category. Verbs, adjectives, and nouns may be easier than conjunctions, articles, and prepositions. Among verbs, adjectives, and nouns, nouns would likely be easiest if frequency is controlled (see Halpern, 1965b). In ambiguous noun–verb tasks, verbs were overselected by participants with fluent aphasia, while nouns were overselected by participants with nonfluent aphasia (Goldberg & Goldfarb, 2005).

Grammar and syntax. There is a hierarchy of grammatical difficulty that affects all the aphasias. In any modality, the harder the grammar, the more difficulty the patient with aphasia has. For example, present-tense sentences (e.g., *The boy catches the ball*) are easier to comprehend than past-tense sentences (e.g., *The boy caught the ball*) or future-tense sentences (e.g., *They both will catch the ball*). Sentences that use the agent-action-object order (e.g., *The mother hugs the baby*) are easier than sentences that do not use this order (e.g., *The policeman was kicked by the robber*). Sentences that are simplified syntactically by expansion (e.g., *The woman was tall and the man was short*) are easier than grammatically compact sentences (e.g., *The woman was taller than the man*).

Other morphologic or syntactic features indicate that comprehension or expression of the affirmative is easier than the negative, singular easier than plural, and plural easier than possessive (e.g., *horses vs. horse's*).

These are just a few examples of how grammatical complexity can affect the patient with aphasia. The type of aphasia (Broca's, Wernicke's, etc.) can also influence the hierarchy of difficulty involved with grammar and syntax.

Context. Context can be simply described as the information received or expressed within the whole communicative setting. A patient receiving or expressing information can do this with silence, single words, sentences, or discourse (running or normal conversation). Currently, discourse seems to be the best way to provide context. Along with context, discourse can also provide redundancy, predictability, and extralinguistic cues, all of which help derive information that will facilitate language received or expressed in the individual with aphasia.

In this vein, the authors (both SLPs whose only language is English) remember a patient with aphasia whose only language was Russian. Part of the team treating this patient was a bilingual (Russian and English) nurse who, under the guidance of the SLP, was able to evaluate the patient's language. The patient was severely impaired in all the language modalities and certainly in need of language therapy. Because there was no bilingual (Russian and English) SLP available, it was decided that one of the authors would work with the patient with the help of the patient's wife who was fluent in both Russian and English.

Treatment started with auditory commands such as "look up," "look down," "turn your head," and so forth. The wife would say these phrases in Russian and the SLP would write down the pronunciation of each word using phonetic symbols. Apparently the SLP's pronunciation of Russian was terrible because she constantly said "no good" and proceeded to correct the SLP.

This scenario went on for a number of words and phrases, when suddenly the patient raised his arm and hand and held it in the "stop" position (as would a traffic cop). He then moved his hand in a "calming" gesture indicating to his wife that "It's OK, leave him alone, it's not so bad." The patient, who was severely impaired in all the language modalities, apparently picked up the extralinguistic cues (facial expression, body movements, prosody of the speakers) that caused him to understand what was going on.

Stress. This factor appears to be tied to word order and saliency. Kimelman (1991) found that stressed target words alone within a paragraph did not bring better auditory comprehension in listeners with aphasia. The author postulated that better auditory comprehension was probably due to the prosodic cues that preceded the stressed target words.

Saliency is characterized by stress and phonological prominence and by informational and personal significance. Not only will adults with aphasia do better with auditory comprehension when stress is employed, but they will also be more successful when asked to repeat sentences that contain salient features (e.g., "Sink or swim, he said" is easier for the patient to repeat than "He said, sink or swim"). Many patients need a salient word at the beginning of the utterance in order to initiate speech.

Order of difficulty. The clinician should begin with familiar, easy tasks, then proceed to less familiar and more difficult ones, and end with tasks that result in a great deal of success. This order contrasts with the presentation of test material on the PICA, where the rationale is to assess more difficult and complex stimuli first, when the patient is presumably fresher, and proceed to easier stimuli when the patient is more tired. Thompson (2007), in her review, emphasized the approach that espouses training complex structures to promote generalized improvement of simpler, linguistically related structures.

Psychological and physical factors. Patients do better when not suffering from tension or fatigue. Tompkins, Marshall, and Phillips (1980) found that mornings are better than afternoons for scheduling therapy. It is also important to discuss timing of therapy with regard to medication schedule. Certain drugs that lower blood pressure, for example, cause fatigue an hour or so after ingestion.

Pattern of auditory deficit. Brookshire (1974) noted that in comprehending sentences, patients can show any of the following: slow rise time (miss initial portions); noise buildup (miss final portions); retention deficit (length causes problems); information capacity deficit (too many ideas in sentences); and intermittent auditory imperception (understanding of auditory input fluctuates randomly).

Specific Examples of the Stimulation Approach

Following are some suggestions for therapy for deficits in the four language modalities. These suggestions derive from the general literature in aphasia and from the authors' own experiences. Within each modality, the tasks gradually move from easy to more difficult items. Each task listed is only one example of what could develop into any number of other tasks.

Therapy for auditory comprehension deficit (ACD). In the following tasks, the clinician provides the auditory stimulus. The patient responds in the different manners described. In those tasks requiring the use of pictures, the number of pictures can range anywhere from one to six.

Starting with auditory comprehension of single words (ACD 1.B), the clinician can place a single picture (e.g., of a key) or a single object (e.g., the key itself) in front of the patient.

The clinician can identify the picture or the object by pointing to it and naming it several times. After that, the clinician says "key," "Point to the key," or "Show me the key," and beckons for the patient to respond by pointing to the picture or the object.

When convinced that the patient understands, the clinician can introduce another stimulus word (e.g., *spoon*) and work with only that word in the manner described above. The next step would be putting the two pictures or the two objects (e.g., key and spoon) side by side. The clinician proceeds by saying one of the two stimulus words and having the patient indicate the correct picture or item.

If the patient is correct according to whatever criterion the clinician uses (e.g., correct 90% or better over 20 trials), then the clinician can introduce additional stimulus words in the same manner. If the patient is not correct at the level of two stimulus words, the clinician should return to a single stimulus word and introduce some of the other modalities to reinforce the auditory modality (e.g., showing the printed stimulus word, having the patient write it, and/or having the patient say it in addition to hearing it from the clinician).

Many of these procedures described as a starting point for auditory comprehension can be converted into a starting point for reading comprehension (e.g., instead of saying the stimulus word to the patient, the clinician can match the printed stimulus word to the picture or the object, as in RCD 3.A, and proceed as outlined for auditory comprehension).

ACD 1.
A. Commands involving the body (e.g., "Look up, look down, stand up, sit down, close your eyes, open your eyes, turn around, stick out your tongue, smile, take off your glasses, put on your glasses," etc.).
B. Point to picture matching single-word stimulus.
C. Point to own body parts or clothing matching single-word stimulus (e.g., *nose, shirt*).
D. Point to items in room matching single-word stimulus (e.g., *lamp, door*).

ACD 2.
A. Point to picture showing antonym to single-word stimulus (e.g., *up–down*).
B. Point to picture showing semantic association for single-word stimulus (e.g., *table–chair*).
C. Point to picture corresponding to single-word nouns (e.g., *pen, carpet*).
D. Point to picture corresponding to single-word adjectives (e.g., *tall, fat*).
E. Point to picture corresponding to single-word verbs (e.g., *smiling, walking*).
F. Point to picture corresponding to single-word prepositions (e.g., *on, in*).

ACD 3.
Follow commands to open, close, show, raise, hold, hum, shake, tap, rub, straighten, look, give, blink, put, scratch, move, touch, pucker, turn, nod, stick out, pick, make, or gesture (using self with and without objects).

ACD 4.
A. Point to a printed letter or number.
B. Point to a printed word.
C. Point to a picture or object in order to complete a sentence (e.g., "Please pass the salt and ___").
D. Point to a picture or object whose name is spelled (e.g., "T-A-B-L-E").

ACD 5.
A. Point to a picture or object described by function (e.g., "Point to the item used for drinking").
B. Point to a picture or object grouped by location (e.g., "What do you find in a living room?").

ACD 6.
A. Point to two or three nouns (e.g., *lamp, chair, window*).
B. Point to two or three verbs (e.g., *walking, reading, sleeping*).
C. Point to two or three items described by function (e.g., *drinking, cutting, writing*).

D. Point to two or three items grouped by location (e.g., "What do you find in a bedroom, living room, and kitchen?").

ACD 7.   A. Point to three or four items (e.g., pictures, self, environment).

B. Point to item described by varying number of descriptors (e.g, "Point to the small, red square").

C. Point to item best described by a sentence (e.g., "Point to the picture of people relaxing." There will be a picture of people relaxing on a beach among other very different pictures).

D. Follow two object location commands (e.g., "Put the pencil in front of the book").

E. Follow two verb commands (e.g., "Point to the book, pick up the pencil").

F. Follow two verb time commands (e.g., "Before touching the comb, pick up the cup").

(The following section requires yes/no responses from the patient.)

ACD 8.   A. Questions about pictures (e.g., "Is the girl walking?").

B. Questions involving general information (e.g., "Was Washington the sixteenth president?").

C. Questions involving auditory retention span (e.g., "Are peaches, apples, pears, chickens, and bananas all fruits?").

D. Questions involving semantic discrimination (e.g., "Do you play tennis with a bat?").

E. Questions involving phoneme discrimination (e.g., "Do men wear shirts and pies to work?").

F. Questions involving specific and general information from sentences and from short and long paragraphs.

(The following section requires oral or written expression, or reading comprehension responses from the patient.)

ACD 9.   A. Listen to short or long paragraphs or stories and answer questions about them.

B. Listen to short or long paragraphs or stories and retell them.

Therapy for reading comprehension deficit (RCD). In the following tasks, the clinician provides the visual stimulus in varying conditions. The patient responds to the visual stimulus in the different manners described. Many of the items suggested for auditory comprehension deficit can be converted into therapy tasks for reading comprehension deficit.

RCD 1.   A. Match identical pictures.

B. Match geometric forms (e.g., ❑ ▼ O • with O ❑ • ▼).

C. Match printed letters, words, phrases, and sentences.

D. Match similar pictures in the same category (e.g., palm, fir, and maple trees).

(The following section requires some of the patient's auditory comprehension and oral expression abilities.)

RCD 2.   A. Identify named letters to printed choices.

Beeson, Rising, Kim, and Rapecsak (2010) used a two-stage treatment protocol to strengthen sublexical skills (phonological treatment) and to train interactive use of lexical and sublexical information to improve spelling performance (interactive treatment) with two participants who both exhibited characteristics of phonological alexia and agraphia. Results showed that both participants improved phonological processing abilities and reading/spelling via the sublexical route. They also improved spelling of real words and were able to detect and correct most residual errors using an electronic spelling aid.

B. Identify named words to printed choices.

C. Identify multiple named words to printed choices.

D. Name individual printed letters.

E. Read in unison with the clinician.

RCD 3. A. Match printed word to picture or object.

B. Match printed word to picture using antonyms (e.g., *up–down*).

C. Match printed word to picture using semantic associations (e.g., *table–chair*).

D. Match printed phrase to picture (e.g., *brushing hair*).

RCD 4. A. Read simple phrase and complete (e.g., *Cats and ___ [oceans, dogs, lamps]*).

B. Read complex phrase and complete (e.g., *A car [travels, auto, fires] fast*).

C. Arrange printed words into a phrase (e.g., *of, soup, bowl*).

D. Arrange printed words into categories (e.g., *animals, fruits, cities*).

RCD 5. A. Read simple sentence and complete (e.g., song lyrics, *The bells are ___*; or nursery rhymes, *Jack and Jill went up the___*).

B. Read complex sentence and complete (e.g., *The horse has 4___ [legs, ears, tails]*).

RCD 6. A. Match printed sentence to picture (e.g., *The door is open*).

B. Read simple sentence and give yes/no response (e.g., *Is ten less than four?*).

C. Read complex sentence and give yes/no response (e.g., *If the water is boiling, is the water cold?*).

D. Read sentence—choice (e.g., *A state in the U.S. is___ [Spain, June, Texas]*).

E. Read sentence—homonyms (e.g., *On his shoes, he wore rubber___ [heels, heals]*).

F. Read sentence—verbs (e.g., *Mom is___[doing, do] the dishes*).

G. Read sentence—plurals (e.g., *My friend has two ___ [son, sons]*).

H. Read sentence—synonyms (e.g., *Another word for big is __ [large, thin, small]*).

I. Read sentence—antonyms (e.g., *The opposite of tall is ___ [fat, long, short]*).

J. Read sentence—comparative (e.g., *He is [tall, taller, tallest] than she is*).

K. Read sentence—time (e.g., *Look at the window, after you point to the floor*).

RCD 7. Follow commands (see ACD 3 for examples).

RCD 8. A. Read a short-to-long paragraph and give yes/no responses.

B. Read a short-to-long paragraph and give multiple-choice responses.

(RCD 9 and 10 require oral or written responses from the patient.)

RCD 9. A. Read single word or sentence and define.

B. Read sentence containing *wh* questions and respond in any manner (*What? Where? When? Why? Whose? Which?*).

C. Read a proverb and tell what it means.

RCD 10. Read a short or long paragraph, or a story, and retell it.

Therapy for oral expression deficit (OED). In the following tasks, the clinician provides stimuli in varying conditions. The patient responds orally. Many of the items suggested for auditory and reading comprehension deficit can be converted into therapy tasks for oral expression deficit.

Some suggestions for correcting erroneous responses are given in the section titled "Specific Examples for Correcting an Incorrect Response." This section follows the section titled "Therapy for Written Expression Deficit (WED)."

OED 1. A. Repeat after clinician, read aloud, or recite automatic language (e.g., numbers, days of week, months of year, alphabet).
   B. Sing in unison with clinician or alone (e.g., "Happy Birthday," "Three Blind Mice," etc.).
   C. Say nursery rhymes in unison with clinician, repeat after clinician, or say alone (e.g., "Jack and Jill," "Humpty Dumpty," etc.).
   D. Repeat after clinician single words, phrases, sentences.

(In OED 2 and 3, the clinician says most of the phrase or sentence and the patient completes it.)

OED 2. A. Complete phrase with familiar paired associates (e.g., "bacon and ____").
   B. Complete phrase with familiar paired antonyms (e.g., stop and ____").
   C. Complete sentence with initial phonemic cue (e.g., "You blow your n ____").
   D. Complete familiar sayings (e.g., "Have a good ____").
   E. Complete song lyrics (e.g., "Row, row, row your____").
   F. Complete nursery rhymes (e.g., "Jack and Jill went up the ____").

OED 3. A. Complete sentence using nouns (e.g., "We sleep in a ____").
   B. Complete sentence using adjectives (e.g., "The sky is ____").
   C. Complete sentence using verbs (e.g., "When hungry, you should ____").
   D. Complete sentence using prepositions; clinician shows pictures or objects (e.g., "The spoon is ____ the cup").
   E. Complete sentence using antonyms (e.g., "He isn't fat; he's ____").
   F. Complete sentence using proverbs (e.g., "Don't put all your eggs in one ____").

OED 4. A. Name pictures, objects, or body parts.

   Schwartz and Halpern (1973) found that naming of body parts may be affected by the physical impairment of the patient with aphasia.

   Recently, Marshall and Freed (2006) described personalized cuing as similar to the mnemonic devices that non-brain-damaged individuals use to remember important everyday information such as an ATM code or computer password. When this method is used with individuals with aphasia, the patient and the SLP work together to create a cue that will help the recall of a difficult-to-name word. Establishing an association between the word (e.g., *coffee*) and another word (*jam*) or phrase ("I love Starbucks"), drawing upon past expressions ("a trip to the country of Colombia"), using visual language (steam coming from a cup of coffee) or using any other informational link are other helpful strategies.

   After the cue has been established, the patient is taught to recall the target word (*coffee*) by repeatedly pairing the cue and the target word. The interaction between the patient and the clinician during the creation of the cue with the target word makes the patient an active participant in the process that will help in the naming ability.

   B. Complete sentence using convergent stimuli (e.g., "A bee makes ____").

C. Complete sentence using divergent stimuli; clinician shows pictures or objects (e.g., "I see a ___").
D. Name through function (e.g., "Name an appliance used for cooking").
E. Name through comparison (e.g., "Name an animal that's faster than a turtle").
F. Name through categories (e.g., "Name a fruit").
G. Name through semantic association (e.g., "Name as many things as you can that are white").

Boyle (2004) used a semantic feature analysis treatment for one person with anomic aphasia and one person with Wernicke's aphasia and found that confrontation naming of treated nouns improved and generalized to untreated nouns for both participants. Kiran and Thompson (2003) provide support for a semantically based treatment, focused on the featural detail of category items, for training naming in patients with fluent aphasia, as did Kiran (2008) with nonfluent aphasia. Kiran et al. (2011) extended previous work by examining the notion of semantic complexity within goal-derived (*ad hoc*) categories in individuals with aphasia. As predicted, they found that training atypical examples in the semantic category generalized to typical examples, whereas training typical examples did not show generalization to untrained atypical examples. Ochipa, Maher, and Raymer (1998) reported that naming through semantic association was a successful intervention strategy in anomia.

Kiran (2002), in reference to the treatment of naming deficits in individuals with aphasia, reviewed work showing that training more complex, atypical items within a semantic category (e.g., *ostrich* in the category of *birds*) advances access to simpler, typical items within the category (e.g., *sparrow*). The opposite training paradigm does not operate as effectively. That is, training simpler items has no effect on more complex ones. Rider, Wright, Marshall, and Page (2008) found that using semantic feature analysis (SFA) with three adults with nonfluent aphasia resulted in an improvement in confrontational naming ability and may benefit word retrieval in discourse production of closed-set contexts. When using SFA, the patient is prompted with questions to provide information about distinctive features associated with a target that is difficult to retrieve. As an example, if the patient has difficulty in retrieving the word *clock*, the patient might be prompted to provide information related to its location (on the wall), use (telling time), sound (tick-tock), or other prominent features. Kiran and Johnson (2008) noted that their previous work using natural categories with fuzzy boundaries (e.g., birds) was successful in treatment of naming deficits for participants with aphasia. Their present study was done to see if using more rigid categories (e.g., shapes) would have the same success in the treatment of naming deficits of three participants with aphasia. Results of the their present study indicated that acquisition and generalization effects within well-defined categories (e.g., shapes) are overshadowed by their inherent abstractness, rendering those difficult categories to train and of questionable utility in terms of real-world or clinical value.

Edmonds and Babb (2011) examined the effect of verb network strengthening treatment (VNEST) on individuals with moderate-to-severe aphasia.

Their research questions addressed pre- to posttreatment changes on probe sentences containing trained verbs (e.g., "The carpenter is *measuring* the stairs") and semantically related untrained verbs (e.g., "The nurse is *weighing* the baby"). As they predicted, the participants did not show the same extent of improvement that was observed in participants with more moderate aphasia (Edmonds, Nadeu, & Kiran, 2009). Nonetheless, they concluded that the findings suggested that VNEST may be appropriate for persons with moderate-to-severe aphasia, especially with a small adaptation to the treatment protocol that will be retained for future iterations of VNEST.

OED 5.   A. Say words that start with certain letters (general, male and female names, fruits, cities, etc.).
         B. Say associated words after clinician gives word (especially useful when related to patient's special interest).
            Goldfarb and Halpern (1981) found that in word association tasks, participants with aphasia had more difficulty in providing paradigmatic responses (words belonging to the same grammatical class, e.g., *hum* and *sing*) than syntagmatic responses (a grammatical continuation, e.g., *hum* and *tune*). Characteristics of the stimulus word that caused the most problems in evoking paradigmatic responses were high level of abstraction, short length, grammatical category of verbs, and infrequent occurrence.
         C. Say words that rhyme, (e.g., "hot–___").
         D. Say antonyms (e.g., "up–___").
         E. Say synonyms (e.g., "car–___").

OED 6.   A. Answer *wh* questions, in single words or sentences (e.g., "What barks?").
         B. Complete sentence using an adjective and noun (e.g., "Santa is wearing a ___").
         C. Formulate sentences in response to pictures.
         D. Formulate sentences in response to manipulated objects using prepositions (e.g., after placing a spoon [in, beside, in front of, behind, on, etc.] an object, the clinician asks, "Where is the spoon?").
         E. Formulate sentences in response to questions about self (e.g., age), family (e.g., names of children), general information (e.g., president of U.S.).
         F. Formulate sentences using various parts of speech (e.g., nouns, verbs).
         G. Formulate a sentence using two particular words (e.g., *find, radio*).
         H. Formulate a sentence using three particular words (e.g., *path, park, walk*).
         I. Formulate a sentence beginning or ending with selected words or phrases (e.g., "I eat," "when," "if," "she").

OED 7.   A. Define words or sentences in response to auditory and/or visual stimuli.
         B. Explain the functions of items or persons (e.g., *pen, razor, tailor*).
         C. Describe what is happening in a picture.
         D. Describe the activity of the clinician as he or she moves objects about.
         E. Explain what to say in certain situations (e.g., "You are tired, so you say ___").
         F. Ask questions to find out information.

OED 8.   A. Explain more than one meaning of word and then put that word in a sentence (e.g., *spring*).
         B. Explain the meaning of phrases (e.g., "blowing off steam").
         C. Explain how items are different (e.g., *pencil–crayon*).
         D. Explain how items are similar (e.g., *bus, bicycle, car*).

    E. Answer general questions (e.g., "Why do people go to school?").

    F. Explain why statements do not make sense (e.g., "Apples and carrots are fruits").

OED 9.   A. Explain each step in a particular activity (e.g., "How would you make eggs for breakfast?").

    B. Describe everything possible about pictures or objects (e.g., physical properties, uses).

    C. Converse generally about selected topics (e.g., favorite TV programs, movies).

        Cherney, Halper, Holland, and Cole (2008) described computer software that was developed specifically for training conversational scripts, and illustrate its use with three individuals with aphasia. The authors found that all measures (content, grammatical productivity, and rate of production of script-related words) improved for each participant on every script. They concluded that computer-based script training potentially may be an effective intervention for persons with chronic aphasia. Holland, Halper, and Cherney (2010) examined the content of 100 short scripts, coconstructed by persons with aphasia (PWAs) and a clinician. The PWAs subsequently learned the scripts by interacting with a computerized virtual therapist. The goal of this study was to provide clinicians with ideas regarding content for treatment that is meaningful to PWAs. In this study 33 PWAs chose to speak about their life experiences, chose to reconnect with their families, and tended to focus on communication that help them to negotiate mundane normal life. The authors concluded that independent of how this content is used in treatment, materials should emphasize matters of high personal relevance to those treated.

    D. Formulate summaries of short and long paragraphs (read or heard).

OED 10.   A. Explain what an expression means (e.g., "The movie was so-so.").

    B. Explain what a proverb means (e.g., "Don't put all your eggs in one basket").

    C. Unscramble words of a proverb and then tell what it means (e.g., "Over don't milk cry spilled").

    D. Have an open-ended conversation on unrestricted topics.

    E. Retell a radio or TV broadcast or familiar story.

    F. Take a side on a debatable question (e.g., capital punishment).

    G. Explain the ideas of well-known people (e.g., Abraham Lincoln, Franklin D. Roosevelt).

    H. Explain the meaning of metaphors (e.g., "She's the apple of his eye") and similes (e.g., "Happy as a clam").

Therapy for written expression deficit (WED). In the following tasks, the clinician provides stimuli in varying conditions. The patient responds in writing. Many of the items suggested for other modalities, especially oral expression deficit, can be converted into therapy tasks for written expression deficit.

Some suggestions for correcting erroneous responses are given in the section titled "Specific Examples for Correcting an Incorrect Response." This section follows the tasks for written expression deficit. Although geared for correcting oral expression responses, many of the suggestions can be adapted for correcting written expression responses, For instance, Example 1 could easily apply to naming ability (WED 3.A). Instead of calling for an oral response, the clinician could call for a written response.

WED 1. A. Trace or copy (lines, geometric forms, numbers, letters).

B. Trace or copy words.

C. Write letters, numbers, words, phrases, and sentences to dictation.

WED 2. A. Fill in missing letters or words with or without associated picture stimuli (e.g., *She is writing a lette-*, *She is writing a* ___).

Beeson, Rising, Kim, and Rapecsak (2010) used a two-stage treatment protocol to strengthen sublexical skills (phonological treatment) and to train interactive use of lexical and sublexical information to improve spelling performance (interactive treatment) with two participants who both exhibited characteristics of phonological alexia and agraphia. Results showed that both participants improved phonological processing abilities and reading/spelling via the sublexical route. They also improved spelling of real words and were able to detect and correct most residual errors using an electronic spelling aid.

B. Put (write) words into proper categories from choices that are mixed up (e.g., clothing, sports, fruits).

C. Find two words embedded in one word and write them (e.g., *mailman*).

WED 3. A. Write names of pictures, body parts, or objects.

B. Fill in the blank to make another word (e.g., *fort* ___).

C. Write associated word for stimulus word.

WED 4. A. Complete sentences using verbs (e.g., *Children like to* ___ *in the sandbox*).

B. Complete sentences using nouns (e.g., *On Sunday, he read the* ___).

C. Complete sentences using adjectives (e.g., *He wore a red and* ___ *tie*).

D. Complete sentences using prepositions (e.g., *Jack jumped* ___ *the candlestick*).

E. Complete sentences using antonyms (e.g., *The policeman signaled stop and* ___).

WED 5. A. Complete series with words in same category (e.g., *Paris,* ___; *apple,* ___; *carrot,* ___).

B. Write words in alphabetical order.

C. Write several examples for each topic (e.g., items that are round, items that sail).

D. Write words in correct order (e.g., *Quiet be, cup a coffee of*).

E. Rewrite sentences (e.g., *That boy are going to school*).

F. Write a sentence using a particular word.

G. Sentence completion—divergent (e.g., I *see* ___).

WED 6. A. Write functional information (e.g., name, address, age).

B. Write answers to questions (e.g., "What can you do with an empty bottle?").

C. Fill out forms (e.g., bank, insurance, government).

WED 7. A. Write sentences in response to pictures or objects.

B. Complete a story with additional sentences.

C. Complete a crossword puzzle.

WED 8. A. Write as much as possible about a particular topic (e.g., *vacation*).

B. Write a summary of a paragraph that the clinician has narrated.

C. Write a paragraph in response to pictures, objects, or clinician's activity.

D. Write responses to divergent tasks (e.g., "Write three things every good citizen should do"; write the meaning of proverbs).

Specific Examples for Restimulating After an Incorrect Response

Following are some specific examples of how the speech-language pathologist might restimulate after an incorrect response. If the patient fails, any one or combination of the following procedures, as reviewed by Goldfarb and Halpern (1989), might be used to restimulate him or her. The following procedures can also be adapted for the written expression deficit tasks suggested in WED 3 and WED 4.

Example 1

Task: Name a picture of *bread*.

1. Integral stimulation ("Watch me and listen to me"): clinician says, "bread," patient repeats.
2. Cueing: clinician shapes own articulators for "b" sound, clinician provides an eating gesture.
3. Association: clinician says, "You eat it, make toast, put butter on it," etc.
4. Completion: clinician says, "I will put butter on the ___; in the bakery, I buy ___."
5. Multimodality: saying and writing *bread*; saying and seeing the printed word *bread*; saying, seeing the printed word, and writing *bread*.
6. Repetition: patient repeats the target response (e.g., three times in a row to make sure it sticks).
7. Rhyming: clinician says, "Sounds like tread, shred, head."

Example 2

Task: Provide the last word to complete a high associative open-ended sentence (or, with some modifications, turn it into a confrontational naming task).

Cues: initial phoneme, sentence completion, semantic association, and printed word.

Program: Present 25 trials, using all 4 cues noted above. When the patient achieves a criterion level of 80% correct responses for 25 trials over three consecutive sessions, cues will be deleted in order, first the printed word, then the initial phoneme, and finally the semantic association cue.

Examples: Although a minimum of 25 different sentences are required for each session, only 2 are used here as examples. The program is presented on four levels. Failure of the patient to achieve criterion level indicates that the speech-language pathologist should return to a previous level for a particular sentence.

Level 1. Hold a flash card in front of the patient with *DOOR* printed in 1-inch block letters. About five seconds may be optimal. Say to the patient, "Someone is knocking at the d ___." Use a similar orthographic cue for "Wash your hands with soap and w ___."

Level II. Present sentences as on Level I, but eliminate the flash cards.

Level III. Present sentences as on Level II, but eliminate the phonemic cue.

Level IV. Present open-ended sentences that do not include semantic association, such as "I don't like___," "I see a ___," or "There is a ___."

For specifics and a further elaboration of this method of aphasia therapy, the reader is referred to Brookshire (2007), Coelho et al. (2008), Darley (1972, 1982), Rosenbeck, LaPointe, and Wertz (1989), Santo Pietro and Goldfarb (1995), Schuell, Jenkins, and Jimenez-Pabon (1964), and Wepman (1951).

PACE Therapy

Some forms of aphasia therapy favor an overall communication approach. One such procedure is Davis and Wilcox's (1981) PACE (Promoting Aphasics' Communicative Effectiveness). This form of therapy is based on the following four principles:

1. The speech-language pathologist and patient participate equally as senders and receivers of messages (taking turns selecting a picture and conveying the message between them).
2. There is an exchange of new information between the clinician and the patient (keep pictures face down).
3. The patient has a free choice of communication modes in sending the message (use of verbal and nonverbal modalities).
4. When receiving a message from the patient, the clinician provides feedback based on whether or not the message was conveyed (a patient may be linguistically inept but communicatively superb).

The clinician can go first by picking up a picture (e.g., a man shaving) from a group of pictures that were face down. The clinician has to describe the picture verbally or through gesture. The patient has to receive this information and indicate that he understands. The patient then takes his or her turn at picking up a picture and describing it to the clinician. Pictures can show individuals who are shaving, brushing their teeth, eating, saluting, waving, and so forth, and can either be professionally made or come from magazines or newspapers. Davis and Wilcox (1981) advocate using PACE as an adjunct to traditional therapy because it gives the patient experience in overall communication.

Functional Communication Therapy

Another overall communication approach is Functional Communication Therapy (FCT) (Aten, 1994). The following tasks are used to elicit any manner of response (verbal, gesture) from the patient: saying name ("Your first name is ___"), greetings, ordering coffee and meals in a restaurant, reciting address and telephone number, naming family members, listing occupation and hobbies, or naming branch of service, where they grew up, make of car, favorite foods, how they like foods cooked, favorite movies, favorite TV shows, favorite vacations.

Variations of PACE and FCT can easily be adapted for patients with specific capabilities and deficits. For example, the speech-language pathologist can present a single printed word to the patient (reading comprehension) with the spoken instruction (auditory comprehension) to tell what the word means using any form of communication (oral expression, gesture, pointing). Lyon (1992) and Simmons-Mackie (2008) reviewed the various forms of communication in natural settings for adult patients with aphasia.

Therapy for Global Aphasia

Treatment for patients with global aphasia is based on the premise that they can learn a number of skills including matching, copying, and imitation. The main justification for training patients in these sublanguage areas is that it could lead to functional communication (see Collins, 1991; Peach, 2008).

For the global patient, the following unique forms of therapy are suggested:

1. The clinician should use stimuli that offer the best chance of a correct response, such as sentence completion ("The bells are ___"), automatic speech (e.g., counting, reciting the days of the week), singing, repeating after the clinician, etc.

Wallace and Canter (1985) found that severely involved patients do better with personally relevant items, and Van Lancker and Klein (1990) found that patients with global aphasia do better with familiar personal names. McKelvey, Hux, Dietz, and Beukelman (2010) found that eight participants with severe aphasia preferred using personally relevant, contextualized photographs rather than other types of photographs/images to represent words; and performed more accurate word–picture matching when presented with target words associated with personally relevant, contextualized photographs than target words associated with noncontextualized or nonpersonalized photographs/images. Clinically, this supports the communication attempt of people with aphasia who cannot communicate effectively using natural speech alone. Hux, et al. (2008) stated that for augmentative and alternative communication (AAC) purposes, practitioners need to consider the partner-dependent, transitional, or partner-independent status of the communication attempts of individuals with aphasia. Specific AAC strategies and techniques for people with aphasia include the use of augmented input, high- and low-tech communication books and devices, drawing, written choice communication, and gestures.

2. Auditory comprehension of body commands appears easier than other auditory comprehension tasks. Commands that can be used are, "Stand up," "Sit down," "Turn around," "Take off your glasses," "Put on your glasses," "Put on the light," "Turn off the light," "Look up," "Look down."

3. Card games such as 21 or Casino might be used to elicit language or a gesture. Patients can match, sequence, pick up, turn over, put, or arrange cards according to color, suit, or number.

4. Patients can visually match forms, figures, postures, and letter tiles.

5. Patients can trace, copy, and write forms, numbers, letters, and words.

6. The patient can match pantomime with a picture or imitate a gesture made by the clinician (e.g., waving, saluting).

7. Adaptations of PACE (Davis & Wilcox, 1981) and Functional Communication Therapy (FCT) (Aten, 1994), along with Visual Action Therapy (VAT) (Helm-Estabrooks, Fitzpatric, & Barresi, 1982), can be used to elicit some form of communication from the patient. VAT is described as a nonverbal method for patients with severe aphasia. With objects and line drawings of objects such as a hammer, screwdriver, cup, razor, salt shaker, and so forth, the patient is taught to trace, match, and demonstrate the object's use through pantomime. Although VAT is centered on a nonverbal approach, gains in auditory comprehension have been noted by Helm-Estabrooks et al. (1982).

8. Another method is visual communication therapy (Gardner, Zurif, Berry, & Baker, 1976), which is designed to teach the global patient artificial language using a system of arbitrary symbols that represent syntactic and lexical components.

9. A copy and recall treatment (CART) protocol for writing has been shown to be effective with participants who have severe aphasia (Beeson, Rising, & Volk, 2003).

One of the goals in working with global patients is to find that language breakthrough which, for example, might move the patient from a global to a Broca's category. Repeated stimulation in letter- and word-matching with letter tiles might lead to formulative letter-spelling with tiles, or repeated auditory comprehension of body commands might lead to other forms of auditory comprehension. When there is a little opening or breakthrough, the clinician wants to "send in all the troops" with more advanced forms of therapy. Reviews of therapy for the global patient can be found in Collins (1983, 1991) and Peach (2008).

Group Therapy

Kearns (1994) and Kearns and Elman (2008) have included and reviewed five approaches for group therapy with patients who have aphasia. In the first approach, the group setting acts as a vehicle for direct language treatment. Whatever is used in individual therapy is now used in the group. For example, patients may be asked to identify various objects around the room in response to auditory and reading comprehension stimuli ("Point to the chair"), or patients may be asked to name objects around the room through oral or written expression.

The second approach for group therapy involves indirect language treatment. In a loosely structured manner, activities such as general conversation, role playing, field trips, discussion of current events or other topics of interest, and general social interchange (e.g., coffee and cake servings, playing cards or checkers) are instituted.

The third approach calls for the use of sociolinguistic treatment groups. Patients engage in social functional language activities as derived from types of therapy such as PACE, FCT, and so forth.

The fourth approach is the transition group that gears the patient for going from the clinical situation to the real-life situation. These groups meet for a limited and specific period of time prior to the patient's discharge from therapy.

The fifth approach is the maintenance group, where the patient attends stroke clubs or other groups for the disabled. These groups are very social in nature with a good deal of indirect language stimulation activities.

Marshall (1993) found that weekly attendance at group therapy that focused on functional situations was successful for patients with mild aphasia. Reviews of group therapy can be found in Brookshire (2007), Darley (1982), and Kearns and Elman (2008).

Programmed Instruction Therapy

Another general approach to aphasia treatment is programmed instruction. Holland (1970) has noted that programmed instruction is one example of applying learning principles to education. A program is created wherein the principles of shaping and reinforcement are used in a learning task. Shaping involves moving in small, carefully controlled steps toward closer and closer approximation of the criterion behavior. Reinforcement consists of affirmative statements as to the adequacy of a response, or merely the forward movement or progression through a program based upon a correct response. Goldfarb (2006b) described operant conditioning and programmed instruction in alternative and augmentative communication in the treatment of aphasia.

Language-Oriented Treatment

Language-Oriented Treatment (LOT) (Shewan & Bandur, 1986) is an example of a specific treatment approach for patients who have aphasia that includes the principles of programmed instruction. LOT is based on the premise that in aphasia, the language system itself and access to the language system can both be disturbed. This is a view of aphasia not as a loss of language, but rather as an impairment of specific components of language (phonologic, syntactic, semantic, or any combination of these).

An example of the language system itself being impaired would be a patient who makes syntactic errors in oral expression and in auditory comprehension. An example of impairment in the access to the language system would be a patient who can write a word but cannot say it. The content of LOT is based upon a psycholinguistic approach that reflects knowledge about language, its organization, its processing, and its recovery from brain damage. The specific areas in LOT involve the following modalities: (1) auditory processing, (2) visual processing, (3) gestural and combined gestural-verbal conversation, (4) oral expression, and (5) graphic expression. Bandur and Shewan (2008) present a further review of LOT.

A shortcoming of LOT lies in the authors' description of facilitation techniques, scaled from least to most effective, which does not differentiate among types and severity of aphasia. For example, a phonemic cue, which was listed among the more effective, should be used only with adults who have nonfluent (such as Broca's) aphasia, and not for those with greater impairment in auditory processing, such as those with fluent (e.g., Wernicke's, conduction, anomic) aphasia. In addition, the facilitation technique of delay is effective only for those with mild impairments, and not for those with more severe impairments.

Base-Ten Programmed Stimulation Method

In a unique combination of the stimulation and programmed instruction approaches, LaPointe (1977) developed the Base-Ten Programmed Stimulation Method. Included in this method are the programmed operant procedures of clearly defined tasks, baseline performance measurement, and session-by-session progress plotting of the patient with aphasia. This is combined with the numerous features of the stimulation approach designed to elicit many responses from patients with aphasia.

With the programmed stimulation approach, speech and language tasks are composed of 10 stimulus items, which are scored and plotted during 10 therapy sessions. This method also includes compensatory-facilitative and self-cueing strategies that are useful for some patients with aphasia in oral expression and auditory comprehension.

Other Therapy Approaches

Other approaches to aphasia therapy include Melodic Intonation Therapy (MIT) (Sparks, 2008), and the Voluntary Control of Involuntary Utterances (VCIU) (Helm & Barresi, 1980), both of which are described later in this text in the discussion of therapy in the section on dysarthria. The Helm Elicited Language Program for Syntax Stimulation (HELPSS) (Helm-Estabrooks, 1981) is an approach designed to stimulate access to syntactical knowledge in patients with agrammatism or paragrammatism. This program is for use with patients who have nonfluent aphasia and includes training of 11 sentence types with a story completion format. Recently, Thompson et al. (2003) found that patients with agrammatic aphasia could benefit in sentence comprehension and sentence production when the direction of treatment is from more complex to less complex constructions. Thompson and Shapiro (2007), in reference to the treatment of syntactic deficits in individuals with aphasia, summarized the benefits of training complex rather than simple sentence structure.

Rothi, Musson, Rosenbek, and Sapienza (2008) introduced a collection of consensus statements regarding the application of neuroplasticity principles to rehabilitation of dysphagia, dysarthria, apraxia, and aphasia. They defined neuroplasticity as functional reorganization/compensation within residual neural tissue, mediated by changes in neural circuitry.

Klein and Jones (2008) reviewed 10 principles of experience-dependent neural plasticity and considerations in applying them to the damaged brain. The 10 principles of experience-dependent neural plasticity are listed and described as follows:

1. Use it or lose it (failure to drive specific brain functions can lead to functional degradation).
2. Use it and improve it (training that drives a specific brain function can lead to an enhancement of that function).

3. Specificity (the nature of the training experience dictates the nature of the plasticity).
4. Repetition matters (induction of plasticity requires sufficient repetition).
5. Intensity matters (induction of plasticity requires sufficient training intensity).
6. Time matters (different forms of plasticity occur at different times during training).
7. Salience matters (the training experience must be sufficiently salient to induce plasticity).
8. Age matters (training-induced plasticity occurs more readily in younger brains).
9. Transference (plasticity in response to one training experience can enhance the acquisition of similar behaviors).
10. Interference (plasticity in response to one experience can interfere with acquisition of other behaviors).

Ludlow et al. (2008) identified potential opportunities for the principles of neural plasticity to apply to clinical research on the rehabilitation of neurogenic speech motor control disorders. These disorders include the various forms of dysarthria and apraxia of speech secondary to stroke, nerve injury, neurodegenerative disease, brain tumors, or trauma. Idiopathic disorders such as spasmodic dysphonia, oral-mandibular dystonia, and essential tremor affecting the head and neck were also discussed.

Raymer et al. (2007) reported on a new form of aphasia therapy called *constraint-induced language therapy* (CILT). Research has shown that sensory, motor, and cognitive activities can stimulate and activate the mature nervous system and bring about neuroplastic changes, often called *cortical reorganization* (Tank, Vsoratte, & Elbert, 2002, as cited in Raymer et al., 2007). Further investigations reported that forced use and intensive practice of a particular task can bring about behavioral and neural changes.

As one example of how CILT can work in aphasia therapy, Raymer et al. (2007) cited Pulvermüller et al. (2001), who compared the verbal responses of 10 stroke-induced individuals with aphasia who were given CILT, with 7 stroke-induced individuals with aphasia who were given traditional forms of therapy. The CILT group was forced into giving only verbal responses (all compensating measures such as gesturing or drawing were suppressed) and a massed practice schedule (31.5 hours of treatment over a 2-week period). The traditional group was allowed to use compensatory measures and the schedule was 33.9 hours of treatment over a 3- to 5-week period. Although the CILT group made significantly more verbal improvement than the traditional group, the study did not show whether the suppression of compensatory measures or the massed practice was the more positive influence.

Raymer et al. (2007) noted other studies in aphasia, voice, and memory and attention that used CILT. Although the authors are optimistic about CILT, they still say that further research is needed to make sure that it is efficacious for aphasia therapy. A review of CILT and other forms of neural language intervention can be found in Nadeau, Gonzalez, and Rosenbek (2008).

Raymer et al. (2008) in their review defined neuroplasticity and reviewed studies that demonstrate neural changes associated with aphasia recovery and treatment. The authors then summarized basic science evidence from animals, human cognition, and computational neuroscience that is relevant to aphasia treatment research. They then turned to the aphasia treatment literature in which evidence exists to support several of the neuroscience principles.

For example, Raymer et al. (2008) reviewed research that is based upon the notion that the potential rehabilitation of the affected limb is detrimentally influenced by the compensatory use of the unaffected limb through a process of learned nonuse. Constraint-induced movement therapy (CIMT) has been shown to result in improved bimanual performance in some patients with chronic poststroke hemiplegia. The key principles of CIMT are massed practice, constraint of the unaffected limb with forced use of the affected limb, and behavioral shaping of the response. These principles have been applied to the rehabilitation of chronic aphasia.

Pulvermüller et al. (2001), as cited in Raymer et al. (2008), found that when individuals with chronic aphasia received intensive massed practice with oral language over a two-week period, restricting responses only to spoken language in a variety of interactive communication tasks, this intensive training was associated with significant improvements on standard tests and self-ratings of communication in daily living. Raymer et al. (2008) and Cherney et al. (2008) reviewed other studies that used constraint-induced language therapy (CILT).

A number of computer systems for use with specific aphasic problems have been reviewed by Katz (2008) and Katz and Wertz (1997); these include programs for verbal word finding, verbal sentence construction, auditory comprehension, single-word visual recognition, single-word reading comprehension, homophone recognition, written spelling, and written word finding.

In their study, Katz and Wertz (1997) found that computerized reading treatment for adults with chronic aphasia showed the following: (1) the tasks could be administered with minimal assistance from a clinician; (2) improvement on the computerized reading treatment tasks generalized to noncomputer language performance; (3) improvement resulted from the language content of the software and not stimulation provided by a computer; and (4) the computerized reading treatment was efficacious.

Conversational Partners

In an approach called "conducting conversation," Boles (1998) reported on the success of including the spouse in aphasia treatment. When conversing with her husband (the patient with aphasia), the spouse was instructed by a speech-language pathologist to reduce her speaking rate (fewer words per minute), reduce her percentage of talking turns, and to make fewer topic shifts. Discourse data taken after two weeks, three weeks, and four months showed that the patient had a successful increase in words per minute and talking turns, and fewer breakdowns in conversation.

Oelschlaeger (1999) reported on the participation of a conversation partner in the word searches of a person with aphasia. Thirty-eight videotaped conversational sequences from eight naturally occurring conversations of one couple were analyzed. Results showed that participation was determined by interactional techniques (e.g., direct or downward gaze) and interactional resources (e.g., information derived from the partners' shared life experience). The author provided examples of the successful use of interactional techniques and resources and their clinical implications.

Kagan et al. (2001) reported on a form of therapy called "Supported Conversation for Adults with Aphasia" (SCA). This approach is based on the tenet that the inherent competence of individuals with aphasia can be shown through the skill of a conversation partner. This study concluded that training volunteers as conversation partners using a 1-day workshop and 1.5 hours of hands-on experience was associated with an improvement in the communication of volunteers and their partners with aphasia, even when the individuals with aphasia received no direct treatment.

Avent (2004) presented "Reciprocal Scaffolding Treatment" (RST), which is group treatment whereby a skilled partner with aphasia is provided with a setting to use pre-CVA knowledge and vocabulary during routine reciprocal training interactions with a group of children or novices. The individual with aphasia instructs the novices in a skill, and the novices provide natural language models for the patient. These authentic interactions can be beneficial to both groups.

Hengst et al. (2005) studied the reported speech of seven individuals with aphasia and their communication partners. The discourse practice of restating or reenacting talk (of others or oneself) that occurred at another place and/or time is known as *reported speech*. Since all seven subjects with aphasia showed gains in their discourse abilities, the use of reported speech could be added to a framework of therapy in aphasia. In an earlier study, Hengst (2003) showed how four persons with aphasia and their conversation partners worked together to complete the same task during a functional communication setting.

Simmons-Mackie, Kingston, and Schultz (2004) showed how a person with severe aphasia enlisted a speaking partner to speak for her. This nonaphasic speaking partner served as a "spokesperson" for messages that were authored by the person with aphasia.

Recently, Nobis-Bosch et al. (2011) stated that the aim of their study was to demonstrate the efficacy of supervised self-training for individuals with aphasia. Linguistic and communicative performance in structured dialogues represented the main study parameters. They concluded that supervised home training works, and that it is an effective tool for bolstering linguistic and communicative skills of individuals with aphasia

A review of the conversational partners approach in aphasia therapy can be found in Simmons-Mackie (2008).

The third goal of therapy is to encourage the patient and the caretaker(s) to continue the rehabilitative process outside of the clinical setting.

Family Attitudes

One of the prognostic variables mentioned earlier noted that if the family of the patient has the proper attitude and provides encouragement, then the prognosis is better. Most families desire the best for the patient who has aphasia and would do anything to make him or her communicatively normal. Because of their feelings for the patient, family members might look at the patient's language abilities unrealistically.

On a number of occasions, the authors have had family members sit in during a therapy session. After watching and listening to a 30- to 45-minute session where the patient showed little or no response to the most basic auditory comprehension stimuli, the family member will say, "But he (the patient) understands everything." Or, after observing a diagnostic or therapy session that is devoted partially or fully to oral expression, the family member will say, "She is too stubborn to talk" or "She thinks it's too simple and that's why she doesn't want to talk."

Spousal Attitudes

Helmick, Watamori, and Palmer (1976) found that spouses of patients with aphasia view the patients' communication as less impaired than it actually is. Zraick and Boone (1991) noted that the attitudes most frequently expressed by spouses were that the spouse with aphasia was demanding, temperamental, immature, worrisome, and nervous. This was not typical of the control subjects. Spouses of patients with nonfluent aphasia showed most of the above attitudes, and spouses of fluent patients showed the fewest of these attitudes. Spouses of the nonfluent group viewed the patients as less independent, less compliant, and less sociable than their fluent patient counterparts. The authors postulated that this may be due in part to the nonfluent patients' absence of words and/or struggle to speak, or possibly to the presence of hemiplegia.

Lomas et al. (1989), in reporting on their development of the Communicative Effectiveness Index (CETI), which measures functional communication of the patient with aphasia, also reviewed some of the literature on spousal attitudes toward the patient. Those authors noted some discrepancies in agreement about impairment between spouse (or significant other) and patient, and between speech-language pathologist and spouse. As an infuriating example, one of the authors tried to justify speech-language therapy to a patient's spouse, who said, "She can cook. She can clean. Why does she need to talk?"

Santo Pietro and Goldfarb (1995) reviewed an investigation done by Gordon-Adams (1985) on the self-reported behaviors and perceptions of wives of adults with aphasia. The findings included the following:

1. Resignation
2. Avoidance of painful issues
3. Resentment of new authority in the household and fear of new responsibility
4. Enjoyment of new authority and reluctance to surrender it to a rehabilitated patient
5. Focus on the patient's problems rather than on the caretaker's own problems or on solutions to the problems
6. Infantilization of the patient
7. Feelings of uniqueness and isolation
8. Difficulty in discussing sexual problems
9. Difficulties due to lack of understanding of aphasia, such as (1) perception that the patient is mentally incompetent or doesn't try hard enough, (2) idea that the patient's ability to use stereotypical responses is a good prognosis for language recovery, (3) intolerance and shock at the patient's use of profanity or of paraphasia, such as substitution of "mom" for "wife"
10. Interpretation of intermittency of a patient's language competence as willfulness

Home Treatment by Caretakers

Home treatment by caretakers can be very effective if conducted under the proper conditions. Marshall et al. (1989) found that nonprofessionals carefully monitored and trained (by speech-language pathologists) can provide effective home treatment for the patient with aphasia. To help put into effect what Marshall et al. found, Santo Pietro and Goldfarb (1995) suggested a number of "do's" and "don'ts" for caretakers of patients with aphasia. These suggestions are meant to help overcome many of the problems mentioned above.

DO's for Caretakers:

1. Do keep talking to the patient.
2. Do get the patient's attention before speaking.
3. Do talk slowly, to allow the patient time to process your message.
4. Do use short, one-idea, easy-to-process sentences.
5. Do establish the context of your message before you begin to expand on it (e.g., say, "Let's talk about tonight's supper" before starting a discussion of whether you should eat at home or go to a restaurant).
6. Do give patients with aphasia time to formulate what they want to say.
7. Do be an attentive listener and look for cues in the patient's tone of voice, facial expressions, and behavior to help you comprehend the message.
8. Do be empathetic and not sympathetic (e.g., say, "I am aware of how frustrated you must feel," not, "Oh, you poor thing!").
9. Do adjust the communication schedule to the best time of day.

10. Do attend to any additional communication problems the patient may have along with the aphasia (e.g., hearing and visual difficulties, medication needs).
11. Do allow the patient access to activity in the house and in the world.
12. Do allow the patient to continue any chores or responsibilities that remain manageable (e.g., gardening, caring for pets, cleaning).
13. Do foster success whenever possible. If the patient says or does something well (e.g., saying a name, dressing, answering the phone), be generous with your praise.

DON'Ts for Caretakers:

1. Don't finish the patient's sentences unless the patient wants it.
2. Don't cut the patient off or interrupt when he or she is speaking. This may cause the aphasic patient to lose his or her train of thought.
3. Don't "fill in" the silence. The patient may need that time to process.
4. Don't turn your face away from the aphasic patient when you are speaking. The patient may need facial cues to help comprehend what you are saying.
5. Don't "talk down" to the aphasic patient. The patient will become highly sensitive to metalinguistic messages and will be insulted and "turned off" if you appear condescending.
6. Don't say things you do not want the aphasic patient to hear, assuming he or she will not understand. Quite often, he or she will.
7. Don't talk about the patient as if he or she were not here or were already dead (e.g., "He used to be a brilliant architect").
8. Don't talk only about activities of daily living.
9. Don't eliminate such activities as the theater, music, restaurants, and sporting events from the patient's daily lifestyle. All of us need stimulation, restoration for the soul, and fun in life to maximize and enhance communication.
10. Don't allow the patient with aphasia to become isolated. Communication is a social undertaking.

Lyon and Shadden (2001) present a comprehensive review that includes family and spousal attitudes, and home treatment by caretakers of individuals with aphasia.

A Final Note

Occasionally, a caretaker will tell the speech-language pathologist what sort of speech therapy the patient needs. The suggested therapy usually centers on the patient's oral expression. This happens when the clinician decides at the beginning of therapy, or after exhaustive amounts of therapy for oral expression deficit have not worked, to concentrate on the other modalities.

Speech-language pathologists should explain to the caretaker (and even doctors, nurses, and so on, who think the same way) that working on the patient's oral expression would not be beneficial, whereas bolstering the other modalities would be more helpful. Apparently, to some caretakers and other health professionals, oral expression is the only way in which language is measured. When they hear the patient speak, it's like an instant assessment of normalcy. Clinicians know differently and must explain this to the caretaker and others.

Advanced Study

State-of-the-art neuroscience research involving clinical brain imaging for aphasia often includes functional magnetic resonance imaging (fMRI) and event-related potentials (ERP)

(Perkins et al., 2007). The main principle of fMRI is that magnetic properties of oxygenated blood are different from those of deoxygenated blood. Changes in brain function or physiology are detected and are associated with performance on language, cognitive, sensory, and motor tasks. The blood oxygenation level dependent (BOLD) technique generates images sensitive to the oxygenation level of blood, and is used in brain mapping studies of language lateralization, word generation, and sentence comprehension.

When a neuron fires, it creates an electrical field that travels along its axon. By firing simultaneously, neurons in the CNS create an electrical field that can be detected outside the skull. For recording such activity, an electrode net is used, with equally spaced electrodes positioned on the surface of the skull (Raphael et al., 2007). A stimulus played into a participant's ear will evoke a response at the cortex that will be recorded by these electrodes. Each resulting waveform shows the averaged electrical activity recorded for one second after the presentation of a word. The response to a given stimulus is described in terms of the negative and positive peaks and their latencies.

Auditory event-related potentials (ERPs) have been used to measure hemispheric processing in patients with aphasia (Hagoort et al., 1996; Kojima & Kaga, 2003; Seliger et al., 1989). The N400 (negative peak occurring 400 milliseconds after the stimulus) is used as a measure of associative and semantic comprehension tasks, while P600 has been associated with syntactic processing.

Regional cerebral blood flow (rCBF) is an indirect measure of metabolism. It is based on the assumption that neural activity in a cortical region causes an increased demand for nourishment. The corresponding increase in blood flow rate indicates increased metabolic activity. However, there is a potential problem of claiming one is looking at brains by looking at veins. Accuracy of localizing neural activity is limited. As is the case with fMRI, part of the functional signal arises not from brain capillaries and parenchyma, presumably at the site of activation, but instead from larger draining veins.

CASE DESCRIPTION

RM, a 38-year-old, right-handed former bank executive with an MBA degree, presented with a history of left hemisphere aneurysm and cerebral hemorrhage, suffered on his 34th birthday, with resultant right hemiparesis and moderate nonfluent (Broca's) aphasia characterized by reduction of available vocabulary, effortful language production, impaired expressive syntax, a stereotypical utterance ("more or less"), and inconsistent evidence of semantic paraphasias, such as "sleeping" for "in a coma" and "read" for "speak."

Good morning. My name is RM. I am Forest Hills Gardens with a house. Normally I started September 1st. I was working Irving Trust Company at night. Four hundred people. I was the boss. Data processing. A lot of girls, like a hundred girls, clean up. These are things I can't say exactly. Clean up, more or less. Wall Street.

So more or less, I went to sleep. The only problem, it didn't sleep until more or less a month. I was in St. John's Hospital, and I couldn't talk. And, more or less to myself, "What happened?" I couldn't walk. I was useless. Completely. At least I woke up, and somebody woke me up, supposedly. And little things, probably more or less, I just woke up. I can remember there was a girl, supposedly, inside. And when I woke up, I was trying to get out. But this woman told me, "Don't move." And I still haven't met the girl, but, luckily, somehow, I got here. And why I'm running means something that because of myself. I have no idea. So when I woke up and I looked, I couldn't understand. But there was one time I just woke up, more or less.

Right now I'm talking about the doctors. I'm at St. John's Hospital sleeping. Then, all of a sudden, I wake up, and I can't talk. I can't talk at all. You have a doctor, O'Brien. He was the man, for years we played volleyball, at Ocean Club, Atlantic Ocean. We played a long time, like June, July, and August. So he's talking to me, and he says, "You have your problem, Bob, but you have to go into a hospital. We've been looking for places, but we're not sure. Each day, I'll see you, and if we know anything, I'll tell you."

Also another doctor, Dr. Charlie M-a-r-d-i, he also Ocean Club. He didn't play volleyball, but he's very close with my mother, and brothers and all together. In fact, when I get married to Margie, we had the doctor, Charlie and his wife Susan. We also had a judge there, because Margie and I get married, talk about November 20th. He was the man at St. John's Hospital. He was in charge. Really, I was sleeping. Margie called Charlie, and for sure, Charlie was very quick. He was here. That was the old story.

Normally, Charlie and Don, they always talk to me. Thank God. I couldn't talk, but there are people who are nice. Both of them had found out that Lenox Hill was much better, because you have to cut a little bit, and you have to come back to read again. They didn't tell me exactly, but they had to cut a little bit. Then I slept.

Now we're talking about Lenox Hill. They moved me, I'd say October 15th or something like that. I'd seen Don, and, "They gonna move. Much better. They gonna be much better, Bob." So I said goodbye.

They drove us Lenox Hill. And is another doctor. He says hello. Margie talked to him. It was like three days. They just checking everything. So he began to cut a little bit. The doctor was there, and I'd say six men, they're also doctors, probably. And maybe three girls, nurses. And I was awake. They started cutting in the middle. The veins, it was only a little bit, five minutes. I don't know what it was, but I was dying. STOP! I was just screaming like [screaming noises]. So the doctors kept moving, and they talk to each other. They said, "I don't think you can do that." So the doctor was getting. Mine, he didn't cut. There were two doctors, they were cutting. They said to me, "Take it easy, Bob. No problem." But I was still going [screaming noises].

So it stopped. So to myself, "Why do they cut me?" So I was back at the hospital, and, thank God, my wife was always there, telling me what's gonna happen, or something like that. This doctor, he was in Forest Hills. I don't know his name. I should find out. But the story is, I'll tell you exactly. Each time I'd see him, I said, "Please tell me." I couldn't talk, but he always ran. That doesn't make sense. This guy is a doctor, he's a worker, too. I have an MBA. He wouldn't even say what kind of problem. This was the doctor. Sometimes I'd see him and ran, try to run. Thank God, November, two years ago, he died. And it's sad, because it's so many people. It's bad, because we're talking about nice doctors, Don, Charlie. This is a doctor, was money. He got everything. He won't even talk to me. And I'm happy that he died. Which is sad, half for me, but I'm glad that he died.

Discussion Questions: Theory

1. Is aphasia language without thought or thought without language?

2. Is aphasia a loss or reduction of efficiency in the comprehension and production of language symbols?

3. How does the polytypic nature of aphasia classification affect differential diagnosis?

4. What is the role of regional cerebral blood flow (rCBF) in establishing brain–behavior relationships following a stroke?

5. What are some advantages and shortcomings of current neural imaging techniques with regard to diagnosis of aphasia?

Discussion Questions: Therapy

1. Why should we implement speech-language therapy for aphasia when there is usually spontaneous recovery after a stroke?

2. How can we apply set theory (the intersection of Set A + Set B = Set C, or $A \cap B = C$) to the clinician–client relationship?

3. How do the intersections of the person with aphasia, the communication partner, and the environment (as seen in the Venn diagrams in this section) inform our therapy planning and procedures?

4. When Schuell described the notion of "the adequate stimulus," what do you think she meant?

5. Should therapy be modality-specific, shutting off distraction from other modalities, or multimodality, offering increased opportunity for sensory reception? Why?

Assignment: Write a multiple-choice question with five options. Explain why the key option is correct, and why the distractors or decoys are incorrect. Avoid using forms such as, "All of the following are (in)correct *except*" in the stem, and "All (or none) of the above" in the options.

Example: Aphasia syndromes represent an aphasia type at only one arbitrary point in time, but aphasia is a migratory disorder. Which migration might happen in aphasia?
   a. Broca's to Wernicke's to anomic
   b. Jargon to conduction to anomic
   c. Transcortical motor to global to Broca's
   d. Anomic to jargon to Wernicke's
   e. Transcortical sensory to Broca's to anomic

The correct answer is *b*: a severe form of fluent aphasia migrates to less severe forms of fluent aphasia; *a* is incorrect because aphasia cannot migrate from nonfluent to fluent forms; *c* is incorrect because transcortical motor aphasia, global aphasia, and Broca's aphasia are associated with different lesion sites; *d* is incorrect because aphasia cannot migrate from a mild to a more severe form, and then to a more mild form; *e* is incorrect because aphasia cannot migrate from fluent to nonfluent forms.

References

Abou-Khalil, R., & Abou-Khalil, B. (2003). Cortical stimulation mapping and speech production. *Neurophysiology and Neurogenic Speech and Language Disorders, 13*(3). (Special Interest Division 2 Newsletter, 10–15). Rockville, MD: American Speech-Language-Hearing Association.

American Speech-Language-Hearing Association. (1994). *Functional assessment of communication skills for adults.* Bethesda, MD: Author.

Aten, J. (1994). Functional communication treatment. In R. Chapey (Ed.), *Language intervention strategies in adult aphasia* (5th ed.) (pp. 292–303). Baltimore, MD: Williams & Wilkins.

Avent, J. (2004). Reciprocal scaffolding treatment for aphasia. *Neurophysiology and Neurogenic Speech and Language Disorders, 14*(2). (Special Interest Division 2 Newsletter, 15–18). Rockville, MD: American Speech-Language-Hearing Association.

Bandur, D., & Shewan, C. (2008). Language-oriented treatment: A psycholinguistic approach to aphasia. In R. Chapey (Ed.), *Language intervention strategies in aphasia and related neurogenic communication disorders* (5th ed.) (pp. 756–798). Baltimore, MD: Lippincott Williams & Wilkins.

Basso, A., Capitani, E., & Vignolo, L. (1979). Influence of rehabilitation on language skills in aphasic patients: A controlled study. *Archives of Neurology, 36,* 190–196.

Basso, A., Lecours, A., Moraschini, S., & Vanier, M. (1985). Anatomoclinical correlations of the aphasias as defined through computerized tomography: Exceptions. *Brain and Language, 26,* 201–229.

Beeson, P., Rising, K., Kim, E., & Rapcsak, S. (2010). A treatment sequence for phonological alexia/agraphia. *Journal of Speech, Language, and Hearing Research, 53,* 450–468.

Beeson, P., Rising, K., & Volk, J. (2003). Writing treatment for severe aphasia: Who benefits? *Journal of Speech, Language, and Hearing Research, 46,* 1038–1060.

Beeson, P. M., & Robey, R. R. (2006). Evaluating single-subject treatment research: Lessons learned from the aphasia literature. *Neuropsychology Review, 16,* 161–169.

Benson, D. F. (1979). *Aphasia, alexia, agraphia.* New York, NY: Churchill-Livingston, Inc.

Benson, D. F., & Ardila, A. (1996). *Aphasia: A clinical perspective.* New York, NY: Oxford University Press.

Benton, A., & Hamsher, K. (1978). *Multilingual aphasia examination.* Iowa City, IA: Benton Laboratory of Neuropsychology.

Beukelman, D., Yorkston, K., & Waugh, P. (1980). Communication in severe aphasia: Effectiveness of three instruction modalities. *Archives of Physical Medicine and Rehabilitation, 61,* 248–252.

Bhatnagar, S. C. (2008). *Neuroscience for the study of communicative disorders* (3rd ed.). Philadelphia, PA: Lippincott Williams & Wilkins.

Boles, L. (1998). Conducting conversation: A case study using the spouse in aphasia treatment. *Neurophysiology and Neurogenic Speech and Language Disorders, 8*(3). (Special Interest Division 2 Newsletter, 24–31). Rockville, MD: American Speech-Language-Hearing Association.

Borkowski, J., Benton, A., & Spreen, O. (1967). Word fluency and brain damage. *Neuropsychologia, 5,* 135–140.

Boyle, M. (2004). Semantic feature analysis treatment for anomia in two fluent aphasia syndromes. *American Journal of Speech-Language Pathology, 13,* 236–249.

Boyle, M., & Coelho, C. (1995). Application of semantic feature analysis as a treatment for aphasic dysnomia. *American Journal of Speech-Language Pathology, 4,* 94–99.

Bracy, C., & Drummond, S. (1993). Word retrieval and non-fluent dysphasia: Utilization of pictogram. *Journal of Communication Disorders, 26,* 113–128.

Brodsky, M., McNeil, M., Doyle, P., Fossett, T., Timm, N., & Dark, G. (2003). Auditory serial position effects in story retelling for non-brain-injured participants and persons with aphasia. *Journal of Speech-Language-Hearing Research, 46,* 1124–1137.

Brookshire, R. (1974). Differences in responding to auditory materials among aphasic patients. *Acta Symbolica, 5,* 1–18.

Brookshire, R. (1994). Group studies of treatment for adults with aphasia: Efficacy, effectiveness, and believability. *Neurophysiology and Neurogenic Speech and Language Disorders, 4.* (Special Interest Division 2 Newsletter, 5–13). Rockville, MD: American Speech-Language-Hearing Association.

Brookshire, R. (2007). *Introduction to neurogenic communication disorders* (7th ed.). St. Louis, MO: Mosby.

Brookshire, R., & Nicholas, L. (1997). *Discourse comprehension test.* Bloomington, MN: BRK Publishers.

Butfield, A., & Zangwill, O. (1946). Re-education in aphasia: A review of 70 cases. *Journal of Neurology, Neurosurgery, and Psychiatry, 9,* 75–79.

Cherney, L., Halper, A., Holland, A., & Cole, R. (2008). Computerized script training for aphasia: Preliminary results. *American Journal of Speech-Language Pathology, 17,* 29–34.

Cherney, L., Patterson, J., Raymer, A., Frymark, T., & Schooling, T. (2008). Evidence-based systematic review. Effects of intensity of treatment and constraint-induced therapy for individuals with stroke-induced aphasia. *Journal of Speech, Language, and Hearing Research, 51,* 1282–1299.

Cherney, L., & Robey, R. (2008). Aphasia treatment: Recovery, prognosis, and clinical effectiveness. In R. Chapey (Ed.), *Language intervention strategies in aphasia and related neurogenic communication disorders* (5th ed.) (pp. 186–202). Baltimore, MD: Lippincott Williams & Wilkins.

Code, C., Hemsley, G., & Herrmann, M. (1999). The emotional impact of aphasia. *Seminars in Speech and Language, 20,* 19–31.

Coelho, C., Sinotte, M., & Duffy, J. (2008). Schuell's stimulation approach to rehabilitation. In R. Chapey (Ed.), *Language intervention strategies in aphasia and related neurogenic communication disorders* (5th ed.) (pp. 403–449). Baltimore, MD: Lippincott Williams & Wilkins.

Collins, M. (1983). Global aphasia: Knowledge in search of understanding. *Communication Disorders, 8,* 125–137.

Collins, M. (1991). *Diagnosis and treatment of global aphasia.* San Diego, CA: Singular.

Crary, M., Haak, N., & Malinsky, A. (1989). Preliminary psychometric evaluation of an acute aphasia screening protocol. *Aphasiology, 3,* 611–618.

Damasio, H. (2008). Neural basis of language disorders. In R. Chapey (Ed.), *Language intervention strategies in aphasia and related neurogenic communication disorders* (5th ed.) (pp. 20–41). Baltimore, MD: Lippincott Williams & Wilkins.

Damecour, C., & Caplan, D. (1991). The relationship of depression to symptomatology and lesion site in aphasic patients. *Cortex, 27,* 385–401.

Darley, F. (1972). The efficacy of language rehabilitation in aphasia. *Journal of Speech and Hearing Disorders, 37,* 3–21.

Darley, F. (1982). *Aphasia.* Philadelphia, PA: Saunders.

David, R., Enderby, P., & Bainton, D. (1982). Treatment of acquired aphasia: Speech therapists and volunteers compared. *Journal of Neurology, Neurosurgery, and Psychiatry, 45,* 957–961.

Davis, G. A., & Wilcox, J. (1981). Incorporating parameters of natural conversation in aphasia treatment. In R. Chapey (Ed.), *Language intervention strategies in adult aphasia* (pp. 169–193). Baltimore, MD: Williams & Wilkins.

Deal, J., & Deal, L. (1978). Efficacy of aphasia rehabilitation; preliminary results. In R. Brookshire (Ed.), *Clinical aphasiology conference proceedings* (pp. 66–67). Minneapolis, MN: BRK Publishers.

del Toro, C., Bislick, L., Comer, M., Velozo, C., Romero, S., Rothi, L., & Kendall, D. (2011). Development of a short form of the Boston Naming Test for individuals with aphasia. *Journal of Speech, Language, and Hearing Research, 54,* 1089–1100.

DeRenzi, E., & Ferrari, C. (1978). The reporters test: A sensitive test to detect expressive disturbances in aphasics. *Cortex, 14,* 279–293.

DeRenzi, E., & Vignolo, L. (1962). The token test: A sensitive test to detect receptive disturbances in aphasics. *Brain, 85,* 665–678.

DiSimoni, F., Darley, F., & Aronson, A. (1977). Patterns of dysfunction in schizophrenic patients on an aphasia test battery. *Journal of Speech and Hearing Disorders, 42,* 498–513.

Duffy, J., & McNeil, M. (2008). Primary progressive aphasia and apraxia of speech. In R. Chapey (Ed.), *Language intervention strategies in aphasia and related neurogenic communication disorders* (5th ed.) (pp. 543–564). Baltimore, MD: Lippincott Williams & Wilkins.

Edmonds, L., & Babb, M. (2011). Effect of verb network strengthening in moderate-to-severe aphasia. *American Journal of Speech-Language Pathology, 20,* 131–145.

Ellis, C. (2009). Does race/ethnicity really matter in adult neurogenics? *American Journal of Speech-Language Pathology, 18,* 310–314.

Elman, R., & Bernstein-Ellis, E. (1999). The efficacy of group communication treatment in adults with chronic aphasia. *Journal of Speech-Language-Hearing Research, 42,* 411–419.

Fitch-West, J., Sands, E., & Ross-Swain, D. (1998). *The Bedside Evaluation Screening Test* (2nd ed.) (BEST). Austin, TX: Pro-Ed.

Freed, D., & Marshall, R. (1995). The effect of personalized cueing on long-term naming of realistic visual stimuli. *American Journal of Speech-Language Pathology, 4*, 105–108.

Freed, D., Marshall, R., & Nippold, M. (1995). Comparison of personalized cueing on the facilitation of verbal labeling by aphasic subjects. *Journal of Speech and Hearing Research, 38*, 1081–1090.

Fridriksson, J., & Holland, A. (2001). Final thoughts on management of aphasia in the early phases of recovery following stroke. *American Journal of Speech-Language Pathology, 10*, 37–39.

Gandour, J., Holasuit Petty, S., & Dardarananda, R. (1988). Perception and production of tone in aphasia. *Brain and Language, 35*, 201–240.

Gardner, H., Zurif, E., Berry, T., & Baker, E. (1976). Visual communication in aphasia. *Neuropsychologia, 14*, 275–292.

Gerber, S., & Gurland, G. (1989). Applied pragmatics in the assessment of aphasia. *Seminars in Speech and Language, 20*, 263–281.

Glista, S. (2006). Educating and supporting individuals with aphasia and their families. *Neurophysiology and Neurogenic Speech and Language Disorders, 16*(4). (Special Interest Division 2 Newsletter, 25–31). Rockville, MD: American Speech-Language-Hearing Association.

Goldberg, E., & Goldfarb, R. (2005). Grammatical category ambiguity in aphasia. *Brain and Language, 95*, 293–303.

Goldfarb, R. (2006a). Diagnosis. In R. Goldfarb (Ed.), *Ethics: A case study from fluency* (pp. 13–26). San Diego, CA: Plural.

Goldfarb, R. (2006b). Operant conditioning and programmed instruction in aphasia rehabilitation. *Journal of Speech-Language Pathology and Applied Behavior Analysis, 1*, 55–65.

Goldfarb, R., & Amsel, L., 1982. The St. Albans stroke club. *Aging, 32*, 38–39.

Goldfarb, R., & Halpern, H. (1981). Word associations of time-altered auditory and visual stimuli in aphasia. *Journal of Speech and Hearing Research, 24*, 233–246.

Goldfarb, R., & Halpern, H. (1989). Impairments of naming and word finding. In C. Code (Ed.), *The characteristics of aphasia* (pp. 33–52). New York, NY: Taylor & Francis.

Goodglass, H., & Kaplan, E. (1983). *Boston diagnostic aphasia examination* (2nd ed.). Philadelphia, PA: Lea & Febiger.

Goodglass, H., Kaplan, E., & Barresi, B. (2001). *Boston diagnostic aphasia examination* (3rd ed.). Philadelphia, PA: Lippincott Williams & Wilkins.

Gordon-Adams, E. (1985). *Group counseling experiences and the self-reported behaviors and perceptions of wives of adult aphasics* (Unpublished doctoral dissertation). Columbia University, New York, New York.

Hagoort, P., Brown, C. M., & Swaab, T. Y. (1996). Lexical-semantic event-related potential effects in patients with left hemisphere lesions and aphasia, and patients with right hemisphere lesions without aphasia. *Brain, 119*, 627–649.

Halliday, M., & Hasan, R. (1976). *Cohesion in English*. London, UK: Longman.

Halpern, H. (1965a). Effect of stimulus variables on dysphasic verbal errors. *Perceptual and Motor Skills, 21*, 291–298.

Halpern, H. (1965b). Effect of stimulus variables on verbal perseveration of dysphasic subjects. *Perceptual and Motor Skills, 20*, 421–429.

Halpern, H., Darley, F., & Brown, J. (1973). Differential language and neurologic characteristics in cerebral involvement. *Journal of Speech and Hearing Disorders, 38*, 162–173.

Halpern, H., Keith, R., & Darley, F. (1976). Phonemic behavior of aphasic subjects without dysarthria or apraxia of speech. *Cortex, 12*, 365–372.

Halpern, H., & McCartin-Clark, M. (1984). Differential language characteristics in adult aphasic and schizophrenic subjects. *Journal of Communication Disorders, 17*, 289–307.

Hartman, J., & Landau, W. (1987). Comparison of formal language therapy with supportive counseling for aphasia due to vascular accident. *Archives of Neurology, 44*, 646–649.

Hegde, M. (1998). *A coursebook on aphasia*. San Diego, CA: Singular.

Helm, N., & Barresi, B. (1980). Voluntary control of involuntary utterances: A treatment approach for severe aphasia. In R. Brookshire (Ed.), *Clinical aphasiology conference proceedings* (pp. 308–315). Minneapolis, MN: BRK Publishers.

Helm-Estabrooks, N. (1981). *Helm elicited language program for syntax stimulation* (HELPSS). Chicago, IL: Riverside.

Helm-Estabrooks, N., Fitzpatric, P., & Barresi, B. (1982). Visual action therapy for global aphasia. *Journal of Speech and Hearing Disorders, 47,* 385–389.

Helm-Estabrooks, N., Ramsberger, G., Morgan, A., & Nicholas, M. (1989). *Boston assessment of severe aphasia* (BASA). Chicago, IL: Riverside.

Helmick, J., Watamori, T., & Palmer, J. (1976). Spouses' understanding of the communication disabilities of aphasic patients. *Journal of Speech and Hearing Disorders, 41,* 238–243.

Hengst, J. (2003). Collaborative referencing between individuals with aphasia and routine communication partners. *Journal of Speech-Language-Hearing Research, 46,* 831–848.

Hengst, J., Frame, S., Neuman-Stritzel, T., & Gannaway, R. (2005). Using others' words: Conversational use of reported speech by individuals with aphasia and their communication partners. *Journal of Speech-Language-Hearing Research, 48,* 137–156.

Henry, M. L., & Beeson, P. (2006). Primary progressive aphasia and semantic dementia. *Neurophysiology and Neurogenic Speech and Language Disorders, 16*(1). (Special Interest Division 2 Newsletter, 21–27). Rockville, MD: American Speech-Language-Hearing Association.

Holland, A. (1970). Case studies in aphasia rehabilitation using programmed instructions. *Journal of Speech and Hearing Disorders, 35,* 377–390.

Holland, A., Frattali, C., & Fromm. D. (1999). *Communication abilities in daily living-2.* Austin, TX: Pro-Ed.

Holland, A., & Fridriksson, J. (2001). Aphasia management during the early phases of recovery following stroke. *American Journal of Speech-Language Pathology, 10,* 19–28.

Holland, A., Fromm, D., DeRuyter, F., & Stein, M. (1996). Treatment efficacy: Aphasia. *Journal of Speech and Hearing Research, 39,* S27–S36.

Holland, A., Halper, A., & Cherney, L. (2010). Telling your story: Analysis of script topics selected by persons with aphasia. *American Journal of Speech-Language Pathology, 19,* 198–203.

Hough, M. (1993). Treatment of Wernicke's aphasia with jargon: A case study. *Journal of Communication Disorders, 26,* 101–111.

Hough, M., Pierce, R., & Cannito, M. (1989). Contextual influences in aphasia: Effects of predictive and nonpredictive narratives. *Brain and Language, 36,* 325–334.

Hunt, K. (1965). *Grammatical structures written at three grade levels* (Research report #3). Champaign, IL: National Council of Teachers of English.

Hux, K., Weissling, K., & Wallace, S. (2008). Communication-based interventions: Augmented and alternative communication for people with aphasia. In R. Chapey (Ed.), *Language intervention strategies in aphasia and related neurogenic communication disorders* (5th ed.) (pp. 814–836). Baltimore, MD: Lippincott Williams & Wilkins.

Kagan, A., Black, S., Duchan, J., Simmons-Mackie, N., & Square, P. (2001). Training volunteers as conversation partners using "supported conversation for adults with aphasia" (SCA): A controlled trial. *Journal of Speech-Language-Hearing Research, 44,* 624–638.

Kaplan, E., Goodglass, H., & Weintraub, S. (1983). *The Boston naming test.* Philadelphia, PA: Lea & Febiger.

Katz, R. (2008). Computer applications in aphasia treatment. In R. Chapey (Ed.), *Language intervention strategies in aphasia and related neurogenic communication disorders* (5th ed.) (pp. 852–873). Baltimore, MD: Lippincott Williams & Wilkins.

Katz, R., & Wertz, R. (1997). The efficacy of computer-provided reading treatment for chronic aphasic adults. *Journal of Speech-Language-Hearing Research, 40,* 493–507.

Kearns, K. (1985). Response elaboration training for patient-initiated utterances. In R. Brookshire (Ed.), *Clinical aphasiology conference proceedings* (pp. 196–204). Minneapolis, MN: BRK.

Kearns, K. (1994). Group therapy for aphasia: Theoretical and practical considerations. In R. Chapey (Ed.), *Language intervention strategies in adult aphasia* (3rd ed.) (pp. 304–321). Baltimore, MD: Williams & Wilkins.

Kearns, K. P. (2005). Back to the future with single-subject experimental designs in aphasia treatment research. *Neurophysiology and Neurogenic Speech and Language Disorders, 15*(3). (Special Interest Division 2 Newsletter, 14–21). Rockville, MD: American Speech-Language-Hearing Association.

Kearns, K., & Elman, R. (2008). Group therapy for aphasia: Theoretical and practical considerations. In R. Chapey (Ed.), *Language intervention strategies in aphasia and related neurogenic communication disorders* (5th ed.) (pp. 376–400). Baltimore, MD: Lippincott Williams & Wilkins.

Keenan, J., & Brassell, E. (1975). *Aphasia language performance scales.* Murfreesboro, TN: Pinnacle Press.

Kennedy, M. R. T., & Chiou, H-H. (2005). Assessment tools for adolescents and adults in languages other than English. *Neurophysiology and Neurogenic Speech and Language Disorders, 15*(2). (Special Interest Division 2 Newsletter, 20–23). Rockville, MD: American Speech-Language-Hearing Association.

Kertesz, A. (2006). *The Western aphasia battery—Enhanced.* San Antonio, TX: Harcourt Assessment.

Kertesz, A., Lau, W., & Polk, M. (1993). The structural determinants of recovery in Wernicke's aphasia. *Brain and Language, 44,* 153–164.

Kimelman, M. (1991). The role of target word stress in auditory comprehension by aphasic listeners. *Journal of Speech and Hearing Research, 34,* 334–339.

King, J., & Hux, K. (1996). Attention allocation in adults with and without aphasia: Performance on linguistic and nonlinguistic tasks. *American Journal of Medical Speech-Language Pathology, 4,* 245–256.

Kiran, S., Sandberg, C., & Sebastian, R. (2011). Treatment of category generation and retrieval in aphasia: Effect of typicality of category items. *Journal of Speech, Language, and Hearing Research, 54,* 1101–1117.

Kiran, S., & Thompson, C. (2003). The role of semantic complexity in treatment of naming deficits: Training semantic categories in fluent aphasia by controlling exemplar typicality. *Journal of Speech-Language-Hearing Research, 46,* 773–787.

Kiran, S., & Johnson, L. (2008). Semantic complexity in treatment of naming deficits in aphasia: Evidence from well-defined categories. *American Journal of Speech-Language Pathology, 17,* 389–400.

Kiran, S., & Thompson, C. (2003). The role of semantic complexity in treatment of naming deficits: Training semantic categories in fluent aphasia by controlling exemplar typicality. *Journal of Speech-Language-Hearing Research, 46,* 773–787.

Kleim, J., & Jones, T. (2008). Principles of experience-dependent neural plasticity: Implications for rehabilitation after brain damage. *Journal of Speech, Language, and Hearing Research, 51,* 5225–5239.

Kohnert, K. (2005). Cognitive-linguistic interactions in bilingual aphasia: Implications for intervention. *Neurophysiology and Neurogenic Speech and Language Disorders, 15*(2). (Special Interest Division 2 Newsletter, 9–14). Rockville, MD: American Speech-Language-Hearing Association.

Kojima, T., & Kaga, K. (2003). Auditory lexical-semantic processing impairments in aphasic patients reflected in event-related potentials (N400). *Auris Nasus Larynx, 30,* 369–378.

LaPointe, L. (1977). Base-10 programmed stimulation: Task specification scoring and plotting performance in aphasia therapy. *Journal of Speech and Hearing Disorders, 42,* 90–105.

LaPointe, L., & Eisenson, J. (2008). *Examining for aphasia* (4th ed.) (EFA-4). Austin, TX: Pro-Ed.

LaPointe, L., & Horner, J. (1980). *Reading comprehension battery for aphasia.* Tigard, OR: C.C. Publications.

Lincoln, N., Mulley, G., Jones, A., McGurik, E., Lendrem, W., & Mitchell, J. (1984, June). Effectiveness of speech therapy for aphasic stroke patients: A randomized controlled trial. *The Lancet, 350,* 1197–1200.

Lomas, J., Picard, I., Bester, S., Elbard, H., Finlayson, A., & Zoghaib, C. (1989). The communicative effectiveness index: Development and psychometric evaluation of a functional communication measure for adult aphasia. *Journal of Speech and Hearing Disorders, 54,* 113–124.

Lorenzen, B., & Murray, L. (2008). Bilingual aphasia: A theoretical and clinical review. *American Journal of Speech-Language Pathology, 17,* 299–317.

Lowell, S., Beeson, P., & Holland, A. (1995). The efficacy of a semantic cueing procedure on naming performance of adults with aphasia. *American Journal of Speech-Language Pathology, 4,* 109–114.

Lyon, J. (1992). Communication use and participation in life for adults with aphasia in natural settings: The scope of the problem. *American Journal of Speech-Language Pathology, 1,* 7–14.

Lyon, J., & Shadden, B. (2001). Treating life consequences of aphasia's chronicity. In R. Chapey (Ed.), *Language intervention strategies in aphasia and related neurogenic communication disorders* (4th ed.) (pp. 297–315). Baltimore, MD: Lippincott Williams & Wilkins.

Marshall, R. (1993). Problem-focused group treatment for clients with mild aphasia. *American Journal of Speech-Language Pathology, 2,* 31–37.

Marshall, R., & Freed. D. (2006). The personalized cueing method: From the laboratory to the clinic. *American Journal of Speech-Language Pathology, 15,* 103–111.

Marshall, R., Wertz, R., Weiss, D., Aten, J., Brookshire, R., Garcia-Bunuel, L., . . . Goodman, P. (1989). Home treatment for aphasic patients by trained non-professionals. *Journal of Speech and Hearing Disorders, 54,* 462–470.

Marshall, R., & Wright, H. (2007). Developing a clinician-friendly aphasia test. *American Journal of Speech-Language Pathology, 16,* 295–315.

Mayer, J. (2003). The role of fMRI in aphasiology: Interface between technology, theory, and clinical care. *Neurophysiology and Neurogenic Speech and Language Disorders, 13*(4). (Special Interest Division 2 Newsletter, 4–7). Rockville, MD: American Speech-Language-Hearing Association.

McKelvey, M., Hux, K., Dietz, A., & Beukelman, D. (2010). Impact of personal relevance and contextualization on word-picture matching by people with aphasia. *American Journal of Speech-Language Pathology, 19*, 22–33.

McNeil, M., & Prescott, T. (1978). *Revised token test*. Baltimore, MD: University Park Press.

McNeil, M., Small, S., Masterson, R., & Fossett, T. (1995). Behavioral and pharmacological treatment of lexical-semantic deficits in a single patient with primary progressive aphasia. *American Journal of Speech-Language Pathology, 4*, 76–87.

Meikle, M., Wechsler, E., Tupper, A., Benenson, M., Butler, J., Muihall, D., & Stern, G. (1979). Comparative trial of volunteer and professional treatments of dysphasia after stroke. *British Medical Journal, 2*, 87–89.

Milman, L., Holland, A., Kaszniak, A., D'Agostino, J., Garrett, M., & Rapcsak, S. (2008). Initial validity and reliability of the SLCAN: Using tailored testing to assess adult cognition and communication. *Journal of Speech, Language, and Hearing Research, 51*, 49–69.

Mlcoch, A., & Metter, J. (2008). Medical aspects of stroke rehabilitation. In R. Chapey (Ed.), *Language intervention strategies in aphasia and related neurogenic communication disorders* (5th ed.) (pp 42–63). Baltimore, MD: Lippincott Williams & Wilkins.

Moineau, S., Dronkers, N., & Bates, E. (2005). Exploring the processing continuum of single-word comprehension in aphasia. *Journal of Speech-Language-Hearing Research, 48*, 884–896.

Molrine, C., & Pierce, R. (2002). Black and white adults' expressive language performance on three tests of aphasia. *American Journal of Speech-Language Pathology, 11*, 139–150.

Murray, L., Holland, A., & Beeson. P. (1997). Auditory processing in individuals with mild aphasia: A study of resource allocation. *Journal of Speech-Language-Hearing Research, 40*, 792–808.

Murray, L., & Holland, A. (1998). Spoken language of individuals with mild fluent aphasia under focused and divided-attention conditions. *Journal of Speech-Language-Hearing Research, 41*, 213–227.

Myers, P., & Blake, M. (2008). Communication disorders associated with right-hemisphere damage. In R. Chapey (Ed.), *Language intervention strategies in aphasia and related neurogenic communication disorders* (5th ed.) (pp. 963–987). Baltimore, MD: Lippincott Williams & Wilkins.

Nadeau, S., Gonzalez Rothi, P., & Rosenbek, J. (2008). Language rehabilitation from a neural perspective. In R. Chapey (Ed.), *Language intervention strategies in aphasia and related neurogenic communication disorders* (5th ed.) (pp. 689–734). Baltimore, MD: Lippincott Williams & Wilkins.

Nicholas, L., & Brookshire, R. (1993). A system for quantifying the informativeness and efficiency of the connected speech of adults with aphasia. *Journal of Speech and Hearing Research, 36*, 338–350.

Nicholas, L., & Brookshire, R. (1995a). Comprehension of spoken narrative discourse by adults with aphasia, right-hemisphere brain damage, or traumatic brain injury. *American Journal of Speech-Language Pathology, 4*, 69–81.

Nicholas, L., & Brookshire, R. (1995b). Presence, completeness, and accuracy of main concepts in the connected speech of non-brain-damaged adults and adults with aphasia. *Journal of Speech and Hearing Research, 38*, 145–156.

Nobis-Busch, R., Springer, L., Sadermacher, I., & Huber, W. (2011). Supervised home training of dialogue skills in chronic aphasia: A randomized parallel group study. *Journal of Speech, Language, and Hearing Research, 54*, 1118–1136.

Ochipa, C., Maher, L. M., & Raymer, A. M. (1998). Neurogenic language case studies: One approach to the treatment of anomia. *Neurophysiology and Neurogenic Speech and Language Disorders, 8*(3). (Special Interest Division 2 Newsletter, 18–23). Rockville, MD: American Speech-Language-Hearing Association.

Odekar, A., & Hallowell, B. (2005). Comparison of alternatives to multidimensional scoring in the assessment of language comprehension in aphasia. *American Journal of Speech-Language Pathology, 14*, 337–345.

Oelschlaeger, M. (1999). Participation of a conversation-partner in the word searches of a person with aphasia. *American Journal of Speech-Language Pathology, 8*, 62–71.

Ostuni, E., & Santo Pietro, M. J. (1991). *Getting through: Communicating when someone you care for has Alzheimer's disease*. Vero Beach, FL: Speech Bin.

Pak-Hin Kong, A. (2011). The main concept analysis in Cantonese aphasic oral discourse: External validity and monitoring chronic aphasia. *Journal of Speech, Language, and Hearing Research, 54*, 148–159.

Paradis, M. (1987). *The assessment of bilingual aphasia*. Hillsdale, NJ: Lawrence Erlbaum.

Patterson, J., & Chapey, R. (2008). Assessment of language disorders in adults. In R. Chapey (Ed.), *Language intervention strategies in aphasia and related neurogenic communication disorders* (5th ed.) (pp. 64–160). Baltimore, MD: Lippincott Williams & Wilkins.

Peach, R. (2001). Further thoughts regarding management of acute aphasia following stroke. *American Journal of Speech-Language Pathology, 10,* 29–36.

Peach, R. (2008). Global aphasia: Identification and management. In R. Chapey (Ed.), *Language intervention strategies in aphasia and related neurogenic communication disorders* (5th ed.) (pp. 565–594). Baltimore, MD: Lippincott Williams & Wilkins.

Perkins, C. J., Korgaonkar, M. S., Fiore, S. M., Squires, N., Goldfarb, R., McCloskey, K. M., & Wagshul, M. E. (2007, May 2). *Functional evaluation of aphasia recovery for stroke patients using fMRI and ERP.* Paper presented at the American Academy of Neurology, Boston.

Piaget, J. (1966). *The language and thought of the child.* Lisbon, NH: The World Publishing Co.

Poeck, K., Huber, W., & Willmes, K. (1989). Outcome of intensive language treatment in aphasia. *Journal of Speech and Hearing Disorders, 54,* 471–479.

Porch, B. (1981). *Porch index of communicative ability.* Palo Alto, CA: Consulting Psychologists Press.

Porch, B. (2007). Comments on "Comparison of alternatives to multidimensional scoring in the assessment of language comprehension in aphasia," by [A.] Odekar and [B.] Hallowell (2005). *American Journal of Speech-Language Pathology, 16,* 84–86.

Ramsberger, G., & Marie, B. (2007). Self-administrated cued naming therapy: A single participant investigation of a computer-based therapy program replicated in four cases. *American Journal of Speech-Language Pathology, 16,* 343–358.

Raphael, L. J., Harris, K. S., & Borden, G. J. (2007). *Speech science primer* (5th ed.). Philadelphia, PA: Lippincott Williams & Wilkins.

Raymer, A., Beeson, P., Holland, A., Kendall, D., Maher, L., Martin, H., . . . Rothi, L. (2008). Translational research in aphasia: From neuroscience to neurorehabilitation. *Journal of Speech, Language, and Hearing Research, 51,* S259–S275.

Raymer, A. M., Maher, L. M., Patterson, J., & Cherney, L. (2007). Neuroplasticity and aphasia: Lessons from constraint-induced language therapy. *Neurophysiology and Neurogenic Speech and Language Disorders, 17*(2). (Special Interest Division 2 Newsletter, 12–17). Rockville, MD: American Speech-Language-Hearing Association.

Reuterskiold, C. (1991). The effects of emotionality on auditory comprehension in aphasia. *Cortex, 27,* 595–604.

Rider, J., Wright, H., Marshall, R., & Page, J. (2008). Using semantic feature analysis to improve contextual discourse in adults with aphasia. *American Journal of Speech-Language Pathology, 17,* 161–172.

Roberts, P. (2008). Aphasia assessment and treatment for bilingual and culturally diverse patients. In R. Chapey (Ed.), *Language intervention strategies in aphasia and related neurogenic communication disorders* (5th ed.) (pp. 245–275). Baltimore, MD: Lippincott Williams & Wilkins.

Robey, R. (1994). The efficacy of treatment for aphasic persons: A metaanalysis. *Brain and Language, 47,* 582–608.

Robey, R. (1998). A meta-analysis of clinical outcomes in the treatment of aphasia. *Journal of Speech, Language, and Hearing Research, 41,* 172–187.

Rosenbek, J., LaPointe, L., & Wertz, R. (1989). *Aphasia: A clinical approach.* Boston, MA: Little, Brown.

Ross, K. B. (2005). Assessing quality of life with aphasia: An annotated bibliography. *Neurophysiology and Neurogenic Speech and Language Disorders, 15*(4). (Special Interest Division 2 Newsletter, 15–18). Rockville, MD: American Speech-Language-Hearing Association.

Ross, K., & Wertz, R. (2003). Discriminating validity of selected measures for differentiating normal from aphasic performance. *American Journal of Speech-Language Pathology, 12,* 312–319.

Rothi, L., Musson, N., Rosenbek, J., & Sapienza, C. (2008). Neuroplasticity and rehabilitation research for speech, language, and swallowing disorders. *Journal of Speech, Language, and Hearing Research, 51,* S222–S224.

Santo Pietro, M., & Goldfarb, R. (1995). *Techniques for aphasia rehabilitation: Generating effective treatment* (TARGET). Vero Beach, FL: The Speech Bin.

Sapir, S., & Aronson, A. (1990). The relationship between psychopathology and speech and language disorders in neurologic patients. *Journal of Speech and Hearing Disorders, 55,* 503–509.

Sarno, J. (1991). The psychological and social sequelae of aphasia. In M. Sarno (Ed.), *Acquired aphasia* (pp. 499–519). New York, NY: Academic Press.

Sarno, M. (1969). *Functional communication profile.* New York, NY: Institute of Rehabilitation Medicine.

Sarno, M. (1991). Recovery and rehabilitation in aphasia. In M. Sarno (Ed.), *Acquired aphasia* (pp. 521–582). New York, NY: Academic Press.

Sarno, M., Silverman, M., & Sands, E. (1970). Speech therapy an language recovery in severe aphasia. *Journal of Speech and Hearing Research, 13*, 607–623.

Schuell, H. (1972). *The Minnesota test for the differential diagnosis of aphasia.* Minneapolis, MN: University of Minnesota Press.

Schuell, H., Jenkins, J., & Jimenez-Pabon, E. (1964). *Aphasia in adults: Diagnosis, prognosis, and treatment.* New York, NY: Hoeber Medical Division, Harper.

Schulte, E., & Brandt, S. (1989). Auditory verbal comprehension impairment. In C. Code (Ed.), *The characteristics of aphasia* (pp. 53–74). Philadelphia, PA: Taylor & Francis.

Schwartz, D., & Halpern, H. (1973). Effect of body-image stimuli on verbal errors of dysphasic subjects. *Perceptual and Motor Skills, 36*, 994.

Schwartz, M. (1984). What the classical aphasia categories can't do for us, and why. *Brain and Language, 21*, 3–8.

Seliger, M., Prescott, T. E., & Shucard, D. W. (1989). Auditory event-related potential probes and behavioral measures of aphasia. *Brain and Language, 36*, 377–390.

Sheehy, L. M. (2006). Crossed aphasia: A review of the syndrome. *Neurophysiology and Neurogenic Speech and Language Disorders, 16*(1). (Special Interest Division 2 Newsletter, 11–16). Rockville, MD: American Speech-Language-Hearing Association.

Shewan, C. (1980). *Auditory comprehension test for sentences.* Chicago, IL: Biolinguistics Clinical Institute.

Shewan, C. (1988). The Shewan spontaneous language analysis (SSLA) system for aphasic adults: Description, reliability, and validity. *Journal of Communication Disorders, 21*, 103–138.

Shewan, C., & Bandur, D. (1986). *Treatment of aphasia: A language-oriented approach.* San Diego, CA: College Hill Press.

Shewan, C., & Kertesz, A. (1984). Effects of speech and language treatment on recovery from aphasia. *Brain and Language, 23*, 272–299.

Shuster, L. I. (2007). Clinical brain scanning: An update. *Neurophysiology and Neurogenic Speech and Language Disorders, 17*(2). (Special Interest Division 2 Newsletter, 17–20). Rockville, MD: American Speech-Language-Hearing Association.

Silver, L., & Halpern, H. (1992). Word-finding abilities of three types of aphasic subjects. *Journal of Psycholinguistic Research, 21*, 317–348.

Simmons-Mackie, N. (2008). Social approaches to aphasia intervention. In R. Chapey (Ed.), *Language intervention strategies in aphasia and related neurogenic communication disorders* (5th ed.) (pp. 290–317). Baltimore, MD: Lippincott Williams & Wilkins.

Simmons-Mackie, N., Kingston, D., & Schultz, M. (2004). "Speaking for another": The management of participant frames in aphasia. *American Journal of Speech-Language Pathology, 13*, 114–127.

Sklar, M. (1973). *Sklar aphasia scale.* Los Angeles, CA: Western Psychological Services.

Sparks, R. (2008). Melodic intonation therapy. In R. Chapey (Ed.), *Language intervention strategies in aphasia and related neurogenic communication disorders* (5th ed.) (pp. 837-851). Baltimore, MD: Lippincott Williams & Wilkins.

Spreen, O., & Benton, A. (1969). *Neurosensory center comprehensive examination for aphasia.* Victoria, Canada: University of Victoria Neuropsychology Laboratory.

Stocker, B., & Goldfarb, R. (1995). *The Stocker probe for fluency and language* (3rd ed.). Vero Beach, FL: The Speech Bin.

Swindell, C., & Hammons, J. (1991). Poststroke depression: Neurologic, physiologic, diagnostic, and treatment implications. *Journal of Speech and Hearing Research, 34*, 325–333.

Thompson, C. (2007). Complexity in language learning and treatment. *American Journal of Speech-Language Pathology, 16*, 3–5.

Thompson, C., & Shapiro, L. (2007). Complexity in treatment of syntactic deficits. *American Journal of Speech-Language Pathology, 16*, 30–42.

Thompson, C., Shapiro, L., Kiran, S., & Sobecks, J. (2003). Syntactic complexity in treatment of sentence deficits in agrammatic aphasia: The complexity account of treatment efficacy (CATE). *Journal of Speech-Language-Hearing Research, 46*, 591–607.

Thompson, C., Shapiro, L., Roberts, M. (1993). Treatment of sentence production deficits in aphasia: A linguistic-specific approach to wh- interrogative training and generalization. *Aphasiology, 7*, 111–133.

Tompkins, C. (1991). Redundancy enhances emotional inferencing by right- and left-hemisphere damaged adults. *Journal of Speech and Hearing Research, 34*, 1142–1149.

Tompkins, C., Gibbs Scott, A., & Scharf, V. (2008). Research principles for the clinician. In R. Chapey (Ed.), *Language intervention strategies in aphasia and related neurogenic communication disorders* (5th ed.) (pp. 163–185). Baltimore, MD: Lippincott Williams & Wilkins.

Tompkins, C., Marshall, R., & Phillips, D. (1980). Aphasic patients in a rehabilitation program: Scheduling speech and language services. *Archives of Physical Medicine and Rehabilitation, 66*, 252–257.

Towne, R., & Banick, P. (1989). The effect of stimulus color on naming performance of aphasic adults. *Journal of Communication Disorders, 22*, 397–405.

Tseng, C., McNeil, M., & Molenkovic, P. (1993). An investigation of attention allocation deficits in aphasia. *Brain and Language, 45*, 276–296.

Ulatowska, H., Freedman-Stern, R., Doyel, A., & Macaluso-Haynes, S. (1983). Production of narrative discourse in aphasia. *Brain & Language, 19*, 317–334.

Ulatowska, H., Wertz, R., Chapman, S., Hill, C., Thompson, J., Keebler, M., . . . Auther, L. (2001). Interpretation of fables and proverbs by African Americans with and without aphasia. *American Journal of Speech-Language Pathology, 10*, 40–50.

Van Lancker, D., & Klein, K. (1990). Preserved recognition of familiar personal names in global aphasia. *Brain and Language, 39*, 511–529.

Vignolo, L. (1964). Evolution of aphasia and language rehabilitation: A retrospective exploratory study. *Cortex, 1*, 344–367.

Wagenaar, E., Snow, C., & Prins, R. (1975). Spontaneous speech of aphasic patients: A psycholinguistic analysis. *Brain and Language, 2*, 281–303.

Wallace, G., & Canter, G. (1985). Effects of personally relevant language materials on the performance of severely aphasic individuals. *Journal of Speech and Hearing Disorders, 50*, 385–390.

Webb, W., & Adler, R. (2008). *Neurology for the speech-language pathologist* (5th ed.). St. Louis, MO: Mosby.

Weisenburg, T., & McBride, K. (1935). *Aphasia.* New York, NY: Hafner.

Wepman, J. (1951). *Recovery from aphasia.* New York, NY: Ronald Press.

Wepman, J. (1976). Aphasia: Language without thought or thought without language? *Asha, 18*, 131–136.

Wepman, J., & Jones, L. (1961). *The language modalities test for aphasia.* Chicago, IL: Education Industry Service.

Wernicke, C. (1874). *Das aphasische symptomenkomplex* [The aphasia symptom complex]. Breslau, Germany: Cohn & Weigart.

Wertz, R. (1992). A single case for group treatment studies in aphasia. In *Aphasia treatment: Current approaches and research opportunities* (NIH Publication No. 93-3424). Bethesda, MD: National Institutes of Health.

Wertz, R. T. (2005). Department of Veterans Affairs cooperative studies on aphasia revisited. *Neurogenic Speech and Language Disorders, 15*(3). (Special Interest Division 2 Newsletter, 6–13). Rockville, MD: American Speech-Language-Hearing Association.

Wertz, R., Collins, M., Weiss, D., Kurtzke, J., Friden, T., Brookshire, R., . . . Resurreccion, E. (1981). Veterans administration cooperative study in aphasia: A comparison of individual and group treatment. *Journal of Speech and Hearing Research, 24*, 580–594.

Wertz, R., Weiss, D., Aten, J., Brookshire, R., Garcia-Bunuel, L., Holland, A., . . .Goodman, R. (1986). A comparison of clinic, home, and deferred language treatment for aphasia: A VA cooperative study. *Archives of Neurology, 43*, 653–658.

Wiegersma, S., Post, H., Veldhuijsen, M., & DeVries, L. (1988). Encoding of frequency of occurrence by aphasia patients: Attentional or linguistic deficits. *Cortex, 24*, 433–441.

Wright, H., & Shisler, R. (2005). Working memory in aphasia: Theory, measures, and clinical implications. *American Journal of Speech-Language Pathology, 14*, 107–118.

Yorkston, K., & Beukelman, D. (1980). An analysis of connected speech samples of aphasic and normal speakers. *Journal of Speech and Hearing Disorders, 45*, 27–36.

Zraick, R., & Boone, D. (1991). Spouse attitudes toward the person with aphasia. *Journal of Speech and Hearing Research, 34*, 123–128.

Communication Disorders Associated with Right Hemisphere Damage

Definition

Right hemisphere damage (RHD) can cause problems in cognition, communication, or both. Problems in cognition would include the areas of attention, perception, orientation (time, place, and person), neglect, constructional impairment, anosognosia, prosopagnosia, and confabulation. Problems in communication would include the areas of language (particularly the semantic and pragmatic components) and speech (particularly the prosody component). Many times deficits in cognition can lead to deficits in language. Effects of RHD do not seem to be different if the individual is left-handed or right-handed (Mackenzie & Brady, 2004).

Symptoms

Cognition Deficits

(For a definition and discussion of the terms *attention*, *perception*, and *orientation*, see the introduction and the sections on communication disorders associated with dementia and traumatic brain injury).

Neglect

Neglect is defined as a failure to report, respond, or orient to novel or meaningful stimuli presented to the side opposite to a brain lesion, that cannot be attributed to either an elemental sensory or motor defect (Filley & Kelly, 1990; Heilman, 1994). Severe neglect is more frequently associated with right than with left hemisphere lesions (Mesulam, 1990). Most patients with neglect have lesions of the parietal lobe, but neglect can also be associated with lesions of the frontal lobe, the cingulate gyrus (part of the limbic lobe or system), the temporal lobe, and the thalamus. The diseases that can cause neglect include stroke, tumors, trauma and degenerative disorders, or any condition that can damage the right hemisphere.

Priftis et al. (2008) presented a line of numbers from one through nine, with "five" in the middle, and asked patients with RHD to discriminate either the number on the left (one) or the one on the right (nine) from the one in the middle (five). There was more of a delay, based on P3b brain waves, in cognitive processing of the targets to the left of the number line compared to targets on the right. The delay of P3b indicates a neural signature of the disorder of representational space. However, in patients who had RHD without neglect, there was no effect of represented number position (Vuilleumier, Ortigue, & Brugger, 2004).

The neuropsychological mechanisms that have been assumed to account for neglect include disorders of attention (Hugdahl, Wester, & Asbjornsen, 1991; Robertson et al., 1994), motor intention-exploration (Heilman et al., 1985, as reported by Benson & Ardila, 1996), and spatial representations (perception) (Chieffi, Carlomagno, Silveri, & Gainotti, 1989; Gutbrod, Cohen, Maier, & Maier, 1987). Neglect can occur through the visual, auditory, tactile, or olfactory modality, singly or in combination, with the visual modality being the most frequently affected.

Myers and Blake (2008) have noted that left hemispatial neglect can cause visual, auditory, and communication problems. Visual problems are manifested when the patient, while viewing things on the left side, disrupts or omits the following: drawing, connecting dots, filling in states on a map, setting a clock, eating food from a tray, and attending to people in a room. In addition, a patient with left spatial unilateral neglect may perceive relative leftward overextension of a line, indicating that representational space is distorted (Geminiani et al., 2004). This may also affect perception of movement on the left side. Auditory problems on the patient's left side are shown by the patient's ignoring a ringing phone, people talking, or a bell or buzzer sounding. Individuals with RHD have a larger mean absolute error in sound localization than do those with left hemisphere damage (LHD), which may be explained by the inattention theory of hemispatial neglect (Sonoda, Mori, & Goishi, 2001). Communication problems are evident when the patient has left-sided problems in reading, and in spelling and punctuation when writing. For example, Stemmer, Giroux, & Joanette (1994) found that RHD subjects were deficient in the production and evaluation of requests when compared to control subjects. The authors postulated that attention and visuospatial abilities could cause the deficiencies. According to Benson and Ardila (1996), the reading problem can be called a *neglect alexia* or a *spatial alexia*, and the writing problem a *spatial agraphia*.

Constructional Impairment

Constructional impairment is quite common with both LHD and RHD patients. Due to problems in attention, perception, and neglect, the RHD patient will have difficulty drawing or copying geometric designs (e.g., Benowitz, Moya, & Levine, 1990), reproducing stick figures, creating designs with colored blocks, or reproducing three-dimensional constructions using wooden blocks. The RHD patient's reproductions will reflect a distorted and disorganized arrangement, whereas the LHD patient will show a primitive type of arrangement, but one very much like the model. Swindell, Holland, Fromm, and Greenhouse (1988) found that when drawing a person, the LHD patients could make drawings that looked like a person and included appropriate facial characteristics, whereas the RHD patients made drawings that were disjointed and contained inappropriate characteristics.

Limb Apraxia

Adults who have RHD with left hemiparesis tend to have greater motor programming difficulties (apraxia) with a poorer functional outcome compared to those with LHD. Whether or not a body-related cognitive disorder plays a role in the difficulty is unclear, which prompted a study (Borde, Mazaux, & Barat, 2006) of reproduction of passive meaningless gestures. Four groups of ten adults—each of which had RHD with neglect, had RHD without neglect, had LHD, or were neurotypical controls—had meaningless gestures passively applied by the examiner on the ipsilesional or contralesional upper limb, and all participants were asked to reproduce the gesture with the ipsilesional nonparetic limb. Results were as follows: those participants with LHD performed about as well as the neurotypical controls, while those with RHD with and without neglect were significantly impaired relative to the other groups, regardless of whether the gestures were applied on the contralesional or ipsilesional limb. The performance of those RHD patients with and without neglect did not differ from each other, and was observed to be defective whether the participants had their eyes open or closed. Borde et al. (2006) drew the following conclusions:

1. RHD is associated with a perceptual multimodal integration disorder, rather than a modality-related sensory disorder.
2. The LH is dominant for visual imitation of meaningless gestures as well as for symbolic gestures.
3. RHD is associated with a disorder of bilateral, perceptual, multimodal integration of knowledge about the individual's own body.

Anosognosia and Prosopagnosia

Patients with right hemisphere damage can exhibit the cognitive deficits of anosognosia and prosopagnosia.

Anosognosia is an abnormal condition characterized by a real or feigned inability to perceive a defect, especially paralysis, on one side of the body, possibly attributable to a lesion in the right parietal lobe of the brain (*Mosby's*, 1994). The individual may deny the existence of the affected part or may feel a depersonalization toward the affected part of the body. The condition may be associated with confabulation, inattention, or disturbed orientation of the body schema. Damasio (1994) noted that individuals with anosognosia have more than just a left-sided paralysis of which they are not aware; they also have a defect in reasoning and decision making, and a defect in emotion and feeling.

Prosopagnosia is an inability to recognize faces, even one's own face (*Taber's*, 1997). The individual will recognize persons known by other features such as sound of voice, stride, body weight and size, or clothing. The condition is attributable to a lesion in the right temporal-occipital area of the brain.

Confabulation

The patient with right hemisphere damage typically will show few or no problems in auditory and reading comprehension, or in oral and written expression, as the adult aphasic patient would (e.g., Cappa, Papagno, & Vallar, 1990). The RHD patient might show irrelevant language where the response does not relate to the stimulus or contains confabulations (the fabrication of experiences or situations, often recounted in a detailed and plausible way, to fill in and cover up gaps in the memory, apparently without any intent to deceive), and/or propagation (an increased amount of irrelevant language that many times connects or includes mention of the patient's illness and its relation to the environment in an erroneous manner).

Hough (1990) found that RHD patients confabulated more and strayed more from a central theme than did LHD patients and persons without brain damage. Sohlberg and Ehlhardt (1998) have noted that, based on observations of behavior, confabulation can be classified as spontaneous or provoked. Spontaneous confabulations are uttered without apparent incitement and are often fantastic or implausible. Provoked confabulations tend to happen as a reaction to questioning and often are tied to some real event. Additional information on confabulation and propagation can be found in the section on communication disorders associated with traumatic brain injury.

As an example of confabulation, one RHD patient responded in the following manner to the inquiry as to whether he did his assignment: The patient explained that he was unable to do the assignment because he was ill with a toothache all weekend and had to see a dentist, whom he identified as one of the authors. He further indicated that his sole complaint and the reason he continued to see the author were problems with his teeth. A conversation with family members revealed that his teeth were in fact in very good shape and that he had neither required a dentist nor complained of a toothache for quite some time.

Communication Deficits

Language Abilities

A sampling of studies reveals that the RHD patient can have difficulty with drawing inferences (implied information), abstract words, story arrangement, comprehension of spoken narrative discourse, and pragmatic abilities.

Inferences. Brownell, Potter, Bihrle, and Gardner (1986) found that RHD patients were deficient in inferential reasoning, and Brownell, Simpson, Bihrle, Potter, and Gardner (1990) observed that the appreciation of metaphoric and nonmetaphoric alternative meanings of single words was impaired in RHD subjects. McDonald and Wales (1986) found that RHD patients did more poorly than the control group in processing inferences.

Myers and Brookshire (1996) found that 24 RHD subjects, particularly those with high levels of neglect, were significantly impaired relative to the 30 non-brain-damaged (NBD) subjects in generating accurate inferences from pictures, but not in their ability to recognize and identify pictured elements.

Tompkins, Bloise, Timko, and Baumgaertner (1994) observed that 25 RHD and 25 LHD subjects showed deficiencies in working memory and tasks requiring inference revision, the RHD group especially with the task that involved the most demanding comprehension processes. No meaningful association within the above conditions was observed for normally aging subjects.

Lehman-Blake and Tompkins (2001) investigated for predictive inferencing (or inferences) about outcomes of events in 13 adults with RHD and 11 adults without brain damage (NBD). Results showed that adults with RHD generated target predictive inferences in contexts with recent mention of strongly biasing inference-related information. They also showed maintenance of inferences over time, but to a lesser degree than participants in the NBD group. Overall, individuals with better auditory comprehension or larger estimated working memory capacity tended to maintain inferences better than did the other participants.

Blake (2009a) replicated and extended a previous study of inferencing in which some adults with RHD generated but did not maintain predictive inferences over time (Lehman-Blake & Tomkins, 2001). In the current study of 14 adults with RHD and 14 with NBD, participants read short narratives that suggested a predictive inference. Reading times were obtained to assess inference generation, maintenance, and integration. Results from the current study provide further evidence that adults with RHD can generate inferences, even those that are not essential for comprehension.

Winner, Brownell, Happe, Blum, and Pincus (1998) found that 13 RHD patients performed worse than 20 neurotypical control participants when asked to distinguish lies from jokes, confirming their known difficulty with discourse interpretation.

On the other hand, a few other studies indicated different results. Tompkins (1990) found that RHD subjects performed similarly to LHD and neurotypical control subjects in the automatic condition (discouraging the use of any associative strategies) and when provided with specific processing strategies, indicating that they retained some knowledge of metaphoric word meanings. When left to glean strategies for themselves, both brain-damaged groups had difficulty. In another study, Tompkins, Boada, and McGarry (1992) observed that no significant differences among typically aging, RHD and LHD groups existed in the processing of familiar idioms.

Abstract and concrete words. Goulet and Joanette (1994) found that in a sentence completion task requiring abstract or concrete words, the use of both kinds of words was more impaired in RHD subjects than in neurotypical participants.

Story arrangement. Schneiderman, Murasugi, and Saddy (1992) observed that RHD subjects had more difficulty with story arrangement than did LHD and NBD subjects.

Comprehension of spoken narrative discourse. Using an earlier version of their *Discourse Comprehension Test* (see the section on aphasia), Nicholas and Brookshire (1995) found that in the comprehension of spoken narrative discourse, 20 RHD subjects had more correct responses when questions assessed main ideas than when they assessed details, and more correct responses when questions assessed stated information than when they assessed implied information. In addition, stated information had stronger effects on their comprehension of details than on their comprehension of main ideas.

The ability of adults with RHD to suppress or inhibit context-inappropriate interpretations has been shown to be an important predictor of narrative discourse comprehension (Tompkins et al., 2000, 2001, 2002). For example, a spoken probe word (e.g., "cards") should bias the meaning of a lexically ambiguous word at the end of a sentence (e.g., "spade"), but should result in a relatively slower response when the last word was unambiguous (e.g., "shovel"). Limited resource allocation in divided-attention tasks (e.g., when the participant was also required to report whether the probe word had one or two syllables) could also affect comprehension.

Tompkins et al. (2004) studied the activation failure versus the multiple activation, and discourse comprehension in 37 adults with RHD and 34 adults with NBD. Results indicated that adults with RHD were partially consistent with the multiple activation view. Also, greater activation for contextual interpretations was associated with poorer discourse comprehension performance.

Kennedy (2000) studied eight adults with RHD and seven NBD matched controls in first-encounter conversations. Results showed that all participants produced more topic scenes (conversations) in the maintenance phase than in the initiation or termination phases. However, some participants with RHD produced statements that were out of context. This suggested that adults with RHD may have difficulty suppressing secondary information during discourse comprehension tasks.

To summarize, Meyers and Blake (2008) in their review note that discourse impairments tend to be cognitively based and include deficits in generating a macro structure, integrating information, disambiguating information, and drawing complex inferences based on contextual clues. These impairments may result in reduced levels of informative content in discourse production and reduced sensitivity to shades of meaning in discourse comprehension.

Blake (2009b) noted that it is widely accepted that RHD can cause difficulty with discourse comprehension. Although the underlying source of the comprehension deficits is not clear, one factor that has been implicated is the ability to use contextual cues. The purpose of this study was to evaluate the effect of varying contextual bias on predictive inferencing by adults with RHD. Fourteen adults with NBD and 14 with RHD read stories constructed with either high predictability or low predictability of a specific outcome. The results and conclusion showed that RHD does not abolish the ability to use context, although adults with this impairment may need more time to do the task than adults with NBD.

Pragmatic abilities. Several studies have shown that RHD subjects are deficient in their pragmatic abilities (Bloom, Borod, Obler, & Gerstman, 1993; Foldi, 1987; Kaplan, Brownell, Jacobs, & Gardner, 1990). As an example of a breakdown in pragmatic behavior (not maintaining proper decorum in a communicative setting), one RHD patient responded in the following manner to the direction, "Tell me three things every good citizen should do": "Go to sleep, get up, and take a good ___" (the third item can best be described as a bodily function performed in the bathroom). The patient was so pleased with himself for giving that answer that he proceeded to laugh and act jolly for the next few minutes of the session.

Discourse characteristics of adults with RHD included more tangentiality, egocentrism, and extremes of quantity (either extreme verbosity or paucity of speech) compared to neurotypical controls (Lehman-Blake, 2006). However, only one-third of the speech-language pathologists who examined the clinical relevance of potential differences across groups were able to classify discourse samples accurately according to group.

Speech Abilities

Prosody. Prosody is a component of speech production that includes such features as intonation, stress, rate, rhythm, melody, pitch, volume, spacing between words, and intervals and pauses in conversation, all of which can convey linguistic and emotional (or affective) (e.g., happy, sad, angry, shocked, gloating, neutral) information. The effects of prosody also involve the listener's comprehension of the linguistic and emotional information provided by the speaker. Patients with posterior RHD have the most difficulty. Deficits in affective prosody, a dominant and lateralized function of the right hemisphere, are different following right brain damage than following left brain damage. Ross and Monnot (2008) suggest that affective prosody in the right hemisphere may be analogous to the organization of propositional language in the left hemisphere.

Comprehension and expression of emotional speech. In their review, Myers and Blake (2008) noted that RHD patients may have difficulty in comprehending and expressing emotional speech. Studies have not made it clear whether this emotional inappropriateness is a result of an emotional (or affective) disorder, or of a more general attention deficit that reduces responsiveness to the external environment. Recently, Sherratt (2007) compared 7 adult males with RHD to 10 neurotypical males on two personal experience narratives, one of a negative discourse topic and one of a positive. For the negative topic, the RHD group used fewer appraisal resources, defined as semantic choices to indicate emotions, judgments, and valuations, compared to the control group. Both groups used similar proportions of appraisal resources for the positive topic.

Reduced responsiveness may impede the understanding of extralinguistic cues (facial expression, body language, gestures, and prosody) from which one can infer the emotional atmosphere of situations and narratives. Borod et al. (1989) found that the "flat affect" of schizophrenics most resembled that of RHD subjects (choices included Parkinson subjects [hypokinetic dysarthria] and normal subjects). Perceptual problems in spatial judgment and feature integration may also contribute to a reduction in the ability to recognize emotional facial expression.

Comprehension of emotional (or affective) prosody is tested by having the subject listen to neutral sentences expressed with an emotional overlay, and then identify the mood of the speaker.

Comprehension and expression of linguistic information. RHD can also produce deficits in prosodic *comprehension* and *expression* of linguistic information. Comprehension of linguistic prosody is tested by having the subject listen to prosodic features used to convey (1) different types of sentences (e.g., declarative, interrogative, or exclamatory), (2) different word meanings through use of emphatic stress (e.g., distinguishing "greenhouse" from "green house," and (3) linguistic stress markers that can alter sentence meanings (e.g., "John wants the *red* bike" versus "John wants the red *bike*").

Then again, comprehension difficulties in prosody may be tied to impaired tonal perception and to impaired attention. All in all, studies in RHD prosodic comprehension are not clear on whether the problem is caused by a linguistic, emotional, or cognitive (perception, attention) disturbance.

In his review, Duffy (2005) noted that aprosodia are prosodic impairments in the *interpretation* or *production* of speech that may be uniquely associated with right hemisphere damage. In the production of speech, prosody disturbances may be associated with various lesion sites (e.g., frontal lobe, frontoparietal lobes, and subcortical areas), motor speech disorders (e.g., dysarthria, apraxia of speech), and cognitive and affective deficits (e.g., depression).

The aprosodic speech pattern is often described as flat, indifferent, devoid of expression and emotion, having little spontaneous prosody, computer-like or robotic, monotonous, and lacking the ability to modulate the voice to convey the subtleties of language (e.g., irony, sarcasm). Duffy (2005) also noted that studies of aprosodia have yielded mixed results, and the defining characteristics and nature of the problem underlying aprosodia are still not well understood.

Communication abilities and inference impairment. Myers and Blake (2008) have postulated that most of the language problems of the RHD patient are due to an inference impairment. They defined an inference as a hypothesis about sensory data where that input is not only sensed but also interpreted. Inferences depend on the following processes: (1) attention to individual cues, (2) selection of relevant cues, (3) integration of relevant cues with one another, and (4) association of cues with prior experience.

They further noted that this underlying inference impairment leads to disturbances in the following areas: (1) producing informative content (e.g., RHD patients may produce a lot of words, but much of it is empty speech), (2) integrating narrative information (e.g., RHD patients may lose the gist of what they hear and subsequently what they say), (3) generating alternative meanings (e.g., RHD patients will have problems with understanding figurative language such as metaphors, idioms, and proverbs; irony; sarcasm; humor; a person's motives), (4) comprehending and expressing emotion, and (5) comprehending and producing prosody.

Etiology

The types of focal brain lesions that cause adult aphasia are the same ones that can cause right hemisphere damage. The major causes include cerebrovascular accidents, trauma to the brain, and brain tumors. The lesser causes include abscesses, infectious diseases, and degenerative diseases of the brain.

Damasio (1994) stated that there is an area of the human brain, the complex of somatosensory cortices in the right hemisphere, whose damage compromises reasoning and decision making, emotion and feelings, with a special emphasis in the social and personal domain.

In addition, damage in the somatosensory cortices also disrupts the processes of basic body signaling. Basic body signaling involves receiving signals from throughout the body (muscles, joints, internal organs) and its interconnections with other regions in the somatosensory system. The major players in this scenario are the cortex (frontal, parietal, temporal, and occipital lobes), the somatosensory cortices in the right hemisphere, and the limbic system (e.g., cingulate gyrus, amygdala, hippocampus).

Bhatnagar (2008, Chapters 2, 7, 19, 20) noted that located in the parietal lobe (Brodmann's areas 3, 1, 2, and 5), the primary sensory cortex receives the bodily experienced modalities of touch (pressure, vibration, and proprioception, which is the internal awareness of position, posture, and movement), temperature (cold, heat), and pain. The primary sensory cortex is arrayed in homunculus fashion and runs parallel to the motor cortex homunculus (Brodmann's areas 4 and part of 6). The primary sensory cortex connects with the associational sensory cortex that is located in superior areas of the parietal lobe.

The primary sensory cortex analyzes the information for the conscious perception of touch, temperature, and pain. In the associational sensory cortex, the sensations are analyzed, elaborated on, integrated with previous experience, and then raised to the highest conscious level for cognitive functions.

The following sections list the cognitive problems that can occur because of a brain lesion.

Lesions in the right parietal lobe may result in left side neglect; anosognosia; dressing apraxia; spatial difficulty; topographical difficulties; constructional problems; prosody changes involving intonation (expression and comprehension); semantic difficulties; and changes in pragmatic behavior, drawing inferences, and mood.

Lesions in the right temporal lobe may result in deficits in the recognition of rhythm and music, and with memory. Acute lesions (e.g., strokes) can cause delirium or confusion.

Lesions in the medial temporal lobe area involving the hippocampus (limbic system) and its connections to the cingulate gyrus of the medial frontal lobes can produce problems with memory.

Lesions in the medial surface of the frontal lobe, which has connections to the cingulate gyrus and hippocampus (limbic system), may affect memory, motivation for survival (aggression, flight), drive, emotion, and learning.

Lesions in the dorsolateral portion of the frontal lobes may produce problems in working memory and lesions in scattered areas of the frontal lobes can affect attention.

Lesions in scattered areas of the occipital lobe may cause prosopagnosia.

Diagnosis

Diagnostic procedures for determining the communication disorders associated with right hemisphere damage can involve (1) establishing background information, (2) giving a neurologic evaluation, (3) employing informal tests, and (4) employing formal tests.

Establishing Background Information and the Neurologic Evaluation

These procedures can be found at the beginning of the "Diagnosis" portion of the section on aphasia.

Informal Tests
Cognition Deficits

The participants involved in the diagnosis of *neglect* can include the neurologist, the neuropsychologist, the occupational therapist, and the speech-language pathologist. The speech-language pathologist can get a good idea as to whether neglect is present by doing the following: (1) for visual neglect, asking the patient to draw symmetrical items (clock, figure and face of a human, baseball diamond, football field, connecting dots, filling in a map) and perform reading and writing tasks; (2) for auditory neglect, standing behind the patient and presenting auditory commands (e.g., "Pick up the pencil," "Look at the window," "Snap your fingers," "Tap the table") of equal intensity to each ear.

General observation of the patient's reaching for items, pointing to things, applying lipstick, results of shaving, and wearing of eyeglasses can also be used for determining neglect. The informal diagnosis of neglect is warranted if the patient misses or distorts any or all of the items presented to the left side.

Facial affect can be assessed by having the patient produce a variety of facial expressions on command (e.g., happy, sad, angry, shocked, afraid, neutral). The clinician can produce a variety of facial expressions and then have the patient tell what they represent.

Communication Deficits

Prosody can be tested by having the patient say or listen to inherently neutral sentences (e.g., saying, "Today is Wednesday," or listening to that sentence and producing or recognizing a happy, sad, angry, shocked, neutral, etc., quality). Bloom, Borod, Obler, and Gerstman (1992) observed that RHD subjects had a selective impairment in producing emotional contents. Tompkins (1991a) found that in automatic and effortful processing of emotional intonation, the RHD subjects were slower than LHD subjects.

Pragmatic abilities can be checked by noting the patient's eye contact, topic maintenance, turn-taking, loudness level, awareness of errors, attention, and so forth. Bloom et al. (1993) found that emotional content suppressed pragmatic performance among RHD subjects. Kaplan et al. (1990) observed that RHD individuals were more deficient in picking up pragmatic cues than were matched control subjects.

Language deficits can be evaluated by using any of the tests noted later in this section, or by using selected portions of the aphasia batteries mentioned in "Diagnosis" in the section on aphasia. Questions probing orientation to time, place, and person, and general information can be added (see "Diagnosis" in the section on communication disorders associated with dementia).

One RHD patient, a lawyer and former foreign diplomat attached to his country's mission at the United Nations, had an excellent vocabulary in English. He could give fine definitions of single words and talk about some of his experiences at the UN (the authors were not sure if they were true or not). His problems became apparent when he was asked to respond to time-, place-, and person-orientation stimuli (e.g., "What year [season, month, day of the week] is it?" "What is today's date?" "Where do you live?" "Who do you live with?" "Where are you right now?"). The patient's responses were off not by 1 year, 1 month, or 1 day, but by as much as 10 years, 6 months, or 3 days. He had no concept of where he lived or how long he had lived there, nor could he identify family members. He also exhibited neglect, flat affect, and pragmatic problems in eye contact, turn-taking, and topic maintenance.

To ascertain if the patient digresses (e.g., confabulates) or can integrate ideas, the clinician can ask open-ended questions such as defining proverbs, telling three things that every good citizen should do, defining words, responding to items requiring a sequence of events (e.g., "What would you do if you saw smoke?" "How would you fry an egg?" "How did you get to work?" "What did your workday consist of?" "How do you wash your hair?").

Picture descriptions can be used for evaluating the patient's narrative verbal output. Myers and Blake (2008) describe a procedure whereby narrative verbal output is broken down into interpretive and literal concepts. An interpretive score is arrived at by dividing the total number of concepts by the number of interpretive concepts. Examples are given of interpretive and literal concepts, and data are cited on how non-brain-damaged and RHD patients performed using this analysis. The non-brain-damaged subjects produced almost twice as many interpretive responses as the RHD subjects.

Formal Tests

Cognitive and language abilities can be tested with some of the batteries available for testing the RHD patient. Adamovich and Brooks (1981) described a procedure for testing the communicative abilities of RHD patients. They borrowed portions of tests used in aphasia, visual organization, and learning aptitude.

The *Discourse Comprehension Test* (Brookshire & Nicholas, 1997) assesses both listening and reading comprehension (see "Diagnosis" in the section on aphasia).

The *Evaluation of Communication Problems in Right Hemisphere Dysfunction* (Burns, Halper, & Mogil, 1985) and the *RIC Evaluation of Communication Problems in Right Hemisphere Dysfunction* (RICE–R) (Halper, Cherney, Burns, & Mogil, 1996, cited in Golper & Cherney, 1999) offer protocols for evaluating the RHD patient by (1) interviewing the patient; (2) observing the patient in contact with hospital staff and family members; (3) evaluating attention; eye contact; awareness of illness; orientation to time, place, and person; facial expression; intonation; and topic maintenance; (4) tests of visual scanning and tracking; (5) evaluating written expression; (6) rating pragmatic skills; and (7) a language test using metaphors.

The *Mini Inventory of Right Brain Injury* (MIRBI) (Pimental & Kingsbury, 1989) assesses (1) visual scanning; (2) integrity of gnosis (e.g., object identification); (3) integrity of body image; (4) reading and writing; (5) serial sevens (e.g., subtracting 7 from 100, subtracting 7 from the remainder, and so on); (6) integrity of praxis (e.g., drawing a clock); (7) speech intonation; (8) humor, incongruities, absurdities, figurative language, and similarities; (9) affect; and (10) general behavior.

The *Right Hemisphere Language Battery* (RHLB) (Bryan, 1989) evaluates (1) comprehension of spoken metaphors, (2) comprehension of printed metaphors, (3) comprehension of inferred meaning (reading), (4) appreciation of humor (reading), (5) pointing to a picture by name, (6) production of emphatic stress in spoken sentences, and (7) discourse analysis of spontaneous conversation.

The *Ross Information Processing Assessment* (RIPA-2) (Ross-Swain, 1996) assesses the following 10 areas of communicative and cognitive functioning: (1) immediate memory, (2) recent memory, (3) temporal orientation (recent memory), (4) temporal orientation (remote memory), (5) spatial orientation, (6) orientation to environment, (7) recall of general information, (8) problem solving and abstract reasoning, (9) organization, and (10) auditory processing and retention.

Milman et al. (2008) investigated the initial validity and reliability of the *Scales of Cognitive and Communicative Ability for Neurorehabilitation* (SCCAN) (Milman & Holland, 2007). The SCCAN was designed to provide an overview of impairment and activity limitations across eight cognitive scales (speech comprehension, oral expression, reading, writing, orientation, attention, memory, and problem solving).

Marshall and Karow (2008) have produced an evaluation tool called the *Rapid Assessment of Problem Solving* (RAPS), which is a modification of the well-researched *20 Question Test*. The authors claim that the RAPS is easy to administer and to score, and it is now part of the public domain and may be used by clinicians to assess clients' problem-solving deficits.

Therapy

The first goal of therapy is to inform the patient and the caretaker(s) about the nature and the consequences of the disorder.

The RHD patient can have problems in the processes of attention, perception, neglect, constructional abilities, emotions, inference abilities, prosody, and pragmatic functioning. Cognitive impairment could lead to overall mild language problems and to the specific irrelevant language errors (confabulations and propagations) displayed by the patient.

Although not as clearly delineated as with the aphasia patient, spontaneous recovery (and prognosis) in the RHD patient can show many of the same patterns. In spontaneous recovery for the RHD patient, the major emphasis would be on the retrieval of the nonlanguage functions described in the previous paragraph, and the minor emphasis would be on the overall mild language problems (see "Spontaneous Recovery" in the section on aphasia).

With prognosis (see "Prognosis" in the section on aphasia), the indicators most applicable to the RHD patient would be age, time of entering therapy, neurologic damage, will to improve and acceptance of limitations, family attitude and encouragement, initial evaluation, length and intensity of therapy, and physical condition.

In reaction to their illness, RHD patients can often show anosognosia, which is defined as a lack of awareness, denial, or a tendency to minimize the condition. They can often be overly optimistic and jocular, and at the same time exhibit a lack of motivation. They may also have unrealistic goals (e.g., going back to work); have time, place, and person disorientation; fail to recognize familiar faces; and have grooming deficits. They can be impulsive and have difficulty in getting to or understanding the main point in conversation.

Due to many of the reactions listed above (e.g., overly optimistic, unrealistic goals, jocularity, minimizing the illness) and the mild language problem that can occur, families tend to believe the patient. This belief in a false, rosy picture, coupled with their own hopes for a return to normalcy, can lead to a very unrealistic perception of the patient's true capabilities.

The second goal of therapy is to provide the appropriate treatment approaches and techniques.

Efficacy of Therapy for the Communication Disorders Associated with Right Hemisphere Damage

Efficacy of treatment studies for communication disorders associated with right hemisphere damage are difficult to find in the literature. One possible reason is that the symptoms of RHD are not, relatively speaking, as clear-cut as the symptoms of adult aphasia. In aphasia, the symptoms involve a language breakdown, and all efforts in diagnosis and treatment are concentrated in that one area.

The symptoms in RHD can involve problems in attention, perception, neglect, constructional abilities, emotion, inference ability, prosody, language, and in particular the pragmatic aspects of language. Because of the variety of symptoms, diagnosis and treatment are geared not only toward language but to cognitive and behavioral problems as well.

There is now some question as to whether RHD patients are best treated by the relatively longtime use of the treatment-of-symptoms approach, or by a relatively new, alternative treatment-of-cause approach (to help the symptoms). For example, emotion can be treated with techniques that directly correct the patient's recognition and production of flat affect (emotion).

As an alternative approach to correcting the symptoms of emotion, Myers and Blake (2008) proposed using items designed to increase patient abilities to generate alternative meanings and integrate information. In their opinion, emotional deficits arise from the same source as narrative-level deficits, namely, an underlying inference impairment.

Blake (2007) set out to describe the current treatment research for communication (prosodic, discourse, and pragmatic) deficits associated with RHD and to provide suggestions for treatment selection given the paucity of evidence specifically for this population. She concluded that controlled treatment studies for communication deficits specifically for adults with RHD are limited to aprosodia. For other communication deficits, clinicians may select treatments based on current theories of right hemisphere function and right hemisphere deficits, and treatments developed for other etiologies for which difficulties are similar to those associated with RHD.

The two types of research design that are used to determine the efficacy of treatment in aphasia can be used with the RHD population (see "Efficacy of Aphasia Therapy" in the section on aphasia).

Several programs of treatment (described later in this section) have been identified as being useful by Anderson and Miller (1986), Brookshire (2007), Burns et al. (1985), Myers and Blake (2008), Santo Pietro and Goldfarb (1995), and Tompkins (1995). They include treatment for the following: attention, perception, and neglect problems; constructional impairment; emotional and prosody impairment; pragmatic impairment; integrating information (inference); time, place, and person orientation; anosognosia; prosopagnosia; and general memory deficits.

Therapy for Attention, Perception, and Neglect Problems

Hallowell et al. (2004) reviewed 668 journal articles dealing with aphasia subsequent to left hemisphere damage and related disorders subsequent to traumatic brain injury (TBI) and right hemisphere damage, and found that few authors controlled for or described even basic aspects of vision. No published empirical studies in adult neurogenic language disorders have dealt with the need to describe and control for visual acuity, color perception, visual fields, visual attention, and oculomotor functions. The authors suggested screening visual function by observing eye symmetry, lesions, swelling, or drainage at the time of research participation. It should also be noted if the participant is wearing glasses or contact lenses.

Anderson and Miller (1986), Brookshire (2003), Burns et al. (1985), Myers and Blake (2008), and Tompkins (1995) have suggested many of the following tasks:

1. Clinician should sit on patient's right, move gradually to his or her left, and say to patient, "Look at me."
2. As a self-cueing strategy, patient is taught to say, "Look to the left." In items 3 through 24, the clinician asks the patient to perform the listed task.
3. Look to the right, left, right visual field.
4. Point to objects in the room in his or her right and then left visual field.
5. Name pictures of people, objects, and food, moving from his or her right or left; starting with large items and moving to smaller items.
6. Name body parts in the right and then the left visual field.
7. Touch objects in the left visual field and then name them.
8. Listen to a bell (behind patient, first on right and then on left side) and then reach for it.
9. Listen to the clinician's voice (behind patient, first on right and then on left side) and then point to source.
10. Listen for a specific word within a group of words (spoken in front of and then behind patient, first on right and then on left side).
11. Identify voice and color of clothing of person in left visual field.

12. Look at door on his or her left and count the number of people coming in.
13. Watch TV placed to his or her left.
14. Label body parts in pictures (e.g., left leg, right hand).
15. Answer questions about a calendar, especially its left side.
16. Find locations on left, using a map or busy picture.
17. Read single words, phrases, sentences, and paragraphs on left; this task moves from large to small print, and from concrete to abstract material. Chieffi et al. (1989) found that in lexical comprehension, aphasic subjects failed because of semantic discrimination, whereas the RHD subjects failed because of perceptual discrimination.
18. Scan or sort objects, pictures, or words according to shape, meaning, color, category, and function.
19. Scan or sort alphabet or number tiles, cubes, pictures.
20. Set a clock with movable hands to different times.
21. Do arithmetic that requires columns.
22. Work simple to complex puzzles (e.g., jigsaw, crossword).
23. Follow up and down columns in newspapers.
24. Play easy card games, tic-tac-toe, checkers.
25. Clinician arranges numbers, letters, pictures, and objects in a certain way and then removes them. Patient has to duplicate arrangement.
26. Patient is asked to remember letters, numbers, forms, and words and to write them.
27. Clinician discusses with patient the visual items that need remembering (e.g., writing down times for breakfast, lunch, dinner, therapy, other appointments).
28. Patient is asked to describe from memory what has just been seen in a picture.

Therapy for Constructional Impairment

Tasks designed to help the patient overcome his or her constructional impairment are as follows:

1. Patient is asked to draw lines from A to B to C, and so on, on a paper or a blackboard.
2. Patient is asked to bisect lines that are placed at different angles randomly on a page.
3. Patient is asked to connect the dots to form letters, words, or shapes (see Santo Pietro & Goldfarb, 1995, for examples).
4. Patient is asked to trace a line straight across a page. Then he or she practices writing words and then sentences, keeping them on the line. Patient also uses graph paper for writing words and sentences.
5. Patient is asked to copy simple drawings (e.g., stick figures, geometric forms). It is useful to have the original drawing on lined or graph paper and to ask the patient to copy on the same kind of paper. This will help the patient check for the correct spatial orientation.
6. Patient is asked to draw a daisy, clock, person, and so forth, including the left half.
7. Patient is shown simple drawings of people, objects, shapes, and so forth, and asked to draw them after they have been removed.

Therapy for Time, Place, and Person Orientation

Burns et al. (1985) proposed instructing the patient in most of the following areas for biographical and environmental information, and for estimating time intervals:

1. Patient's name
2. Year, month, day, date, time of day
3. Present location

4. Home address (number, street, section, borough, town, city, state, county)
5. Home phone number
6. Significant family members' names and pertinent data (e.g., married or single, number of children, number of grandchildren)
7. Reason for hospitalization
8. Names of the president and vice president of the U.S., governor of state, mayor of city or town, two U.S. senators from home state
9. Estimated time intervals for getting out of bed and turning off alarm, brushing teeth, showering, putting on makeup or shaving, getting dressed, eating breakfast

Therapy for Anosognosia (Lack of Awareness of Illness and Deficits)

Procedures designed to help the patient overcome a lack of awareness of the illness and deficits are as follows:

1. Clinician informs patient as to what they are working on and why (e.g., "You're not paying attention to anyone who is on your left side").
2. Clinician informs patient in a gentle manner when he or she denies the impairments.
3. Clinician provides a great deal of enthusiastic, positive feedback to patient, because awareness information and training might be perceived as negative.
4. Clinician counsels patient's family about anosognosia (e.g., patient might convince family that nothing is wrong).

Therapy for Prosopagnosia (Facial Recognition Impairment)

Burns et al. (1985) suggested the following procedures for helping the patient to recognize individuals. The clinician simultaneously presents photographs and brief audio recordings (if possible). The patient has to name the person, and the following cues can be used:

1. Male or female?
2. Adult or child?
3. Hair color?
4. Body size?
5. Distinguishing facial features (e.g., scar, size or shape of nose, beard, eye color, voice characteristics, including accent, dialect, habitual use of word or phrase)?

Therapy for General Memory Deficits

If needed, see suggestions for memory deficits noted in the sections on communication disorders associated with dementia and traumatic brain injury.

Therapy for Integrating Information

Anderson and Miller (1986), Burns et al. (1985), Myers and Blake (2008), and Tompkins (1995) have proposed many of the following tasks:

1. Clinician helps patient to understand the daily routine involving medication times and their importance, food selections, and so forth.
2. Clinician helps patient to understand conversations with other professionals (doctors, nurses, etc.).
   In items 3 through 11, the clinician asks the patient to perform the listed task.

3. Tell a story that has sequential events (e.g., making scrambled eggs). Roman, Brownell, Potter, Seibold, and Gardner (1987) found that RHD patients have a relatively well-preserved "script" knowledge. Scripts represent knowledge of the sequence of events in familiar situations (e.g., washing one's hair would involve the following: turning on the water, wetting the hair, applying the shampoo, rinsing, drying, etc.). The familiarity of the sequence of events in frequently occurring situations allows one to make inferences about information that is not directly stated in discourse.

4. Read or listen to a story and then summarize it or answer questions about it (e.g., important newspaper and magazine articles, TV stories). Nicholas and Brookshire (1995) suggested the use of scripts, and main idea and stated information strength as a means of enhancing discourse comprehension.

5. Relate or write a description of a picture, including any emotions portrayed by the picture.

6. Put words into groupings (e.g., five fruits, five cities).

7. Relate what proverbs or analogies mean (e.g., *once in a blue moon*; *don't cry over spilled milk*).

8. Relate how one would get to particular locations (e.g., in current facility, former workplace, well-known landmarks).

9. Figure out, itemize, and arrange charts, graphs, checkbooks, calendars.

10. Figure out arithmetic problems that are given in story form.

11. Read or listen to a controversial story and take a stand on it (e.g., capital punishment, abortion rights, dropping of atom bomb). Rehak et al. (1992) found that RHD patients were strongly influenced by interest level in their ability to process a story.

Santo Pietro and Goldfarb (1995) offer additional items for integrating information. For these items, the clinician asks the patient to do the following:

1. Respond to specified and implied information (e.g., *The boss fired the man for being late. Why did the boss fire the man? Why was the man late?*)

2. Explain metaphors (e.g., *She's the toast of the town.*)

3. Explain similes (e.g., *She's as American as apple pie.*)

4. Rephrase figurative language (e.g., *He saw red.*)

The following four examples of understanding inferences were developed by Fuchs (1981) and elaborated on by Santo Pietro and Goldfarb (1995):

1. Laura had a stomach virus. She ate nothing for three days.
   A. Did Laura have a stomach virus? Did Laura have a sore throat?
   B. Did Laura lose weight? Did Laura gain weight?

2. The teacher bit into the juicy apple. She enjoyed her afternoon snack.
   A. Did the teacher bite into a fruit? Did the teacher bite into a vegetable?
   B. Did the teacher bite into a juicy apple? Did the teacher bite into a dry apple?

3. Barbara swept the kitchen floor. Now it was nice and clean.
   A. Did Barbara use a broom? Did Barbara use a sponge?
   B. Was the kitchen floor swept? Was the bedroom floor swept?

4. The student studied hard for the test. She slept poorly the night before.
   A. Did the student sleep poorly? Did the student sleep soundly?
   B. Did the student feel anxious about the test? Did the student feel confident about the test?

Example 1 is an inference made through *consequence*, whereby subsequent actions or states of being are suggested by an event or series of events. One can infer that Laura lost weight due to the stomach virus and consequent failure to eat for three days.

Example 2 is an inference made through *semantic entailment*, whereby the listener knows that statements valid for the member element may also be valid for the class in general. One can infer that the teacher bit into a fruit because an apple is a member of the general category called fruits.

Example 3 is an inference made through *implied instrument*, whereby tools, containers, vehicles, or other objects are conceptually necessitated by the function or operation of certain verbs. One can infer that Barbara used a broom from the use of the verb *swept*.

Example 4 is an inference made through *presupposition*, whereby prior actions or states of being are suggested by an event or series of events. One can infer that the student felt anxious about the test because sleeping poorly the night before the exam can be a symptom of anxiety.

Therapy for Pragmatic Impairment

Brookshire (2007) has noted that eye contact, turn-taking, and topic maintenance are often treated because they are relatively manageable, and their improvement can have quite an effect on the patient's appropriate use of language. Eye contact is practiced by the clinician's saying to the patient, "Look at me" during conversations. This activity is then followed by an analysis of why it is important to maintain eye contact during conversation (e.g., shows interest, alertness, concentration, politeness, comprehension). Another procedure is to instruct the patient to make eye contact at the beginning and end of his or her own utterances and then to do the same with the utterances of his or her conversational partner. The beginning and end of utterances is a self-cueing device.

Turn-taking is treated by first discussing with the patient why turn-taking is important during conversation with others (e.g., hearing the full message, getting the meaning of the message, what interruptions do). The clinician then instructs the patient to watch videotapes of conversations between two or more persons (e.g., television, movies) and then analyze the turn-taking of the participants. Other techniques include having the patient write a simple script or engage in free conversation with the clinician and analyze the appropriate spots for turn-taking.

Topic maintenance is taught by reading stories in newspapers and magazines, watching videotapes of conversations involving two or more participants, and engaging in structured conversations. The above activities are performed together by the clinician and patient, with an analysis of when the topic is maintained and when it changes or stops.

Myers and Blake (2008) stated that most of the language problems of the RHD patient are due to an inference impairment. They advocate treating the inference problem as a means of ameliorating the pragmatic impairment of the patient.

Therapy for Emotional and Prosody Impairment

There are no set guidelines in the literature for treating emotional and prosodic impairment. However, if a treatment-by-symptom approach is desired, portions of diagnostic material can be used as possible therapy techniques. For example, facial affect can be worked on by instructing the patient to produce a variety of facial expressions (e.g., happy, sad, angry, shocked, gloating, neutral). Prosody can be worked on by having the patient say or listen to inherently neutral sentences (e.g., saying or listening to "Today is Wednesday" and producing or recognizing a happy, sad, angry, shocked, neutral, etc., quality).

Before undertaking these therapy procedures, the clinician should make sure that the patient does not have a true emotional disorder. The clinician can recommend a psychiatrist or psychologist for help in this matter. Borod et al. (1989) found that the flat affect of adults with schizophrenia resembled that of the RHD patient. Myers and Blake (2008) have advocated that training in the comprehension of other contextual cues is likely to be a more effective way of treating emotional and prosodic impairment. Tompkins (1991b) found that the redundancy of stimuli enhanced the emotional inferencing abilities of RHD and LHD adults.

The third goal of therapy is to encourage the patient and the caretaker(s) to continue the rehabilitative process outside of the clinical setting.

Although not as clearly delineated, home treatment by caretakers of RHD patients can benefit from many of the suggestions mentioned for the aphasia patient (see "Home Treatment by Caretakers" in the section on aphasia). The most applicable suggestions for the RHD patient follow (numbering follows that in the section on aphasia).

DO's for Caretakers:

1. Do keep talking to the patient.
2. Do get the patient's attention before speaking.
3. Do talk slowly, to allow the patient time to process your message.
4. Do use short, one-idea, easy-to-process sentences.
5. Do establish the context of your message before you begin to expand on it.
6. Do give the patient time to formulate what he or she wants to say.
7. Do be an attentive listener and look for cues in the patient's tone of voice, facial expressions, and behavior to help you comprehend the message.
8. Do be empathetic and not sympathetic.
9. Do adjust the communication schedule to the best time of day.
10. Do attend to any additional communication problems the patient may have.
11. Do allow the patient access to activity in the house and in the world.
12. Do allow the patient to continue any chores or responsibilities that remain manageable.
13. Do foster success whenever possible. If the patient says or does something well, be generous with your praise.

DON'Ts for Caretakers:

1. Don't finish the patient's sentences unless the patient wants it.
2. Don't cut the patient off or interrupt when he or she is speaking.
3. Don't "fill in" the silence. The patient may need that time to process.
4. Don't turn your face away from the patient. The patient may need facial cues to help him or her comprehend what you are saying.
5. Don't "talk down" to the patient.
6. Don't talk only about activities of daily living.
7. Don't eliminate such activities as the theater, music, restaurants, and sporting events from the patient's daily lifestyle.
8. Don't allow the patient to become isolated. Communication is a social undertaking. Nicholas and Brookshire (1995) recommended that the patient's communication partners be trained by the clinician to use a strategic approach to communication discourse. With the knowledge that RHD patients have strengths in scripts and main idea and

stated information, the communication partner might be encouraged to clearly state the topic or theme early in the discourse. The communication partner can increase the main idea information by presenting it redundantly and connecting it to the theme or central points of the message. The central points of the message could be paraphrased and elaborated on, and then explained as to how they relate to the more peripheral details. Communication partners might be advised to provide important information in a stated (direct) manner, rather than requiring the patient to make inferences through implication. These strategies may be particularly worthwhile when the information to be understood is less familiar to the patient.

Advanced Study: Coprolalia

It is not unusual for individuals with right brain damage, aphasia, TBI, or certain disease states, such as Tourette syndrome, to use swear words excessively. It may be that foul language is no longer inhibited in these conditions, or that such language represents a lower form of verbalization that is released when higher communicative abilities are impaired. We worked with an elderly woman with right hemisphere damage who had this condition. She had previously been a nun, and was mortified by the blasphemous words she produced, followed by the swear words she used to chastise herself.

According to Van Lancker Sidtis (2004), nonpropositional language in typical and disordered communication consists of formulaic expressions, idioms, serial and memorized speech, slang, sayings, clichés, and expletives. LaPointe (2006) found profanity, which he defined as taboo words, swearing, and obscenity, to be present across cultures and periods, and retained even after severe lexical impoverishment in aphasia. Coprolalia, the involuntary, brief, stereotyped vocal tics associated with irresistible urges in Tourette syndrome, is characterized by obsessive use of obscene or scatological language. Vocal tics may be present in about 4 out of 10 British adults with Tourette syndrome (Lees, Robertson, Trimble, & Murray, 1984); other incidence reports of coprolalia in Tourette syndrome range from 4–60%. Coprolalia may not always be associated with vocal tics, as it has also appeared as sign language tics in a prelingually deaf man with Tourette syndrome (Morris, Thacker, Newman, & Lees, 2000).

Brain activity associated with coprolalia has been found in prerolandic and postrolandic language regions, insula, caudate, thalamus, and cerebellum (Stern et al., 2000). A case study of a young woman with traumatic brain injury (Pena-Casanova, Bertran-Serra, Serra, & Bori, 2002) reported that expletives were the only expressions used propositionally in the initial stage of recovery. The authors postulated that the pathophysiological feature of the case was the combination of bilateral anterior and posterior hemispheric lesions, which led to the release of overlearned language controlled by lower brain structures.

Medications which reduce coprolalia are usually of the neuroleptic (antipsychotic) class. Behavioral interventions focus on increasing cortical control or reducing subcortical influences on language production (Lebrun, 1997).

CASE DESCRIPTION

Dr. Edwin Weinstein, a neuropsychiatrist at the Mount Sinai School of Medicine in New York City, who died in 1998 at age 89, was well known for his book on President Woodrow Wilson, as well as his work on jargon aphasia (see, for example, Weinstein & Lyerly, 1976).

Weinstein presented a case study of right hemisphere damage with neglect to the Aphasia Study Group of New York. The patient, a retired full colonel in the army (the rank just below general), had suffered a right hemisphere stroke with resultant left hemiplegia, and was evaluated at Walter Reed National Military Medical Center in Washington, DC.

Dr. Weinstein explained that he began his examination of the wheelchair-borne patient's right side by noting that there did not seem to be any impairment in naming and word retrieval. The patient responded in the courtly way a Southern gentlemen of his stature would, thanking his doctor for the careful examination, and expressing his hope for a rapid recovery. Then Dr. Weinstein examined the patient's left side. Asked about his left arm, which was limp at his side, the patient reported that it was fine. Asked by the doctor to raise his hand, the patient indicated that he did not want to. After further prodding to move his left arm, the formerly courtly gentleman swore at the doctor, saying, "You (expletive deleted) quack, you don't know what you're doing."

Discussion Questions: Theory

1. What is the presumed etiology for different types of neglect?

2. Why are individuals with right hemisphere damage (RHD) more at risk for limb apraxia than those with left hemisphere damage (LHD)?

3. Why is it advisable to assume that the individual with RHD may not be a reliable informant?

4. Why are efficacy-of-treatment studies for communication disorders associated with RHD difficult to find in the literature?

5. Studies in RHD prosodic comprehension are not clear on the cause of the problem. What are some possible causes?

Discussion Questions: Therapy

1. Consider this therapy activity: *The Johnson family was sitting at the pool. They had to run for cover. Was it raining or snowing? How do you know?* What deficit does this task address, and how does it address the deficit?

2. In narrative or story-retelling tasks, should the speech-language pathologist (SLP) focus more on themes or details? Why?

3. What are some ways to test for orientation to time, place, and person?

4. Describe three therapy tasks to reduce pragmatic impairment in RHD.

5. In the case study at the end of the section, what was the problem exhibited by Dr. Weinstein's patient?

Assignment: Write a multiple-choice question with five options. Explain why the key option is correct, and why the distractors or decoys are incorrect. Avoid using forms such as, "All of the following are (in)correct *except*" in the stem, and "All (or none) of the above" in the options.

Example: If a patient with RHD digresses when asked to describe how to change a flat tire, the clinician might suspect:

a. Prosopagnosia
b. Perseveration
c. Anosognosia
d. Confabulation
e. Limb apraxia

The correct answer is *d*, because the clinician asks open-ended questions to see if the patient can integrate ideas, rather than tell tall tales; *a* is incorrect because prosopagnosia is a deficit in recognition of faces; *b* is a persistent response which is no longer appropriate, and is more characteristic of individuals with psychosis; *c* is incorrect because anosognosia is a denial of impairment; and *e* is incorrect because limb apraxia is a motor-programming disorder.

References

Adamovich, B., & Brooks, R. (1981). A diagnostic protocol to assess the communication deficits in patients with right hemisphere damage. In R. Brookshire (Ed.), *Clinical aphasiology conference proceedings* (pp. 244–253). Minneapolis, MN: BRK Publishers.

Anderson, K., & Miller, P. (1986, November). *Clinical management of the right hemisphere damaged patient.* Short course presented at the American Speech-Language-Hearing Association, Detroit, MI.

Benowitz, L., Moya, K., & Levine, D. (1990). Impaired verbal reasoning and constructional apraxia in subjects with right hemisphere damage. *Neuropsychologia, 28*, 231–241.

Benson, D. F., & Ardila, A. (1996). *Aphasia: A clinical perspective.* New York, NY: Oxford University Press.

Bhatnagar, S. (2008). *Neuroscience for the study of communicative disorders.* Philadelphia, PA: Lippincott Williams & Wilkins.

Blake, M. (2006). Clinical relevance of discourse characteristics after right hemisphere damage. *American Journal of Speech-Language Pathology, 15*, 255–267.

Blake, M. (2007). Perspectives on treatment for communication deficits associated with right hemisphere damage. *American Journal of Speech-Language Pathology, 16*, 331–342.

Blake, M. (2009a). Inferencing processes after right hemisphere brain damage: Maintenance of inferences. *Journal of Speech, Language, and Hearing Research, 52*, 359–372.

Blake, M. (2009b). Inferencing processes after right hemisphere brain damage: Effects of contextual bias. *Journal of Speech, Language, and Hearing Research, 52*, 373–384.

Bloom, R., Borod, J., Obler, L., & Gerstman, L. (1992). Impact of emotional content on discourse production in patients with unilateral brain damage. *Brain and Language, 42*, 153–164.

Bloom, R., Borod, J., Obler, L., & Gerstman, L. (1993). Suppression and facilitation of pragmatic performance: Effects of emotional content on discourse following right and left brain damage. *Journal of Speech and Hearing Research, 36*, 1227–1235.

Borde, C., Mazaux, J-M., & Barat, M. (2006). Defective reproduction of passive meaningless gestures in right brain damage: A perceptual disorder of one's own body knowledge? *Cortex, 42*, 8–16.

Borod, J., Alpert, M., Brozgold, A., Martin, C., Welkowitz, J., Diller, . . . Lieberman, A. (1989). A preliminary comparison of flat affect schizophrenics and brain-damaged patients on measures of affective processing. *Journal of Communication Disorders, 22*, 93–104.

Brookshire, R. (2007). *Introduction to neurogenic communication disorders.* St. Louis, MO: Mosby Elsevier.

Brookshire, R., & Nicholas, L. (1997). *Discourse comprehension test.* Bloomington, MN: BRK Publishers.

Brownell, H., Potter, H., Bihrle, A., & Gardner, H. (1986). Inference deficits in right-brain damaged patients. *Brain and Language, 27*, 310–321.

Brownell, H., Simpson, T., Bihrle, A., Potter, H., & Gardner, H. (1990). Appreciation of metaphoric alternative word meanings by left and right brain-damaged patients. *Neuropsychologia, 28*, 375–383.

Bryan, K. (1989). *The right hemisphere language battery.* Leicester, UK: Far Communications.

Burns, M., Halper, A., & Mogil, S. (1985). *Clinical management of right-hemisphere dysfunction.* Rockville, MD: Aspen Systems Corp.

Cappa, S., Papagno, C., & Vallar, G. (1990). Language and verbal memory after right hemispheric stroke: A clinical-CT scan study. *Neuropsychologia, 28,* 503–509.

Chieffi, S., Carlomagno, S., Silveri, M., & Gainotti, G. (1989). The influence of semantic and perceptual factors in lexical comprehension in aphasic and right brain damaged patients. *Cortex, 25,* 591–598.

Damasio, A. (1994). *Descartes' error.* New York, NY: G. P. Putnam's Sons.

Duffy, J. R, (2005). *Motor speech disorders: Substrates, differential diagnosis, and management* (2nd ed.). St. Louis, MO: Mosby.

Filley, C., & Kelly, J. (1990). Neurobehavioral effects of focal subcortical lesions. In J. Cummings (Ed.), *Subcortical dementia* (pp. 59–70). New York, NY: Oxford University Press.

Foldi, N. (1987). Appreciation of pragmatic interpretation of indirect commands: A comparison of right and left hemisphere brain-damaged patients. *Brain and Language, 31,* 88–108.

Fuchs, E. (1981). Comprehension of explicit and implicit information in adult aphasia. (Unpublished doctoral dissertation.) Columbia University, New York, NY.

Geminiani, G., Corazzini, L. L., Stucchi, N., & Gindri, P. (2004). Acceleration perception and spatial distortion in a left unilateral neglect patient. *Cortex, 40,* 315–322.

Goulet, P., & Joanette, Y. (1994). Sentence completion task in right-brain damaged right-handers: Eisenson's study revisited. *Brain and Language, 46,* 257–277.

Gutbrod, K., Cohen, R., Maier, T., & Maier, E. (1987). Memory for spatial and temporal order in aphasic and right hemisphere damaged patients. *Cortex, 23,* 463–474.

Hallowell, B., Douglas, N., Wertz, R. T., & Kim, S. (2004). Control and description of visual function in research on aphasia and related disorders. *Aphasiology, 18,* 611–623.

Heilman, K. (1994). Unpublished memo. Academy of Neurologic Communication Disorders and Sciences (ANCDS). Washington, DC.

Helm-Estabrooks, N. (2001). *Cognitive linguistic quick test.* San Antonio, TX: Psychological Corporation.

Hough, M. (1990). Narrative comprehension in adults with right and left hemisphere brain damage: Theme organization. *Brain and Language, 38,* 253–277.

Hugdahl, K., Wester, K., & Asbjornsen, A. (1991). Auditory neglect after right frontal lobe and right pulvinar thalamic lesions. *Brain and Language, 41,* 465–473.

Kaplan, J., Brownell, H., Jacobs, J., & Gardner, H. (1990). The effects of right hemisphere damage on the pragmatic interpretation of conversational remarks. *Brain and Language, 38,* 315–333.

Kennedy, M. (2000). Topic scenes in conversations with adults with right-hemisphere brain damage. *American Journal of Speech-Language Pathology, 9,* 72–86.

LaPointe, L. L. (2006). Profanity. *Journal of Medical Speech-Language Pathology, 14,* 7–9.

Lebrun, Y. (1997). Subcortical structures and non-volitional verbal behaviour. *Journal of Neurolinguistics, 10,* 313–323.

Lees, A. J., Robertson, M., Trimble, M. R., & Murray, N. M. (1984). A clinical study of Gilles de la Tourette syndrome in the United Kingdom. *Journal of Neurology, Neurosurgery, and Psychiatry, 47,* 1–8.

Lehman-Blake, M., & Tompkins, C. (2001). Predictive inferencing in adults with right hemisphere brain damage. *Journal of Speech, Language, and Hearing Research, 44,* 639–654.

Mackenzie, C., & Brady, M. (2004). Communication ability in non-right handers following right hemisphere stroke. *Journal of Neurolinguistics, 17,* 301–313.

Marcel, A. J., Tegner, R., & Nimmo-Smith, I. (2004). Anosognosia for plegia: Specificity, extension, partiality and disunity of bodily unawareness. *Cortex, 40,* 19–40.

Marshall, R., & Kanow, C. (2008). Update on a clinical measure for the assessment of problem solving. *American Journal of Speech-Language Pathology, 17,* 377–388.

McDonald, S., & Wales, R. (1986). An investigation of the ability to process inferences in language following right hemisphere brain damage. *Brain and Language, 29,* 68–80.

Mesulam, M. (1990). Large-scale neurocognitive networks and distributed processing for attention, language and memory. *Annals of Neurology, 28,* 597–613.

Milman, L., Holland, A., Kazniak, A., D'Agostina, J., Garrett, M., & Rapcsak, S. (2008). Initial validity and reliability of the SCCAN: Using tailored testing to assess cognition and communication. *Journal of Speech, Language, and Hearing Research, 51,* 49–69.

Morris, H. R., Thacker, A. J., Newman, P. K., & Lees, A. J. (2000). Sign language tics in a prelingually deaf man. *Movement Disorders: Official Journal of the Movement Disorder Society, 15,* 318–320.

Mosby's medical, nursing, and allied health dictionary. (1994). St. Louis, MO: Mosby.

Myers, A., & Blake, M. (2008). Communication disorders associated with right-hemisphere damage. In R. Chapey (Ed.), *Language intervention strategies in aphasia and related neurogenic communication disorders* (pp. 963–987). Baltimore, MD: Lippincott Williams & Wilkins.

Myers, P., & Brookshire, R. (1996). Effect of visual and inferential variables on scene descriptions by right-hemisphere-damaged and non-brain-damaged adults. *Journal of Speech and Hearing Research, 39,* 870–880.

Nicholas, L., & Brookshire, R. (1995). Comprehension of spoken narrative discourse by adults with aphasia, right-hemisphere brain damage, or traumatic brain injury. *American Journal of Speech-Language Pathology, 4,* 69–81.

Patterson, J., & Chapey, R. (2008). Assessment of language disorders in adults. In R. Chapey (Ed.), *Language intervention strategies in aphasia and related neurogenic communication disorders* (pp. 64–160). Baltimore, MD: Lippincott Williams & Wilkins.

Pena-Casanova, J., Bertran-Serra, I., Serra, A., & Bori, I. (2002). Uncommonly long sequences of speech automatisms in a young woman with traumatic brain injury. *Journal of Neurolinguistics, 15,* 109–128.

Pimental, P., & Kingsbury, N. (1989). *Mini inventory of right brain injury.* Austin, TX: Pro-Ed.

Priftis, K., Piccione, F., Giorgi, F., Meneghello, F., Umilta, C., & Zorzi, M. (2008). Lost in number space after right brain damage: A neural signature of representational neglect. *Cortex, 44,* 449–453.

Rehak, A., Kaplan, J., Weylman, S., Kelly, B., Brownell, H., & Gardner, H. (1992). Story processing in right-hemisphere brain-damaged patients. *Brain and Language, 42,* 320–336.

Robertson, I., Halligan, P., Bergego, C., Homberg, V., Pizzamiglio, L., Weber, E., & Wilson, B. (1994). Right neglect following right hemisphere damage? *Cortex, 30,* 199–213.

Roman, M., Brownell, H., Potter, M., Seibold, M., & Gardner, H. (1987). Script knowledge in right hemisphere damaged and normal elderly adults. *Brain and Language, 31,* 151–170.

Ross, E. D., & Monnot, M. (2008). Neurology of affective prosody and its functional-anatomic organization in right hemisphere. *Brain and Language, 104,* 51–74.

Ross-Swain, D. (1996). *Ross information processing assessment* (2nd ed.). Austin, TX: Pro-Ed.

Santo Pietro, M. J., & Goldfarb, R. (1995). *Techniques for aphasia rehabilitation: Generating effective treatment (TARGET).* Vero Beach, FL: The Speech Bin.

Schneiderman, E., Murasugi, K., & Saddy, J. (1992). Story arrangement ability in right-brain-damaged patients. *Brain and Language, 43,* 107–120.

Sherratt, S. (2007). Right brain damage and the verbal expression of emotion: A preliminary investigation. *Aphasiology, 21,* 320–339.

Sohlberg, M. M., & Ehlhardt, L. (1998). Case report: Management of confabulation after subarachnoid hemorrhage. *Neurophysiology and Neurogenic Speech and Language Disorders, 8*(2). (Special Interest Division 2 Newsletter, 9–13). Rockville, MD: American Speech-Language-Hearing Association.

Sonoda, S., Mori, M., & Goishi, A. (2001). Pattern of localization error in patients with stroke to sound processed by a binaural sound space processor. *Journal of Neurology, Neurosurgery, and Psychiatry, 70,* 43–49.

Stemmer, B., Giroux, F., & Joanette, Y. (1994). Production and evaluation of requests by right hemisphere brain-damaged individuals. *Brain and Language, 47,* 1–31.

Stern, E., Silbersweig, D. A., Chee, K. Y., Holmes, A., Robertson, M. M., Trimble, M., . . . Dolan, R. J. (2000). A functional neuroanatomy of tics in Tourette syndrome. *Archives of General Psychiatry, 57,* 741–748.

Swindell, C., Holland, A., Fromm, D., & Greenhouse, J. (1988). Characteristics of recovery of drawing ability in left and right brain-damaged patients. *Brain and Cognition, 7,* 16–30.

Taber's cyclopedic medical dictionary (18th ed.). (1997). Philadelphia, PA: F. A. Davis.

Tompkins, C. A. (1990). Knowledge and strategies for processing lexical metaphor after right or left hemisphere brain damage. *Journal of Speech and Hearing Research, 33,* 307–316.

Tompkins, C. A. (1991a). Automatic and effortful processing of emotional intonation after right or left brain damage. *Journal of Speech and Hearing Research, 34,* 820–830.

Tompkins, C. A. (1991b). Redundancy enhances emotional inferencing by right- and left-hemisphere damaged adults. *Journal of Speech and Hearing Research, 34*, 1142–1149.

Tompkins, C. A. (1995). *Right hemisphere communication disorders: Theory and management.* San Diego, CA: Singular Publishing Group.

Tompkins, C. A., Baumgaertner, A., Lehman-Blake, M. T., & Fassbinder, W. (2000). Mechanisms of discourse comprehension impairment after right hemisphere brain damage: Suppression in lexical ambiguity resolution. *Journal of Speech, Language, and Hearing Research, 43*, 62–78.

Tompkins, C. A., Lehman-Blake, M. T., Baumgaertner, A., & Fassbinder, W. (2002). Characterising comprehension difficulties after right brain damage: Attentional demands of suppression function. *Aphasiology, 16*, 559–572.

Tompkins, C. A., Bloise, C., Timko, M., & Baumgaertner, A. (1994). Working memory and inference revision in brain-damaged and normally aging adults. *Journal of Speech and Hearing Research, 37*, 896–912.

Tompkins, C. A., Boada, R., & McGarry, K. (1992). The access and processing of familiar idioms by brain-damaged and normally aging adults. *Journal of Speech and Hearing Research, 35*, 626–637.

Tompkins, C. A., Fassbinder, W., Lehman-Blake, M. T., Baumgaertner, A., & Jayaram, N. (2004). Inference generation during text comprehension by adults with right hemisphere brain damage: Activation failure versus multiple activation. *Journal of Speech, Language, and Hearing Research, 47*, 1380–1395.

Tompkins, C. A., Lehman-Blake, M. T., Baumgaertner, A., & Fassbinder, W. (2001). Mechanisms of discourse comprehension impairment after right hemisphere brain damage: Suppression in inferential ambiguity resolution. *Journal of Speech, Language, and Hearing Research, 44*, 400–415.

Van Lancker Sidtis, D. (2004). When novel sentences spoken or heard for the first time in the history of the universe are not enough: Toward a dual-process model of language. *International Journal of Language and Communication Disorders, 39*, 1–44.

Vuilleumier, P., Ortigue, S., & Brugger, P. (2004). The number space and neglect. *Cortex, 40*, 399–401.

Weinstein, E. A., & Lyerly, O. G. (1976). Personality factors in jargon aphasia. *Cortex, 12*, 122–133.

Winner, E., Brownell, H., Happe, F., Blum, A., & Pincus, D. (1998). Distinguishing lies from jokes: Theory of mind deficits and discourse interpretation in right-hemisphere brain damaged patients. *Brain and Language, 62*, 89–106.

Communication Disorders Associated with Dementia

Definition

In its definition, the *Diagnostic and Statistical Manual of Mental Disorders* (DSM-IV) (American Psychiatric Association, 2000) states that the essential feature of a dementia is the development of multiple cognitive deficits that include memory impairment and at least one of the following: aphasia, apraxia, agnosia, or a disturbance in executive functioning. The cognitive deficits must be sufficiently severe to cause impairment in occupational or social functioning (e.g., going to school, working, shopping, dressing, bathing, handling finances, and other activities of daily living) and must represent a decline from a previously higher level of functioning.

Classical literature refers to dementing diseases named after a researcher using the possessive form. In this text, we delete the possessive, which is the current preferred use. Accordingly, we refer to Alzheimer, Parkinson, and Pick diseases.

The specific communication problems of patients with dementia, especially those with Alzheimer disease, have been well documented (e.g., Bayles, 2003; Grossman et al., 1996; MacDonald, Almor, Henderson, Kempler, & Andersen, 2001), and include loss of auditory comprehension skills, withdrawal from communication encounters, excessive ego-orientation, lack of responsiveness, lack of relevance, lack of cohesion and coherence, and repetitiveness, as well as such cognitive-psychiatric characteristics as loss of short-term episodic memory, paranoia, and anxiety. Individuals with dementia typically use empty speech (semantic impairments are discussed later in this chapter) and stereotypical phrases, and speak with reduced volume. Individuals with Alzheimer disease have a higher rate of hearing loss and vision problems than neurotypical elderly (Weinstein & Amsel, 1986), as well as communication problems caused by depression, chronic illness, physical disability, medication, and the effects of institutionalization, or "learned helplessness."

Symptoms and Etiology

The American Psychiatric Association (2000) describes the multiple cognitive deficits that can exist in dementia. They are presented below with some modifications.

Memory impairment is needed to make the diagnosis of a dementia and is a prominent early symptom (Cummings & Benson, 1992; note that in Pick disease memory is preserved in the early and middle stages of the condition). Persons with dementia become impaired in

Impaired in

their ability to learn new information, and/or they forget previously learned information. They may lose items like wallets and keys, forget food cooking on the stove, and become lost in unfamiliar neighborhoods. In the advanced stages, these individuals can forget their occupation, schooling, birthday, family members, and their own names. (For additional comments on memory see other parts of this chapter and the section on communication disorders associated with traumatic brain injury.)

Sander, Nakase-Richardson, Constantinidou, Wertheimer, and Paul (2007), in their comprehensive review, provided a theoretically based model of memory. Useful for understanding memory performance are the terms *encoding, storage*, and *retrieval*. Encoding refers to the early processing of the material that is to be learned. How well information is encoded can contribute to how well it is stored for later use as eventually recalled. Encoding encompasses a variety of operations that can be performed on material to be learned, including simple repetition through rehearsal, and organizing material in a way that is meaningful (e.g., creating a story; typing it up with a particular theme, topic, or event; or using an acronym).

Storage refers to the way information is held in memory for future use. Retrieval refers to the act of pulling information from storage, typically from long-term store. The authors (Sander et al., 2007) noted that encoding, storage, and retrieval are interactive processes. The way information is encoded can affect the form in which it is stored, which can later affect its retrieval. For example, information that is organized meaningfully and that fits with information that already exists in the long-term store is more likely to be recalled than information that is stored piecemeal.

The following framework comes from Sander et al. (2007), and the neurophysiology within the framework comes from Sander et al. (2007) and Bhatnagar (2008). This all relates to **Figure 5.1**.

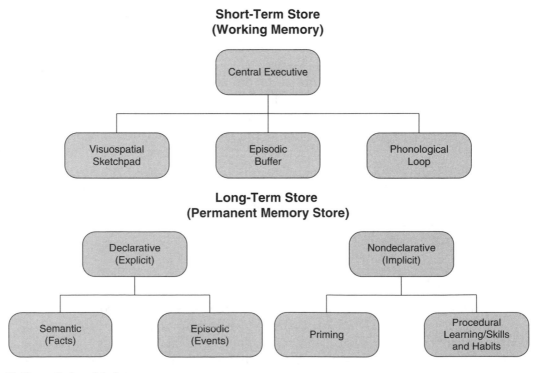

FIGURE 5.1 Theoretical model of memory.
Source: Adapted from Sander et al. (2007), who adapted from Baddeley (2001).

Short-Term Store (Working Memory)

The short-term store temporarily stores information and performs operations that result in the maintenance and transfer into the long-term store, and includes encoding (rehearsal and organization) described previously. The neurophysiology of the short-term store is associated with the dorsolateral prefrontal cortex.

Central Executive: Considered to be primarily responsible for allocating attention to different processes by inhibiting competing information. The neurophysiology of the central executive is associated with the prefrontal areas and the hippocampus (limbic system).

Visuospatial Sketchpad: The subsystem that stores and processes visual information. The neurophysiology of the visuospatial sketchpad is associated with the right hemisphere.

Phonological Loop: The subsystem that stores and processes auditory information. The neurophysiology of the phonological loop is associated with the left hemisphere.

Episodic Buffer: Described as an additional storage system that is responsible for combining verbal and visual information that exceeds the capabilities of the phonological loop or visuospatial sketchpad. The buffer also is hypothesized to integrate information from the long-term store, so that this information can be combined with information from the short-term store to solve problems, form new memories, and direct behavior. The neurophysiology of the episodic buffer is associated with the frontal lobes.

Prospective Memory: Has been hypothesized to be more related to "real-world" functioning, because memory demands are similar to those involved in everyday activities (e.g., keeping an appointment, going shopping for certain items). The neurophysiology of prospective memory is associated with the prefrontal areas and the hippocampus.

Long-Term Store (Permanent Memory Store)

The long-term memory system is composed of separate systems. The *declarative (explicit)* long-term memory system consists of the subsystems *semantic* and *episodic* memory.

Semantic Memory: Consists of knowledge of facts learned over time, such as multiplication tables, vocabulary, spelling, historical events, and appropriate social behaviors.

Episodic (Events) Memory: Consists of knowledge regarding specific personal experiences, such as last year's vacation, or where one was when one learned multiplication tables or spelling. The episodic and semantic subsystems interact. For example, episodic memories often are used as a basis for updating or adding to the knowledge represented in semantic memory. These two systems also interact with processes such as attention, so that patients with attention problems may present as if they have deficits in semantic or episodic memory (e.g., because of failure to attend to instructions or events).

Within long-term memory, the distinction between declarative and nondeclarative memory is that the declarative memory system involves conscious learning (explicit) and recall of information and events, whereas in nondeclarative memory the learning (implicit) occurs in the absence of explicit recall of the learning episodes. The neurophysiology of declarative memory is associated with medial temporal lobe structures including the hippocampus, parahippocampal gyrus, and diencephalic structures such as the medial thalamus, mamillary bodies, basal forebrain, and the frontal lobes. Nondeclarative memory involves experiential *priming*, which refers to the benefits a person receives from previous exposure to information, such as words or pictures, even though the person is unable to recall being exposed to the materials. Nondeclarative also involves preserved learning of *procedural* and *perceptual* skills, such as tracing a path on a turning stylus (maze learning), mirror reading, and acquisition of habits, despite being unable to recall the learning episodes. The neurophysiology of nondeclarative memory is associated with the posterior neocortex.

Aphasia is a language disturbance that affects auditory and reading comprehension and oral and written expression, and can appear in persons with dementia. In the advanced stages of dementia, individuals may be mute or have a deteriorated speech pattern characterized by echolalia (echoing what is heard) or palilalia (repeating sounds or words over and over). (For additional comments on aphasia see the section on aphasia and other parts of this chapter.)

Apraxia is an impairment in the ability to execute motor activities despite intact motor abilities, sensory function, and understanding of the required task, and may appear in individuals with dementia. These persons will be impaired in their ability to pantomime the use of objects (e.g., brushing teeth) or to execute familiar motor acts (e.g., waving goodbye). Problems in cooking, dressing, and drawing may be attributed to apraxia.

Agnosia is a failure to recognize or identify objects despite intact sensory function, and can appear in persons with dementia. Individuals may have normal visual acuity but lose the ability to recognize objects such as pencils or chairs. In the latter stages, they may be unable to recognize family members or even themselves in the mirror. They may have normal tactile sensation but be unable to identify, through touch, objects placed in their hands (e.g., pencil, coin, key).

Executive dysfunction is an impairment in the ability to think abstractly and to plan, initiate, sequence, monitor, and stop complex activities, and may appear in persons with dementia. Impairment in abstract thinking may be shown by difficulty coping with new or novel tasks or the avoidance of situations that require the processing of new and complex information.

Executive dysfunction is also apparent in the reduced ability to shift mental sets (e.g., moving from counting to saying the alphabet, then days of the week, then months of the year), to generate new or novel information (e.g., noting similarities and differences between a doctor and lawyer or a farmer and gardener, or naming as many animals as possible in one minute), or to execute serial motor activities (e.g., imitating simple tapping rhythms with the hand or using the telephone). Executive dysfunction can interfere with the activities of daily life (e.g., ability to work, plan activities, or budget finances). (For additional comments on executive function see the section on communication disorders associated with right hemisphere damage.)

Associated Features and Disorders

Associated features and disorders of dementia can include difficulty with spatial tasks (copying drawings); poor judgment and insight; little or no awareness of memory loss or other cognitive abnormalities; an unrealistic assessment of the person's own abilities and prognosis (e.g., planning to start a new business); an underestimation of risks involved in certain activities (e.g., driving); violence; suicidal tendencies; motor disturbances of gait; disinhibited behavior; neglecting personal hygiene; showing undue familiarity with strangers; disregarding conventional rules of social conduct; dysarthria; anxiety, mood, and sleep disturbances; delusions; hallucinations (mostly visual); delirium (acute confusional state); and a vulnerability to physical stressors (e.g., illness or minor surgery) and psychosocial stressors (e.g., going to hospital, bereavement) (American Psychiatric Association, 2000).

Age and Course

Depending on the etiology, dementia usually occurs late in life, with the greatest proportion of cases appearing in those older than 85 years of age. Dementia may be progressive, static, or remitting. Historically, it implied a progressive or irreversible course, and this section will deal with patients who present that picture.

Types

Dementia is classified as cortical, subcortical, or mixed cortical-subcortical (Cummings & Benson, 1992). Cortical dementia has its major neuropathology in the cerebral cortex. Subcortical dementia has its major neuropathology in the basal ganglia, thalamus, and the brainstem. A mixed dementia has its major neuropathology in both cortical and subcortical structures.

Speech and language problems will vary typically according to the type of dementia. Cortical dementia is characterized by language disorders. Subcortical dementia features speech disorders. Mixed cortical-subcortical dementia presents both language and speech disorders (Benson & Ardila, 1996; Cummings & Benson, 1992).

There are other ways of classifying dementia that are described at the end of this part of the section.

Cortical Dementia

Alzheimer Disease

The condition that typically produces a cortical dementia is Alzheimer disease (AD), which comprises about 50% of all cases of dementia. The neuropathology in the brains of these patients includes *neuritic plaques*, *neurofibrillary tangles*, and *granulovacuolar degeneration* (Cummings & Benson, 1992; Hopper & Bayles, 2008). Neuritic plaques are minute areas of tissue degeneration consisting of granular deposits and remnants of neuronal processes. Neurofibrillary tangles are filamentous structures in the nerve cell body, dendrites, axon, and synaptic endings, which become twisted or tangled. Granulovacuolar degeneration involves fluid-filled cavities containing granular debris that appear within nerve cells.

According to Breen and Gustafson (1978, as cited by Cummings & Benson, 1992; and Brookshire, 2003), the neuritic plaques and neurofibrillary tangles occur most frequently in the temporoparietal-occipital junctions and the inferior temporal lobes. The granulovacuolar degeneration occurs most frequently in the hippocampus (part of the limbic system deep in the temporal lobe), which plays a major role in memory.

Benson and Ardila (1996) have noted that at least two varieties of Alzheimer disease exist, each with clinical features that are clearly distinct from typical aging, and from the other disorders that cause dementia. One variety, familial Alzheimer disease (FAD), presents a relatively early onset (before age 60), a progressive course, and many times a family history of the condition. The second variety, senile dementia of the Alzheimer type (SDAT), is also called sporadic.

Alzheimer disease has a later age of onset, a somewhat more indolent course, and less evidence of a family history. Most clinicians group the two varieties as a single disorder called dementia of the Alzheimer type (DAT).

Alzheimer disease is identified by problems in language, cognition, visuospatial abilities, behavior, and motor problems in the latter stages of the condition. Language problems can include a *restricted vocabulary* that is limited to small talk and stereotyped clichés (Critchley, 1970), *perseveration* (Au, Obler, & Albert, 1991; Bayles, Tomoeda, Kazniak, Stern, & Eagans, 1985; Gewirth, Shindler, & Hier, 1984; Hopper & Bayles, 2008), and *word-finding difficulty* (Au et al., 1991; Huff, Corkin, & Growdon, 1986).

Additional language problems can include *semantic errors* (Abeysinghe, Bayles, & Trosset, 1990; Au et al., 1991; Huff et al., 1986; Santo Pietro & Goldfarb, 1985), *naming problems*

(Au et al., 1991; Hopper & Bayles, 2008; Shuttleworth & Huber, 1988; Smith, Murdoch, & Chenery, 1989), *jargon* (Hopper & Bayles, 2008), *circumlocution* (Au et al., 1991; Hopper & Bayles, 2008), *auditory comprehension deficit* (Au et al., 1991; Eustache et al., 1995; Hopper & Bayles, 2008), *mutism and echolalia* (Obler & Albert, 1981), and *deficits in pragmatic language* (Hopper & Bayles, 2008; Obler & Albert, 1981).

Neils-Strunjas, Groves-Wright, Mashima, and Harnish (2006) presented a critical review of literature on dysgraphia associated with Alzheimer disease (AD). Studies have shown that writing impairment is heterogeneous within the AD population. Identifying patterns of writing impairment at different stages of AD may help to chart disease progression and assist in the development of appropriate interventions.

At least in the earlier stages, *syntactic* (Kempler, Curtiss, & Jackson, 1987; Rochon, Waters, & Caplan, 1994), *spelling* (Nebes & Boller, 1987; Neils, Roeltgen, & Constantinidou, 1995), and *phonologic* (Au et al., 1991; Bayles & Boone, 1982) abilities are more intact, relatively, than other language functions. A review of the nonlanguage symptoms of cortical dementia can be found in Cummings and Benson (1992).

Stages in Alzheimer Disease

There are three stages in Alzheimer disease, as described in the following sections (Au et al., 1991; Bayles, Tomoeda, & Caffrey, 1982; Benson & Ardila, 1996; Cummings & Benson, 1992; Hopper & Bayles, 2008).

Mild stage.   During the mild stage, the patient senses a decline, becomes apologetic, and is reluctant to be tested. Frequently, the patient is disoriented to time, and memory for recent events has begun to fail. The patient relies heavily on overlearned situations and stereotypical utterances, and is often unable to generate sequences of related ideas. In this stage, the patient might resemble the Wernicke patient; however, the Wernicke patient cannot repeat, whereas the patient with dementia often can.

In this stage, the patient with dementia begins to exhibit impairment semantically (slightly reduced vocabulary, word-finding difficulties, increased use of automatisms and clichés) and pragmatically (mild loss of desire to communicate, occasional disinhibitions), whereas syntactically and phonologically he or she is intact.

As an example of increased use of clichés and occasional disinhibitions, one particular patient, who was in the mild stage of dementia, was very effusive in her praise for one of the authors as a therapist (e.g., "You're the tops," "My hat's off to you," "You're peaches and cream"). Her effusiveness was unwarranted because the author had worked with her only for a few routine but appropriate sessions. When her husband was present at our sessions, she would be very benevolent toward him. But as soon as he left, the patient accused him of seeing another woman (e.g., "He's alley catting around," "He's acting like a wild animal"). While she related this in cliché-ridden language, her tone and manner became very aggressive. Other members of the family confirmed that the husband was faithful to his wife throughout their marriage, including this trying period.

Moderate stage.   During the moderate stage, the patient has a more noticeable impairment of memory and time and place orientation, is more perseverative and nonmeaningful, and does not self-correct errors. In this stage, the patient with dementia shows further impairment semantically (significantly reduced vocabulary, naming errors usually semantically and visually related, verbal paraphasias evident in discourse), shows some impairment syntactically (reduction in syntactic complexity and completeness), and shows further impairment pragmatically (declining sensitivity to context, diminished eye contact, egocentricity), but is phonologically generally intact.

Because of difficulty with abstraction, utterances are usually concrete. Repetition begins to break down, and the patient shows circumlocutions and anomic difficulties. Eye contact begins to diminish, and there is a lot of touching of objects, indicating that the pragmatics of communication are inappropriate. Wilson et al. (1982) found that patients with dementia show a deficit in the retention of facial information. The patient with aphasia would probably be adequate in this area.

Advanced stage.   In the advanced stage, patients are very much disoriented to time, place, and person, and fail to recognize family and friends. They are unable to carry out the routines of life and require extensive personal care. Many times they will make spontaneous corrections of syntactic and phonologic errors, but without awareness. They have brief moments when stimuli appear to be comprehended, but for the most part they will neither comprehend nor self-correct any errors.

Their phonology is generally correct; syntax may be disturbed, but not as disturbed as the semantic aspects of language (Bayles, 1982; Bayles & Boone, 1982; Cummings & Benson, 1992; Hopper & Bayles, 2008). It seems that the phonologic and syntactic aspects of language remain relatively unimpaired while the semantic and pragmatic aspects are much impaired. The referential aspects of language are very disturbed but the mechanics of speech production are not, unless subcortical degeneration has taken place. In some cases, the patient could be mute except for jargon (Benson & Ardila, 1996).

In this stage, the patient with dementia shows further impairment semantically (markedly reduced vocabulary, frequent unrelated misnamings, jargon common), further impairment syntactically (many inappropriate word combinations), further impairment pragmatically (nonadherence to conventional rules, poor eye contact, lack of social awareness, inability to form a purposeful intention), and some impairment phonologically (occasional phonemic paraphasias and neologisms, sometimes jargon).

As mentioned previously, a patient in the advanced stages of dementia may have verbalization that sounds very appropriate to the situation. During a speech and language diagnosis, one patient emerged from her flood of inappropriate responses by saying, "Is this necessary?" This most likely chance appropriate response was picked up by her hopeful husband, who thought that this was a sign of neurotypical behavior. The husband was probably convinced otherwise when a few minutes later the seating arrangement shifted and brought the patient too close. She suddenly reached out, grabbed the author's tie, and held on to it for about three or four minutes. It seemed like three or four hours.

Pick Disease

Pick disease is another cortical dementia that can produce a language breakdown (Holland, McBurney, Moossy, & Reinmuth, 1985; Volin, Goldfarb, Raphael, & Weinstein, 1990). The neuropathology of this rare dementia involves the appearance of neuronal abnormalities called *Pick bodies* (dense globular formations) and *Pick cells* (enlarged neurons). In Pick disease, personality and language impairment have an early onset, whereas the cognitive problems come later (Cummings & Benson, 1992). The typical progression of dementia is faster in Pick than in Alzheimer disease, and the brain damage is usually most significant in the frontal lobes. Currently, the diagnosis is more properly "probable Pick disease," as confirmation of evidence of Pick bodies is usually made at autopsy.

Subcortical Dementia

Subcortical dementia (Cummings, 1990) is characterized by a gradual decline in cognitive abilities without any appreciable loss in associational cortical areas (language). The patient has emotional and personality changes, which are typically inertia and apathy. Memory disorders are present, and the patient has a defective ability to manipulate acquired knowledge. There is also a general slowness of information processing through the visual or auditory modality.

Benson and Ardila (1996) have noted that hypophonia is a significant problem in all subcortical dementias. The decreased voice volume usually occurs early, and unless the disease is treated, the hypophonia will progress to total mutism. The speech disturbance is usually dysarthric, whereas the language disturbance tends toward the concrete, and until the terminal stages, is insignificant in comparison to the dysarthria.

Parkinson disease, a degenerative disorder, is the condition that produces the majority of all subcortical dementias. About 20–60% of patients with Parkinson disease will have dementia as part of their syndrome (American Psychiatric Association, 2000). Huntington disease (a hereditary degenerative disorder); progressive supra nuclear palsy (starts with a motor impairment and eventually a mild dementia appears); Wilson disease, which has a juvenile type (onset in youth) and an adult type (onset between 20 and 30 years of age); olivopontocerebellar degeneration (onset between 30 and 50 years of age); and immunodeficiency virus (HIV) are other conditions that can produce subcortical dementia. Neuropathology within subcortical structures of the brain (i.e., basal ganglia, thalamus) is the cause of subcortical dementia.

Vascular Dementia

Vascular dementia (formerly called *multi-infarct dementia*, or MID; also called *fronto-temporal dementia*) can involve multiple infarcts (cell death caused by a loss of blood supply) in cortical, subcortical, or both areas (Cummings & Benson, 1992). Vascular dementia shows the second highest incidence and accounts for between 15% and 20% of dementia cases. Another 15% of dementia cases suffer from both Alzheimer and vascular dementia. Patients with vascular dementia will present a history that includes hypertension, heart disease, strokes, abrupt onset, focal neurologic signs, and a stepwise breakdown in their progression to dementia.

Multiple cortical infarcts can affect the anterior, middle, and/or posterior cerebral arteries, which feed such territories as the perisylvian or extrasylvian (borderzone) areas. These patients can show the symptoms of aphasia and apraxia in their progression to dementia.

Multiple subcortical infarcts are called *lacunar state* (infarcts involving the basal ganglia, thalamus, and internal capsule) or *Binswanger disease* (infarcts involving the subcortical white matter of both hemispheres). These patients can show the symptoms of dysarthria in their progression to dementia.

Mixed Dementia

A mixed dementia would show both cortical and subcortical involvement. Individuals in this grouping would display the language abnormalities stemming from the cortical involvement, and the speech abnormalities (dysarthria, mutism, hypophonia) arising from the subcortical involvement. An example of mixed dementia is Creutzfeldt-Jakob disease, which is a *transmissible spongiform encephalopathy* resulting in cortical and subcortical abnormalities (caused by *prions*; the bovine form is known as "mad cow disease").

According to Cummings and Benson (1992), the major causes of mixed dementia are vascular dementia (multi-infarct dementia), infectious dementia (e.g., HIV encephalopathy), toxic (e.g., drug intoxication) and metabolic (e.g., chronic anoxia), and miscellaneous dementia syndromes (e.g., posttraumatic, tumors).

Other Ways of Classifying Dementia

Ripich and Horner (2004) described the subtypes of neurodegenerative dementias as the following:

Alzheimer Dementia (AD)

Profile: Insidious progressive course of cognitive disability, often may years; onset before or after age 65
Diagnosis: Proliferation of neural plaques and tangles at autopsy
Subtypes: Sporadic (in most cases) or familial (5–10% of cases)
Communication: Language impairment common; semantic system most affected; progression to mutism
Behavior: Depression, insomnia, incontinence, delusions, agitation

Lewy Body Dementia

Profile: Periods of normal cognition alternate with abnormal cognition; progressive course, often rapid
Diagnosis: Lewy bodies (protein deposits in neuronal cell bodies) at autopsy
Subtypes: Attentional impairment, visual hallucinations, Parkinsonism
Communication: Motor speech disorder with hypophonia
Behavior: Periods of delirium (confusion); daytime drowsiness

Vascular Dementia (VaD)

Profile: Abrupt deterioration; course may be stable, improving or worsening (stair-step decline)
Diagnosis: Varied, including multiple infarcts, strategically placed single infarct, small-vessel disease, multiple lacunae, hypoperfusion, or hemorrhage
Subtypes: Predominantly cortical clinical signs, predominantly subcortical signs, extent of brain lesions
Communication: Motor speech disorder prominent; may have simplified grammar and writing; slowness and reduced initiation
Behavior: Depression and mood changes

Frontotemporal Lobar Dementia (FTD)

Profile: Insidious onset, more likely before age 65; progressive course, often slow
Diagnosis: Focal cortical atrophy
Subtypes: FTD-frontal variant (executive dysfunction), FTD-temporal variant (semantic deficits), FTD-nonfluent aphasia variant
Communication: Varies with subtype
Behavior: Wide range, especially frontal lobe variant

Hopper and Bayles (2008) described the classification of dementia as Alzheimer disease; cerebrovascular disease; Lewy body disease; and Parkinson disease, where Lewy bodies are in all patients (both with and without dementia), and patients exhibit procedural memory impairment and declarative memory deficits when cortical lesions exist.

Diagnosis

Diagnostic procedures for determining the communication disorders associated with dementia can involve (1) establishing background information, (2) giving a neurologic evaluation, (3) employing tests for assessing cognition, (4) employing information about differential diagnosis, and (5) employing specific language probes.

Establishing Background Information and the Neurologic Evaluation

These procedures can be found at the beginning of the "Diagnosis" portion of the section on aphasia.

Test for Assessing Cognition

The diagnosis of dementia is usually made after input from the neuropsychologist, the psychologist, the neurologist or psychiatrist, the speech-language pathologist, and other healthcare professionals. There are several tests that can be used for diagnosis. These include *The Global Deterioration Scale of Primary Degenerative Dementia* (GDS) (Reisberg, Ferris, DeLeon, & Crook, 1982), the *Mattis Dementia Rating Scale* (MDRS) (Mattis, 1976), and the *Mini-Mental State Examination* (MMS) (Folstein, Folstein, & McHugh, 1975). For example, the MMS evaluates orientation, learning names, counting backward, spelling backward, recalling names, naming, repeating, auditory and reading comprehension, writing, and copying.

The U.S. Department of Health and Human Services has provided criteria for diagnosing Alzheimer dementia (McKhann et al., 1984). These criteria state that if any two areas among language, memory, visuospatial orientation, and judgment are deficient along with the absence of depression, multiple infarcts, alcoholism, malnutrition, or other diseases, then a diagnosis of Alzheimer disease is warranted.

Kempler et al. (1987) used the following to diagnose Alzheimer dementia: (1) physical examination, (2) neurological examination, (3) neuropsychological evaluation, (4) laboratory evaluation, (5) EEG, (6) EKG, (7) chest x-ray, and (8) computed tomography (CT) scan of the head, plus cognitive dysfunction and absence of focal motor, sensory, cerebellar, and cranial nerve defects.

Ripich and Terrell (1988) employed the following criteria: (1) gradual onset and progression, for at least six months, of sustained deterioration of memory in an alert patient; and (2) impairment in at least three cognitive abilities: orientation, judgment and problem solving, functioning in community affairs, functioning in the house, functioning in personal care.

Fromm and Holland (1989) used the following criteria: (1) deficits in two or more areas of cognition, (2) a progressive worsening of memory and other cognitive functioning, (3) no disturbance of consciousness, (4) onset between the ages of 40 and 90, and (5) the absence of systemic disorders or other brain diseases that could account for the progressive memory and cognitive deficits.

Differential Diagnosis

Substantial differences have been noted in the language output of adults with Alzheimer disease compared to those with multi-infarct or vascular dementia (Bayles & Tomoeda, 1996). With vascular dementia, there may be more varied language changes early on than with Alzheimer disease, wherein some functions remain preserved while others are impaired (Chapman, 1997). Language changes tend to progress more slowly with vascular dementia than with Alzheimer disease. Word finding may be less impaired in early vascular dementia than in Alzheimer disease; later, however, the naming impairment in vascular dementia may result in the production of jargon, neologisms, and literal paraphasias, phenomena not usually present in Alzheimer disease (Chapman, 1997). In vascular dementia, speech becomes more concise because of preservation of substantive words. In contrast, speech in Alzheimer disease becomes empty with an increasing loss of substantives.

Kontiola, Laaksonen, Sulkava, and Erkinjunnti (1990) found that the most complex linguistic functions, those associated with intellectual and mnestic operations, become impaired in Alzheimer disease. In their study, the Alzheimer disease group had special difficulty understanding and constructing complex grammatical structures. In contrast, in vascular dementia, it is the more elementary language functions that break down, those functions associated with symbolic aspects such as word recognition, naming, and repetition.

Patterns of errors differentiated responses of participants with Alzheimer disease and vascular dementia independent of severity of impairment (Goldfarb & Goldberg, 2004). This was especially evident in the greater impairment of participants with Alzheimer disease to produce antonym responses. With regard to multiword responses, both groups showed more impairment in storytelling than feature description, a tendency opposite that observed in adults with aphasia. Participants with Alzheimer and vascular dementia were more impaired for text than for words, although very impaired for both.

The following sections review some of the literature that relates to the differential diagnosis of dementia using language as the prime characteristic.

Dementia Versus Aphasia

Appell, Kertesz, and Fisman (1982) found that patients with Alzheimer disease showed symptoms that resembled those of adults with Wernicke and transcortical sensory aphasia more than those of adults with Broca or transcortical motor aphasia. Bayles and Boone (1982) have noted that patients with dementia in the mild stage exhibit some semantic and pragmatic impairment; in the moderate stage, further semantic and pragmatic impairment, and some syntactic impairment; and in the advanced stage, further semantic, pragmatic, and syntactic impairment, and some phonologic impairment. In contrast, the patient with aphasia at any severity level may be impaired semantically, syntactically, and phonologically (except the patient with Wernicke or transcortical sensory aphasia, whose phonology is mostly intact), but may retain pragmatic behavior that is socially appropriate.

Fromm and Holland (1989) found that patients with Alzheimer disease showed irrelevant, vague, and rambling responses, whereas those with Wernicke aphasia demonstrated comprehension deficit types of responses. Huff, Mack, Mahlmann, and Greenberg (1988) found that adults with aphasia have access to lexical-semantic information, but those with Alzheimer disease have a loss of that information. Murdoch, Chenery, Wilks, and Boyle (1987) also found that the language deficit in Alzheimer disease resembled a transcortical sensory aphasia.

Nicholas, Obler, Albert, and Helm-Estabrooks (1985) found that adults with Alzheimer disease showed more empty phrases and conjunctions, whereas those with Wernicke aphasia produced more neologisms, and verbal and literal paraphasias. Obler, Albert, Estabrooks, and Nicholas (1982) pointed out that more neologisms and verbal paraphasias exist in Wernicke aphasia, whereas individuals with Alzheimer disease show more logical conjunctions and comments.

Pragmatic disturbances in lexical specificity/accuracy were observed in five people with AIDS but without a diagnosis of aphasia or AIDS dementia complex (ADC) (McCabe, Sheard, & Code, 2007). In a case report by the same authors (McCabe, Sheard, & Code, 2008), a man with ADC but without aphasia or dysarthria had similar scores on standardized language tests compared to two matched controls with AIDS but without ADC. However, the man with ADC had severe impairment in pragmatic language skills, particularly in the skills of topic maintenance and informational redundancy.

Hodges, Martinos, Woolams, Patterson, and Adlam (2008) proposed a Repeat and Point test to differentiate between semantic dementia and progressive nonfluent aphasia (PNFA). Participants with semantic dementia were consistently more impaired than controls and participants with PNFA in pointing to a pictorial referent, among a choice of six foils, for a spoken noun. However, participants with PNFA were more impaired in repeating 10 multisyllable concrete nouns.

Naming Ability in Dementia Versus Aphasia

Bayles and Tomoeda (1983) and Martin and Fedio (1983) have noted a naming problem in dementia, which gets worse as the disease progresses. Benson (1979) stated that anomia in adults with aphasia separates them from those with dementia. Individuals with dementia would have no trouble in confrontation naming but would have difficulty in producing words in categories (five fruits, five vegetables, etc.). Adults with aphasia would have problems in both confrontation naming and producing words in categories. Boller et al. (1991) found that language task performance (especially naming) was the best predictor of the course of Alzheimer disease.

Bowles, Obler, and Albert (1987) found that individuals with Alzheimer disease were distinguished by the number of unrelated responses in naming tasks, when compared to healthy younger and aging adults. Critchley (1970) has stated that in cases of dementia, language impairment essentially entails a poverty of language due to an inaccessibility of the speaking, writing, and reading vocabulary. The difficulty in word finding differs from the anomia of patients with aphasia. The patient with dementia does not necessarily show hesitancy in naming objects. Semantic errors in naming do not occur, nor do neologisms and substitutions. On the other hand, these patients find it difficult to name unless the real object is before them. They lapse into a sort of concrete attitude.

There are many reports of naming impairment associated with Alzheimer dementia (Bayles & Tomoeda, 1996; Chenery, Murdoch, & Ingram, 1996; Huff, Corkin, & Growdon, 1986; Kontiola et al., 1990; among others). Chenery et al. (1996) reported that naming difficulty is evidence of a predominant semantic disruption, the character of which is related to the severity of illness. "As the disease progresses, the integrity of the structural store of semantic memories proceeds to break down" (p. 433). As the semantic function becomes increasingly compromised, the ability to name becomes increasingly restricted. Chenery et al. (1996) claimed that the severity of the naming deficit can be used to gauge the severity of dementia of an individual. However, there may be a selective impairment in action naming (compared to object naming) among those with multi-infarct dementia, a finding not observed in patients with Alzheimer disease (Cappa et al., 1998). This finding was independent of severity of dementia or of overall language impairment.

Horner, Heipman, Aker, Kanter, and Royall (1982) and Obler and Albert (1981) have noted that the naming errors of the patient with dementia are more likely due to visual misperceptions than are the naming errors of patients with aphasia, which are mostly of a semantic or phonological nature.

Overall Language Ability Within Types of Dementia Versus Other Disorders

Bayles, Boone, Tomoeda, Slauson, and Kazniak (1989) found that tasks involving memory seemed to differentiate individuals with Alzheimer disease (poorest) from neurotypical elderly and those with aphasia. Dick, Kean, and Sands (1989) noted that young and elderly adults showed a higher recall for internally generated words than did those with Alzheimer disease. The authors attributed this to a semantic memory breakdown in the individuals with Alzheimer disease. Fromm, Holland, Nebes, and Oakley (1991) found that word-reading ability was sensitive to severity in the latter stages of Alzheimer disease. Granholm and Butters (1988) noted that those with Alzheimer disease were worse than those with Huntington disease in encoding semantic relationships.

Kontiola et al. (1990) compared the language abilities of neurotypical elderly to patients with Alzheimer and multi-infarct dementia. They found that the neurotypical elderly participants had the best language abilities, those with Alzheimer disease showed defects in the understanding of grammatical structures, and those with multi-infarct dementia displayed disorders in recognition of words, naming, and repetitions. Verbs are associated with frontal brain structures, and may be relatively better preserved in early stages of the disease. Objects or nouns, associated with temporal lobe structures, might be affected earlier. Alternatively, verbs are semantically more complex than nouns. In comparing 19 patients with mild to moderate Alzheimer disease to 19 neurotypical matched participants (Druks et al., 2006), both the patients and the comparison group responded faster and made fewer errors on object pictures than on action pictures. A study (Masterson et al., 2007) of 23 participants with Alzheimer disease also concluded that verbs are not selectively preserved. However, in a case study of the frontal variant of frontotemporal dementia (d'Hornicthun & Pillon, 2008), the patient's disproportionate verb deficit depended on the type of stimulus used to assess verb processing. Her deficit, observed in descriptions of photographs, disappeared when she responded to videotaped actions or verbal stimuli.

McNamara, Obler, Au, Durso, and Albert (1992) found that patients with Parkinson and Alzheimer diseases had more problems correcting output error than did typically aging participants.

Mentis, Briggs-Whitaker, & Gramigna (1995) compared 12 patients with Alzheimer disease to 12 typical elderly participants and observed significant differences between the two groups. The patients with Alzheimer disease were characterized by a reduced ability to change topics while preserving the discourse flow, difficulty in actively contributing to the propositional development of the topic, and a failure to maintain a topic in a clear and coherent manner. Tomoeda, Bayles, and Boone (1990) found that patients with Alzheimer disease performed more poorly than typical elderly participants in auditory comprehension on tasks involving syntactic complexity.

Kavé and Levy (2003) found that although persons with Alzheimer disease conveyed less information and made more semantic errors than did control participants, their language remained structurally rich. Persons with AD used the same syntactic structures and the same morphological forms as control participants and made very few structural errors. Kavé and Levy (2004) found that despite severe semantic-conceptual deficits in naming, fluency, and comprehension tasks, persons with AD engage in adequate morphologic decomposition of words, in a manner similar to neurotypical speakers of Hebrew.

Rochon, Waters, and Caplan (2000) studied patients with dementia of the Alzheimer type (DAT) and age- and education-matched older volunteers who were tested on a battery of working memory tests as well as on two tests of sentence comprehension. The results suggest that patients with DAT have working memory impairments that are related to their ability to map the meanings of sentences onto expectations of events in the world.

Mahendra, Bayles, and Harris (2005) have noted that episodic memory (EM) deficits are the hallmark of AD. Story-retelling tasks are particularly sensitive to EM impairments and require participants to recall a short story immediately and after a delay. The authors wanted to know whether presentation modality influences story recall in AD participants. Thirty AD participants and 30 healthy elders recalled short stories in (1) auditory, (2) visual, and (3) combined auditory-visual modalities. Recall was assessed immediately as well as after 15- and 30-minute delays. They found that AD participants demonstrated better recall after silently reading a story than after an examiner told the story or after simultaneously hearing and reading the story.

Horley, Reed, and Burnham (2010) studied 20 individuals with moderate DAT and 20 control participants engaged in two expressive and two receptive tasks with randomly presented exemplars of sentences targeting the emotions of happiness, anger, sadness, and surprise. Results showed that in the expressive tasks, objective acoustic measurements revealed significantly less pitch modulation by the patient group, but these measurements showed that they retained the ability to vary pitch level, pitch modulation, and speaking rate as a function of emotion. In the receptive tasks, perception of emotion by the patient group was significantly inferior to the control group.

Speech and Language Probes

In testing for the communication disorders associated with dementia, Hopper and Bayles (2008) have suggested using tasks that are active (nonautomatic) or generative, or that depend on logical reasoning.

Active (nonautomatic) tasks call for mental and linguistic involvement. Examples are describing objects, story retelling, defining concepts, and explaining sentence meaning. Generative tasks call for the conception and production of a series of related ideas or objects in a category. Examples would be naming five fruits, five vegetables, five countries, and so forth, or naming as many words as possible that begin with a certain letter, within a minute's time, as in the *Word Fluency Measure* (Borkowski, Benton, and Spreen, 1967).

Logical reasoning tasks require the participant to arrive at a conclusion based on understanding similarities or differences between two or more items and the ability to use analogy. Examples are explaining the similarities or differences between a doctor and a lawyer or a farmer and a gardener, or defining proverbs (e.g., *Don't count your chickens before they hatch*) as a means of using analogy.

Questions relating to time, place, and person orientation and simple general information can be used along with the procedures described above. Where necessary, the different modalities should be used for eliciting an answer. The following questions were adapted from the *Mayo Clinic Procedures for Language Evaluation* (unpublished test): What day is it? What month? What is today's date? What year? Where are you now? What city? What state? Why are you here? What are the names of significant family members? What is their relationship to you? How many children, grandchildren, and so forth, do you have?

In addition to these orientation questions, the clinician can ask general information questions: When do we celebrate Christmas? What is the capital of the United States? Who is the president of the United States? Before him? Who discovered America? When? How many states are there in the United States? Who was the first president of the United States? Who was president during the Civil War? Who invented Mickey Mouse and Donald Duck? What country is immediately north of the United States? Who was Helen Keller (or Mother Theresa)?

The Arizona Battery for Communication Disorders of Dementia (ABCD) (Bayles & Tomoeda, 1991) is a test for quantifying the communication disorder associated with Alzheimer disease. The battery provides information about linguistic comprehension, linguistic expression, verbal episodic memory, mental status, and visuospatial construction. The ABCD was found to correlate highly with the *Global Deterioration Scale of Primary Degenerative*

Dementia (Reisberg et al., 1982), the *Mini-Mental State Examination* (Folstein et al., 1975), and the Block Design subtest of the *Wechsler Adult Intelligence Scale* (Wechsler, 1981).

As a supplement to the tests mentioned above and to get an overall assessment of the patient's speech and language abilities, one might employ some of the assessment tools used in testing for aphasia. However, the aphasia batteries should be used in whole or in part to round out the picture, not as a definitive diagnostic tool. Homer, Dawson, Heyman, and Fish (1992) noted that it was most difficult to classify patients with Alzheimer disease when using the *Western Aphasia Battery* (Kertesz, 1982). Hopper, Bayles, Harris, and Holland (2001) assessed 57 individuals with a medical diagnosis of dementia. All exhibited deficits in communication and hearing function; however, the majority of participants were rated as having normal or adequate communication and hearing on the Minimum Data Set (MDS), which is a federally mandated assessment tool used to evaluate individuals residing in skilled nursing facilities, a large percentage of whom have dementia. Typically, the MDS is completed by a nurse. The authors concluded that the documented prevalence of communication and hearing problems among nursing home residents with dementia necessitates the involvement of communication specialists in the screening and evaluation of these individuals. Input from speech-language pathologists or audiologists is needed to promote the highest level of communicative functioning possible for nursing home residents with dementia.

A review of the tests used for evaluating dementia can be found in Cummings and Benson (1992); Haynes and Pindzola (2004); Hopper and Bayles (2008); and Huber and Shuttleworth (1990).

Therapy

Traditional models of speech-language therapy are seldom appropriate for patients with dementia. The clinician intent on reteaching a skill with the goal of more "normal" communication is unlikely to have much success with a patient who cannot remember what was just learned. Some of the more effective strategies for individual therapy, described below, include spaced-retrieval training (Brush & Camp, 1998), memory notebooks (Mateer & Sohlberg, 1988), and memory wallets (Bourgeois, 1992). Some effective group communication therapies include reminiscence; exercise, music, and dance; arts and crafts; games such as bingo; religious gatherings; and traditional conversation (Barr, 1988). A review of the literature (Bourgeois, 1991) reveals successful group therapies that are highly structured and organized; generally include some hands-on activity, take place in home-like secure settings, often include serving of food, center on previously enjoyed activities, and encourage demonstration of emotion.

A document from the American Speech-Language-Hearing Association (ASHA, 2005) indicates that speech-language pathologists (SLPs) should know about and apply computerized and other technologies when working with individuals with cognitive-communication disorders. Among the cognitive process to be addressed are helping clients with dementia develop functional skills, compensatory strategies, and support systems. A literature search of about 30 years of electronic databases (Mahendra et al., 2005) yielded a final three articles dealing with computer-assisted cognitive interventions (CACIs), which met the evidence template of purpose of the study. The evidence template should include the following: factors which affect validity; frequency, intensity, and duration of intervention; methodology; treatment outcomes; and documentation of treatment effects (Mahendra et al., 2005, p. 37). CACI was operationally defined as interactive, programmed computer technology used as tools to teach information and skills to individuals with Alzheimer disease.

Preliminary evidence (Mahendra et al., 2005) indicates that individuals with mild to moderate dementia who are optimal candidates for CACIs have impairments in episodic memory, but spared motor learning skills (procedural memory); and have corrected vision and hearing to within normal limits. Anticipated outcomes include improved ability to acquire and retain trained information and skills; generalization to real-world tasks and behaviors; retained information and skills for several weeks; but no change on measurements of global cognitive functioning. In other words, these individuals would not be showing decreased dementia (which is not an expected outcome), but would be making the most of their residual cognitive abilities.

The first goal of therapy is to inform the patient and the caretaker(s) about the nature and the consequences of the disorder.

The patient with dementia will show cognitive impairment directly correlated to the mild, moderate, and advanced stages of the condition. In cortical dementia, the language components are also affected according to the stage. In subcortical dementia, typically there is no characteristic breakdown of language, although speech can be dysarthric. There are dementias that are reversible, which are many times caused by nutritional and metabolic conditions. Most dementias are of the progressive and irreversible type. Because the types of dementia discussed in this section are of the progressive and irreversible type, spontaneous recovery and prognosis obviously play a lesser role. In some cases of Alzheimer and Parkinson disease, the symptoms of dementia can develop over a long period of time. These patients can remain in the mild stage for a number of years.

A review of about 30 years of electronic databases (Zientz, 2007) yielded six studies that specifically assessed the effect of educational interventions in communication strategies on families and caregivers of individuals with Alzheimer disease and dementia. There were five trends that emerged regarding educating caregivers in communication strategies: more successful conversational exchanges, both reduced and increased caregiver burden, improved quality of life, maintenance of language abilities of individuals with Alzheimer disease, and increased understanding by caregivers of communication breakdown and Alzheimer disease in general.

Small, Gutman, Makela, and Hillhouse (2003) found that strategies that caregivers employed for effective communication outcomes with Alzheimer patients were to (1) eliminate distractions, (2) use simple sentences, and (3) use yes/no questions. Small and Peary (2005) found that communication was more successful when caregivers, with their spouses who had Alzheimer disease, used yes/no questions compared to open-ended questions and questions that placed demands on semantic rather than episodic memory.

The literature reviewed (Zientz et al., 2007) was not helpful regarding optimal dose characteristics (frequency, intensity, and duration of treatment), which varied widely. The content of the training programs was predictable: impact of Alzheimer disease on communication; both verbal and nonverbal communication strategies; and opportunities for practice with individualized feedback. Expected outcomes of caregiver education reflected the training: increased knowledge of communication problems in Alzheimer disease, and better use of and satisfaction with communication strategies. The literature did not provide evidence to support conclusions about effects of caregiver training on attitudes, symptoms, or communication skills of individuals with Alzheimer disease.

Regarding how patients with dementia present their illness to their families, Brookshire (2007) reviewed a study by Rabins, Mace, and Lucas (1982) that questioned the families of 55 patients with irreversible dementia to ascertain what they considered the major problems in caring for the patient. These families identified the most serious problems, in order, as physical violence, memory disturbance, catastrophic reactions, incontinence, delusions, making accusations, hitting, and suspiciousness.

It is generally known that speech and language therapy will not achieve long-term improvement in the patient with dementia. However, speech and language therapy can help the patient (and the family) to communicate maximally within the scope of limited abilities. *The second goal of therapy is to provide the appropriate treatment approaches and techniques.*

Efficacy of Therapy for Communication Disorders Associated with Dementia

Although efficacy-of-treatment studies for communication disorders associated with dementia are lacking, clinical reports in the literature (see Bourgeois, 1991) indicate that therapy tasks that enhance memory; time, place, and person orientation; word-finding abilities; functional and daily living activities; and overall language communication between patient and family seem to be helpful for the patient. Typically, treatment is geared toward the behavioral and speech and language disturbances found in the mild, moderate, and advanced stages of the disease. Treatment for anomia is probably most beneficial in the early stages of disease, and is likely to be more effective in an autobiographical context (Henry, Beeson, & Rapcsak, 2008).

Bourgeois (1991) reviewed over 100 communication treatment studies for adults with dementia. She found that a number of treatment techniques have been successfully applied within the general areas of changing the communication environment, controlling stimulus conditions, changing the consequences of appropriate communication, group therapy intervention, and caregivers as communication partners.

Changing the communication environment includes rearranging furniture; adding plants, pictures, and other homey decorations; providing peers, children, and pets as conversational partners; and providing refreshments during group sessions. Controlling stimulus conditions includes external memory aids such as notebooks, calendars, signs, labels, color codes, loudspeaker announcements, verbal prompts, diaries, watches, cue cards, memory wallets, appointment books, seven-day pill dispensers, reality orientation, and the enhancement of stimuli with training, or routine and repetitive exposure.

Altmann, Kempler, and Anderson (2001) found that their results support a model of speech production in which all words are represented by semantic and grammatical features, both of which are vulnerable to failures of activation when there is damage or noise in the system as a result of pathology, trauma, or even divided attention. Nelland, Lubinski, and Higginbotham (2002) found that, although overall narrative comprehension is diminished in those with DAT, individuals appear to retain a mental representation for narratives that facilitates better comprehension of main ideas than of details, as well as better comprehension of stated information than of implied information.

Changing the consequences of appropriate communication includes tangible reinforcers such as candy, cigarettes, and exchangeable tokens; planned ignoring; and praising correct responses. Group therapy intervention includes remotivation therapy, sensory training, resocialization therapy, reminiscence therapy, and life review therapy.

Caregivers as communication partners includes, in the mild stage, early intervention by the caregiver, education about the nature and course of the disease, and training about appropriate approaches to the patient's problem behaviors, with support group participation also recommended. In the moderate stage, caretakers provide reinforcing and stimulating communicative environments for patients.

Typically, treatment is geared toward the behavioral and communication disturbances found in the mild, moderate, and advanced stages of the disease. The therapy tasks that enhance memory; time, place, and person orientation; word-finding abilities; functional and daily living activities; and overall language communication skills can be applied in the mild stage.

In the moderate stage, the caregiver needs to be trained to be the communication facilitator, using appropriate prompts to stimulate correct responses. In the advanced stage, treatment should be caretaker-oriented, and caretakers should be taught how to provide the stimuli that will bring positive changes in the patient's behavior and communication abilities.

Simulated presence therapy (abbreviated in the literature as SimPres) is a patented intervention (SimPres Incorporated, Boston, Massachusetts) enabling a family member or caregiver to make an audiotape about positive events to simulate their presence in the life of an individual with dementia (Bayles et al., 2006). The recording module enables caregivers to tape only the caller's part of a telephone conversation. The familiarity of the audiotape may provide comfort and reduce problem behaviors for an individual with dementia of the Alzheimer type, because of preserved remote memories and positive associations with these memories.

The Academy of Neurologic Communication Disorders and Sciences (ANCDS) writing committee for dementia (Bayles et al., 2006) reviewed over 30 years of literature in 9 databases, as well as manual searches of textbooks and other articles, and identified 5 papers on SimPres. Most participants responded positively to SimPres by smiling, singing, and reducing purposeless body movements. However, small sample sizes and the lack of a control group limited generalization of results. In addition, the data did not provide evidence of how long positive effects lasted, or whether SimPres was better than usual care.

Managing the Memory Deficits of Persons with Mild to Moderate Dementia

Bayles and Tomoeda (2007) summarized some of the basic systems of human memory and how they are affected by the neuropathology of dementia. These authors stated that memory refers to stored knowledge and the processes for making and manipulating stored knowledge. Essential to this are the processes called *activation* and *retrieval*. Two forms of stored knowledge, or long-term memory, are delineated as declarative and nondeclarative or procedural.

Declarative memory is fact memory, composed of semantic memory (knowledge of concepts), episodic memory (knowledge of events), and lexical memory (knowledge of words). When declarative or fact memory is activated into consciousness, it integrates with the working or active memory system. The working or active memory system activates and retrieves information and focuses attention. There are distinct profiles of semantic memory impairment in aphasia and dementia (Antonucci & Reilly, 2008).

Procedural memory involves the learning and implementation of motor skills (e.g., driving, playing tennis, writing). Thinking about driving would involve declarative memory, and performing the act of driving would involve procedural memory. Both declarative and procedural memory systems are typically simultaneously active and are essential parts of the working or active memory system.

During the early and middle stages, AD affects working and declarative memory, but mostly spares procedural memory. The neuropathology of AD causes a proliferation of neuritic plaques, neurofibrillary tangles, and granulovacuolar degeneration in brain areas (hippocampi and basal forebrain) that are specialized for declarative and working memory. These brain areas are important in the formation of new episodic memory (events). Forgetting events that happened recently is an early symptom of AD, but as the disease advances into cortical association areas, the lexical (words) and semantic (concepts) memory systems show more deterioration.

Based on the memory systems described, Bayles and Tomoeda (1996) suggested a plan of memory therapy for AD patients that calls for linguistic manipulations that reduce the demands on episodic and working memory systems. Simplifying the form of language would include speaking in simple and short sentences, speaking slowly, and providing multimodal cues.

Amending the content of language would include talking about the present (use of a daily memory book) and not the difficult-to-remember past or the future; talking about concrete items that the patient can see, hear, touch, and smell; using words with high frequency of occurrence; using proper nouns instead of pronouns (pronouns have difficult-to-remember antecedents); and revising and restating misunderstood language.

Modifying the use of language would include not asking questions that require the patient to search through fact (declarative) memory and recall information (e.g., instead of asking, "What is your favorite TV program?" which requires a memory search, giving a choice of several TV programs, or if the disease is more severe, using a yes/no question such as, "Do you like watching TV?"). AD patients often can produce meaningful language if they are engaging in an activity that they previously enjoyed. Pleasant activities that reduce fear and agitation include making a meal together, singing, and engaging in crafts, simple games, and massage.

A review (Ehlhardt et al., 2008) of 20 years of literature from 6 databases dealt with treatment of acquired memory impairments in adults with neurogenic disorders (acquired brain injury, dementia, and schizophrenia/schizoaffective disorder), with the purpose of developing guidelines for clinical practice. These treatments included use of direct attention training; external aids for memory; behavior modification; executive function treatments; and standardized assessment in traumatic brain injury (TBI). There was a wide range of treatment dosage in the studies, in terms of number and frequency of sessions, length of sessions, and duration of treatment.

The literature supported the effectiveness of some instructional practices in cognitive rehabilitation. Clinical practice recommendations reflected the level of the research evidence (Ehlhardt et al., 2008, p. 8). There were no Class I studies for aphasia and dementia, and only one for schizophrenia. Nearly all studies reflected Class III and IV levels of evidence.

The literature review revealed two broad instructional categories: systematic and conventional methods. The systematic methods included vanishing cues, errorless learning, and spaced retrieval; and the conventional methods included errorful learning, which was also called trial-and-error learning. In vanishing cues, the client is given progressively stronger or weaker cues after recall attempts of the task information or procedures. Guessing is discouraged in errorless learning, where the clinician provides models during the acquisition phase of learning, before the client attempts to respond. Clients practice spaced retrieval by recalling information over expanded intervals of time. In the conventional methods, clients try to recall targeted information or skills without prior models or prompts; the clinician models only if there are errors. Some studies emphasized strategy components, such as verbal elaboration, imagery, prediction and reflection, and evaluative questioning or self-generating responses, while other studies focused on stimulus manipulation, such as varied training examples or prior exposure of the stimulus. There was no single right method for a particular disorder.

In a review of some 30 years of research published in 11 databases, Hopper et al. (2005) found 13 articles (all evaluated as providing Class II or Class III levels of evidence) dealing with spaced-retrieval (SR) training. The original purpose of using SR was to teach face–name associations to individuals with memory impairments. It was later adapted for individuals with dementia, where the interval between recall opportunities is systematically lengthened. Ultimately, the client should demonstrate the ability to recall information in everyday situations (Hopper et al., 2005, p. 28).

The clinically applicable trends across SR studies were positive, in that participants learned some or all of the target information (Hopper et al., 2005, p. 32). Because of methodological shortcomings in the studies, the results should be interpreted with caution. In future studies, participant characteristics should be specified in order to facilitate generalization of findings, and interrater reliability judgment scores should be reported to control for the effect of instrumentation on validity of findings.

A literature search covering 30 years in 8 databases revealed 7 articles, a published manual, and one videotaped presentation dealing with Montessori-based interventions for dementia; 5 articles were analyzed in detail (Mahendra et al., 2006). Well known for its application in teaching children, Montessori methods may be adapted for use with individuals who have dementia. Its main principles include: preparing the environment to provide stimulation and encourage purposeful activities; progressing from simple, concrete activities to more complex, abstract ones; building in success by breaking down tasks and activities into components and cueing one part at a time; sequencing learning through observation and recognition, leading to recall and demonstration; using functional, real-life materials; and incorporating multisensory stimulation through activities (Mahendra et al., 2006, p. 16).

Participants in the five studies (total N = 74) had mild to severe dementia, mainly of the Alzheimer type. Interventions used Montessori principles to maintain or improve behavior, cognitive function, and mood (Mahendra et al., 2006, p. 18). They provided Class II and III levels of evidence in support of using these interventions for people with dementia. Candidates for Montessori-based treatment should have the following characteristics associated with dementia: impaired episodic memory, but capacity for motor learning, verbal communication, and socializing; no history of physical aggression; ability to attend to and participate in intervention; and corrected auditory and visual abilities sufficient to permit participation in sensory discrimination and reading activities.

Additional Activities for the Mild Stage Patient

Reminiscence, or recalling personally experienced past episodes, was reviewed (Kim et al., 2006), with a focus on the role of speech-language pathologists working with individuals with dementia. A review of more than 30 years of publications from 10 databases was supplemented by hand searches of relevant books. The structure of group reminiscence therapy involved a facilitator and individuals with dementia meeting one to three times per week. Outcome measures varied from count of utterances produced, to measures of discourse, to cognitive change based on standardized measures, such as the *Mini-Mental State Exam* (MMSE) (Folstein, Folstein, & McHugh, 1975).

Some trends observed included improved cognitive functioning as assessed by the MMSE; improvements in narrative production, as well as linguistic and verbal behaviors in discourse; and increased well-being in both the individuals with dementia and their caregivers. Appropriate candidates for group reminiscence therapy included individuals with dementia who had episodic memory impairments, severity level from mild to moderate, and adequate functional vision and hearing to receive sensory stimuli.

Listed below are some additional activities that can be employed with the patient who has dementia in the mild stage, and possibly in the moderate stage. The clinician should help orient the patient to time, place, and person in a concrete manner. This can be achieved through the use of visual aids such as calendars, a blackboard for large words and simple drawings, poster cards or large uncluttered pictures, daily newspapers, and photographs of family members and close friends. The clinician should also determine what functions the patient will perform in daily activities. This can include making grocery shopping lists, putting food in categories, identifying the locations and names of supermarkets, practicing money concepts coupled with simple arithmetic, and reading bus schedules (time, destinations, simple arithmetic).

1. Perform simple cooking activities (measuring with quarts, pints, pounds, ounces). Santo Pietro and Goldfarb (1995) provided specific examples for the reading of food labels (popcorn, fish filets, and cereals), maps (city of Baltimore, shopping centers), schedules

(television, recycling), food coupons (brand-name cereals), recipes (soup and stew, cookies), menus (Chinese restaurant), and price lists (airfares).

2. Set clocks and timers (seconds, minutes, hours).
3. Use the telephone for work on numbers in sequence and memory.
4. Use concrete vocabulary centered around everyday activities.
5. Participate in social and group situations to stimulate mental activity.
6. Practice orientation to family placement and relationships by using real family names. Bourgeois (1992) suggested using a naming wallet containing 30 pictures and sentences about familiar persons, places, and events that are difficult for the patient to remember.

Vanhalle, Van der Linden, Belleville, and Gilbert (1998) reported on the successful use of the Spaced Retrieval Strategy (SRS), which consists of retrieving the information to be learned after increasingly longer delays, in helping a 69-year-old patient with Alzheimer disease to recall names.

The third goal of therapy is to encourage the patient and the caretaker(s) to continue the rehabilitative process outside of the clinical setting.

Rehabilitation at Home

Bayles and Boone (1982) and Bourgeois (1991) pointed out that the family and caretakers can make many modifications in the way they communicate with the patient, to facilitate the comprehension and retention of information. Rate of speech, level of syntactic complexity, and the mode of linguistic input may all affect the patient's comprehension. Verbal analogies, fragmented discourse, humor, sarcasm, use of indefinite referents, conversation involving more than two individuals, and open-ended questions are the types of language that are hardest for the patient with dementia. Providing conversational partners (peers, children, etc.) and rewarding appropriate communication with tangible reinforcers (food, etc.) will also facilitate communication.

In addition, those authors and the *Mayo Clinic Health Letter* "Dementia" (1995) suggested counseling the family to do the following:

1. Maintain a simple routine.
2. Maintain a constant environment (dressing, eating, etc.).
3. Be consistent.
4. Minimize distractions.
5. Keep your loved one involved.
6. Reassign household chores.
7. Join support groups for families and/or patient.
8. Give yourself a break for reenergizing.
9. Keep some hobbies that renew your mental or physical health.
10. Expect the patient to deny the problem.
11. Expect the affected individual to become anxious.
12. Simplify verbal interactions.
13. Expect a change in the patient's condition if there is a major change in lifestyle.
14. Avoid arguing with the affected individual.
15. Dispense the patient's medication and make sure the patient eats and exercises properly.
16. Have the patient wear an identification bracelet.
17. Put sensors under the rug in case the patient roams at inappropriate times.
18. Install complicated door locks.

Bayles and Tomoeda (1996) also suggested a plan of memory therapy for AD patients that calls for nonlinguistic manipulations that reduce the demand on episodic memory (events) and capitalize on procedural (motor activity) and recognition memory.

Patients with AD quite often have difficulty in feeding themselves. This functional motor skill can be helped by the following:

1. Feeding the patient in the same place
2. Positioning the food so that it can be seen
3. Eliminating distractions
4. Placing eating utensil in patient's hand
5. Providing a model of the actual eating act
6. Pairing touch with the start of feeding
7. Pacing feeding so that time between bites is about the same
8. Using social reinforcements for self-feeding (e.g., verbal compliments, touching)
9. Providing beverages routinely
10. Using finger food where possible

Orange, Lubinski, and Higginbotham (1996) examined the conversational repair (the efforts of conversational partners to correct and resolve misunderstandings or mishearing) of six neurotypical elderly adults, five participants with early stage dementia of the Alzheimer type (EDAT), and five with middle stage DAT (MDAT), with a family member who acted as a conversational partner. The percentage of conversation involved in repair was significantly higher for MDAT participants versus the control group and EDAT participants. Despite the increase of conversational troubles with DAT onset and progression, the difficulties were repaired successfully a majority of the time. These findings have implications for developing caregiver communication enhancement strategies that are specific to the clinical stage of DAT. The authors provided examples of the trouble sources, repair initiators, repairs, and resolutions of conversational repair.

Orange and Colton-Hudson (1998) reported on how a communication education and training program (1) helped the spouse in coping with her husband's illness (dementia of the Alzheimer type, or DAT), (2) produced fewer instances of communication breakdown between the two, (3) produced greater use of efficient techniques to signal and repair communication problems, (4) showed a decrease in negative emotional responses to challenging behaviors, and (5) produced a positive response to the implementation and completion of the program.

Chapman, Weiner, Packley, Hyman, and Zientz (2004) found that donepezil along with cognitive-communication stimulation produced benefits in areas of discourse abilities, functional abilities, emotional symptoms, and overall global performance in patients with mild to moderate Alzheimer disease.

Rehabilitation in a Facility

Long-term care facilities that provide the consistent routines, familiar environments, and appropriate cultural markers (art, music, dress, language, food, and surrounding decor) that were part of the patients' premorbid lives, can greatly enhance the patients' ability to maintain skills. There is a trend toward designing nurturing environments in long-term care facilities for dementia patients.

Johnson and Bourgeois (1998) reported on how a respite program helped a 90-year-old dementia patient increase her initiation of conversational topics, and how the patient's daughter received temporary relief from caregiving and specific instructions for helping her mother at home. The patient's swallowing and auditory acuity problems were also addressed.

The Breakfast Club (Boczko & Santo Pietro, 1997) is a directed activity in which a small group of persons with Alzheimer disease prepares, serves, and eats breakfast and cleans up afterward. Goals are maintenance of conversation and social skills, and also organization and decision-making skills. There is a structured 10-step protocol that includes greetings, choices of juices and breakfast foods, joint preparation of coffee and breakfast, serving of coffee and breakfast entrée, cleanup, conversation over coffee, and leave-taking. Results of a study (Santo Pietro & Boczko, 1998) showed improvement in the use of language and communication skills, as well as renewed use of procedural memories for preparing, sharing, and eating a meal. Social ritual abilities resurfaced, and patients became calmer, more independent, and able to show social concern for one another.

Additional Memory Helpers

Although the following memory guidelines (Hearst Business Communications, Inc., n.d.) are geared for the typically aging person, they can be adapted quite easily for use with a patient who has dementia in the mild stage.

1. Take time to remember. Train yourself to become more aware by pausing before you go anywhere or say anything. Take a deep breath, clear your throat, relax.
2. Write notes and lists. Whenever you think of something you have to do, try to do it right away. If you can't get to the task, write it down. This is especially useful when there is too much to do and too little time.
3. Establish routines. Set up habits such as storing keys, your pocketbook, and /or your wallet in a certain place each time you put them down.
4. Don't become distracted. Any type of distraction will hinder your ability to recall information. If you tend to do several things at the same time, choose priorities and try to do one thing after the other.
5. Keep mentally active. Play games, join a study group, or take a class to keep your mind alert. For example, start doing crossword puzzles or anagrams, or playing Monopoly.
6. Rehearse information. Before you go to a party or class reunion, review the names of people you will be seeing and visualize them in the context in which you know them.
7. Create a mental picture. "Seeing" something can help you recall a name or other information. For example, develop a mental picture of a store when trying to recall the name of the business.
8. Keep physically active. Exercise seems to have a positive effect on mental abilities; even a little physical activity can help mental awareness.
9. Beware of fatigue. When tired or under stress, pay even more attention to normal daily tasks. If at all possible, postpone doing tasks until fully rested.
10. Don't doubt yourself. Most important, don't question your ability. By doubting yourself, you can make a situation worse by exaggerating every memory lapse.

The caretaker or clinician can follow a few simple rules to help in communicating with an individual who has Alzheimer disease (Goldfarb & Santo Pietro, 2004):

1. Reduce the demands on episodic memory by relying on recognition memory rather than recall memory. Rather than asking, "What did you have for breakfast?" ask, "Did you have the eggs or the pancakes?" Ask choice questions both for information and for behavior management.
2. Label everything in the environment. Everyday sights and objects should be remembered longer if they are kept salient.
3. Reduce distractions before beginning speaking.
4. Use short sentences that do not challenge the individual's memory span.
5. Provide visual support, such as gestures, facial expressions, pictures, and written words.
6. Speak loudly and slowly enough.

7. Refer to long-term memories as often as possible. Build on the clearer memories of early experiences.
8. Listen carefully. Sometimes what sounds initially like nonsense may not be. Individuals with Alzheimer disease often have lucid moments.

Agnosia

As noted at the beginning of this section, the American Psychiatric Association (2000) states that the essential feature of a dementia is the development of multiple cognitive deficits that include memory impairment and at least one of the following: aphasia, apraxia, agnosia, or a disturbance in executive functioning. If auditory or visual agnosia is present, Halpern (1986) has offered some therapy procedures for these conditions.

Agnosia is a disturbance of recognition or identification of sensory stimuli. It is an input modality-bound impairment in which the person has difficulty only with the affected modality, but can perform well through an alternate modality. For example, the person may have difficulty through the auditory modality (auditory agnosia), but no difficulty through the visual modality, as in reading. Bhatnagar (2008) noted that most agnosias require bilateral cortical lesions, cutting off input from the sensory modality (auditory, visual, tactile) to the left hemisphere language centers. In our discussion, we will consider only the auditory and visual modalities, and not the tactile (touch) modality.

Auditory Agnosia

Brookshire (2007) identified auditory agnosia as similar to visual agnosia, in the sense that it may be incomplete or intermittent. He further noted that auditory agnosia indicates damage (usually bilateral) in the auditory association cortex.

Halpern (1986) has suggested that therapy for auditory agnosia might consist of the following:

1. *Discrimination, Recognition, and Association Between Nonlanguage Objects and Sounds*: Using objects that produce sounds that are common in the environment (e.g., bell ringing, horn blowing, hitting with a hammer, knocking on a table), the clinician should blow a horn and then let the patient do likewise. Pictures of a horn and the printed word(s) *horn* or *blowing the horn* can be used to build up an association between the sound and the object producing it. Discrimination can begin when the clinician blows the horn after instructing the patient to listen but not to look. The patient then has to identify the object (horn) that produced the sound from among other objects (hammer, bell, etc.) or pictures of objects.
2. *Discrimination, Recognition, and Association Between Animal Noises with Two- or Three-Dimensional Forms*: Animal noises (mooing of cow, meowing of cat, roaring of lion, barking of dog, etc.) can be imitated by the clinician or produced on a tape and presented to the patient. Let the patient imitate the sound and associate it with a two-dimensional (picture) or three-dimensional (stuffed animal) representation of the animal. The printed word also helps. As before, discrimination can occur when the clinician produces the animal sound (meowing) with the patient not looking. The patient then has to choose from a group of pictures or stuffed animals (cat, lion, dog, etc.) the representation that produced the meow sound. Discrimination, recognition, and association of coughing, sneezing, yawning, humming, and other nonverbal sounds can be accomplished in the manner described above.
3. *Sound Recognition*: The clinician should start off by producing the /a/ sound. The patient should then imitate the production while looking in the mirror. After a number

of attempts, a card with *AH* should be introduced and the association between the auditory sound and the visual representation should be stressed. The next step would be introducing the *EE*, *OH*, and *OO* vowels in a similar manner. Once associations have been built for each of these sounds, discrimination can be achieved by having the clinician or a tape recorder present the /a/ sound auditorily, and subsequently having the patient identify a visual representation of *AH*, *EE*, *OH*, and *OO*.

Visual Agnosia

Brookshire (2007) noted that visual agnosia is typically caused by damage (usually bilateral) in the occipital lobe, in the posterior parietal lobe, or in the fiber tracts connecting the visual cortex to other areas in the brain. He further mentioned that visual agnosias often are incomplete, intermittent, and inconsistent, and patients with visual agnosias usually function reasonably well in daily life.

Halpern (1986) has suggested that therapy for visual agnosia might consist of the following:

1. *Discrimination, Recognition, and Matching of Two- and Three-Dimensional Nonlanguage Forms*: It is best to initiate therapy using three-dimensional objects such as two pencils, two cups, two squares, two triangles, and so forth. The clinician should correctly match an identical pair of these items and simultaneously name them. The patient is then directed to follow suit. Sometimes the mere handling of the three-dimensional object will aid in the correct identification. Subsequently, two-dimensional representations (pictures, drawings, etc.) of the same or different items that were used in the three-dimensional object situation can be employed. The clinician matches an identical pair of items as before, and the patient has to follow suit. After a while, the patient can match two-dimensional items with three-dimensional items. If successful with the above, the patient can then match items that are similar but not identical. These could include different types of cars, different-size triangles, different shapes of houses, and so forth. Discrimination practice can take place by asking the patient to choose the form that is different (e.g., ○○○○■○, etc.).

2. *Repeating and Naming of Those Forms or Objects*: During the above process it is advisable to have the patient repeat after the clinician or name directly the item being worked on. Again, this utilization of several modalities seems to help the patient with agnosia. The clinician can also add pantomime in the directions to the patient (e.g., making a circle with fingers, smoking a cigarette, drinking from a glass, etc.). If it facilitates an appropriate response, the patient can use the same pantomime.

3. *Tracing and Copying of Those Forms or Objects*: Again, the same principle of using multiple modalities is employed. The patient traces or copies the item and simultaneously names it or repeats it after the clinician. After a while, copying can be done from memory (showing the item and then removing it) or from the clinician's direction.

4. *Letter Recognition*: In cases where the patient has a visual letter agnosia or a pure word blindness, large alphabet cards and large magazine pictures (or a large font in a computer-generated presentation) can be used to discriminate and recognize the individual letter. For example, if a task involves the recognition of H, the alphabet cards should spell HAT and be placed under a picture of a hat. Letters that look like the picture or object (S for snake, A for apple, etc.) are especially helpful. Discrimination practice can take place by having the patient choose the letter that is different (e.g., SSSTS, abaaa, etc.) or choose the identical word from a group of words (e.g., SIT from SIP, SIR, SIT, SIN, etc.).

5. *Repeating and Naming*: During letter recognition training, the clinician should name the letter and have the patient simultaneously repeat and name the letter. Again, other modalities are brought into play to facilitate recognition of the letter.

6. *Copying, Tracing, and Pantomime of Letter*: The patient can be asked to trace or copy the letter and simultaneously name it or repeat after the clinician. After this is done successfully, copying can be done from memory (showing the item and then removing it) or from the clinician's direction. The clinician can also add pantomime as an additional aid (e.g., making a real form with fingers or drawing an imaginary form in the air for the letters O, X, V, etc.). Finally, the patient can write the letter after the clinician says it.

Advanced Study

Language use depends on intellectual functioning and memory. Individuals with vascular disease and infarctions in frontal lobes suffer serious intellectual and memory deficits. The frontal lobes are crucial to normal functioning of working memory that plays a significant role in language comprehension, encoding, activation, and retrieval. Small-vessel ischemic diseases, or a frontotemporal form of degeneration, are the most frequent causes of multi-infarct or vascular dementia (Grossman et al., 1996). Positron emission tomography (PET) measurements in neurotypical volunteers, during a graded auditory-verbal memory task, revealed increased memory load correlating with increased regional cerebral blood flow in the cerebellar vermis and hemispheres, thalamus bilaterally, the superior and middle front gyri bilaterally, anterior insular regions bilaterally, anterior cingulated, precuneus, and left and right lateral premotor areas (Grasby et al., 1994, p. 1271). Neurological and behavioral changes, language and communication, and disease progression help to differentiate frontotemporal dementia from Alzheimer disease (Cycyk & Wright, 2008).

MacDonald, Almor, Henderson, Kempler, and Anderson (2001) cautioned against assuming that impairments in working memory underlie comprehension deficits. They found vagueness in the term "working memory," as well as limitations of available working memory tasks. Indeed, they reported that many such tasks bore little relationship to language comprehension. In addition, many tasks were too confusing or difficult for participants with Alzheimer disease. Bayles (2003) also noted a paucity of documentation on how working memory deficits affect communicative functioning. Using five tests of language comprehension and four tests of language expression, Bayles (2003, p. 209) argued that in her participants with Alzheimer dementia, lower scores on language tests resulted primarily from reduced attention span and difficulties focusing attention, encoding, and activating long-term knowledge rather than from loss of linguistic knowledge.

CASE DESCRIPTION

Hours after his family reported him missing, DB, age 78 years, was returned to his home on the Upper East Side of Manhattan, having been reported to the police to be wandering in Harlem alone, lost, and frightened.

DB was a retired research scientist, having led a group decades earlier in the development of nylon. After his diagnosis of Alzheimer disease, he stayed at the home of one of the authors for a few days, accompanied by his wife and caregiver. DB referred to the author's young daughter as "Butch," indicating, "That's quite a little guy you have there," despite his wife's gentle admonition that the child was female. He would spend long periods of time holding a newspaper, without averting his gaze from the same paragraph, and never turning a page. Occasionally, he would become agitated and demand his car keys. His appetite was good, table manners were preserved, and he commented appropriately about what he was eating.

A particularly poignant deficit was that this formerly brilliant scientist no longer engaged in self-care, and needed the assistance of his home attendant to shower.

Discussion Questions: Theory

1. According to the DSM-IV (American Psychiatric Association, 2000), what cognitive-linguistic deficits are required for a diagnosis of dementia?

2. What aspects of memory are impaired in dementia?

3. What aspects of executive function are impaired in dementia?

4. How are the language deficits in dementia similar to and different from those of aphasia?

5. How are cognitive-linguistic deficits of Alzheimer dementia similar to and different from vascular dementia?

Discussion Questions: Therapy

1. Should group therapy be combined with individual therapy, used separately, or not used at all?

2. How can we train a caregiver to be a better communicative partner?

3. What are some benefits and disadvantages in providing speech-language therapy at home, compared to treatment in an institution?

4. What are some specific techniques and goals for improving memory?

5. What are some specific techniques and goals for improving language?

Assignment: Write a multiple-choice question with five options. Explain why the key option is correct, and why the distractors or decoys are incorrect. Avoid using forms such as, "All of the following are (in)correct *except*" in the stem, and "All (or none) of the above" in the options.

Example: In dementia of the Alzheimer type, some communication functions remain preserved while others are impaired. Which functions are preserved in mild to moderate stages?
a. Vocabulary
b. Syntax, phonology, and spelling
c. Naming and word finding
d. Complex linguistic functions
e. Pragmatic language

The correct answer is *b*, because syntax, phonology, and spelling are not impaired until the most advanced stages of Alzheimer dementia; *a* is incorrect because vocabulary is restricted, limited to small talk and stereotyped clichés; *c* is incorrect because there is word-finding difficulty, characterized by empty syntax and an increasing loss of substantive words; *d* is incorrect because there is impairment in complex linguistic functions associated with intellectual and mnestic operations; *e* is incorrect because circumlocutions, auditory comprehension deficit, mutism, and echolalia are associated with deficits in pragmatic language.

References

Abeysinghe, S., Bayles, K., & Trosset, M. (1990). Semantic memory deterioration in Alzheimer's subjects: Evidence from word association, definition, and associate ranking tasks. *Journal of Speech and Hearing Research, 33,* 574–582.

Alpert, M., Rosen, A., & Welkowitz, J. (1990). Interpersonal communication in the context of dementia. *Journal of Communication Disorders, 23,* 337–346.

Altmann, L., Kempler, D., & Andersen, F. (2001). Speech errors in Alzheimer's disease: Reevaluating morphosyntactic preservation. *Journal of Speech, Language, and Hearing Research, 44,* 1069–1082.

American Psychiatric Association. (2000). *Diagnostic and statistical manual of mental disorders* (4th ed.). Washington, DC: Author.

American Speech-Language-Hearing Association. (2005). *Knowledge and skills needed by speech-language pathologists providing services to individuals with cognitive-communication disorders* [Knowledge and Skills]. Available from www.asha.org/policy. doi:10.1044/policy.KS2005-00078.

Antonucci, S. M., & Reilly, J. (2008). Semantic memory and language processing: A primer. *Seminars in Speech and Language, 29,* 5–17.

Appell, J., Kertesz, A., & Fisman, M. (1982). A study of language functioning in Alzheimer's patients. *Brain and Language, 17,* 73–91.

Au, R., Obler, L., & Albert, M. (1991). Language in aging and dementia. In M. Sarno (Ed.), *Acquired aphasia* (pp. 405–423). New York, NY: Academic Press.

Baddeley, A. (2001, November). Is working memory still working? *American Psychologist, 56,* 851–863.

Barr, J. (1988). Group treatment: The logical choice. In B. Shadden (Ed.), *Communication behavior and aging: A sourcebook for clinicians.* Baltimore, MD: Williams & Wilkins.

Bayles, K. (1982). Language function in senile dementia. *Brain and Language, 16,* 265–280.

Bayles, K. (2003). Effects of working memory deficits on the communication functioning of Alzheimer's dementia patients. *Journal of Communication Disorders, 36,* 209–219.

Bayles, K., & Boone, D. (1982). The potential of language tasks for identifying senile dementia. *Journal of Speech and Hearing Disorders, 47,* 210–217.

Bayles, K., Boone, D., Tomoeda, C., Slauson, T., & Kazniak, A. (1989). Differentiating Alzheimer's patients from the normal elderly and stroke patients with aphasia. *Journal of Speech and Hearing Disorders, 54,* 74–87.

Bayles, K., Kim, E., Chapman, S., Zientz, J., Rackley, A., Mahendra, N., . . . Cleary, S. (2006). Evidence-based practice recommendations for working with individuals with dementia: Simulated presence therapy. *Journal of Medical Speech-Language Pathology, 14,* 13–21.

Bayles, K., & Tomoeda, C. (1983). Confrontation naming impairment in dementia. *Brain and Language, 19,* 98–114.

Bayles, K., Tomoeda, C., & Caffrey, J. (1982). Language and dementia producing diseases. *Communication Disorders, 7,* 131–146.

Bayles, K. A., & Tomoeda, C. K. (1996). Principles and techniques for managing the memory deficits of persons with mild to moderate dementia. *Neurophysiology and Neurogenic Speech and Language Disorders,* (Special Interest Division 2 Newsletter, 21–27). Rockville, MD: American Speech-Language-Hearing Association.

Bayles, K., & Tomoeda, C. (2007). *Cognitive-communication disorders of dementia.* San Diego, CA: Plural Publishing.

Bayles, K., & Tomoeda, C. (1991). *Arizona battery for communication disorders of dementia*. Tucson, AZ: Canyonlands Publishing.

Bayles, K., Tomoeda, C., Kazniak, A., Stern, L., & Eagans, K. (1985). Verbal perseveration of dementia patients. *Brain and Language, 25*, 102–116.

Bayles, K., Tomoeda, C., & Trosset, M. (1992). Relation of linguistic communication abilities of Alzheimer's patients to stage of disease. *Brain and Language, 42*, 454–472.

Benson, D. F. (1979). *Aphasia, alexia, agraphia*. New York, NY: Churchill-Livingston, Inc.

Benson, D. F., & Ardila, A. (1996). *Aphasia: A clinical perspective*. New York, NY: Oxford University Press.

Bhatnagar, S. (2008). *Neuroscience for the study of communication disorders*. Baltimore, MD: Lippincott Williams & Wilkins.

Boczko, F., & Santo Pietro, M. J. (1997). The Breakfast Club and related programs. In B. Shaddon & M. Toner (Eds.), *Aging and communication: For clinicians by clinicians*. Austin, TX: Pro-Ed.

Boller, F., Becker, J., Holland, A., Forbes, M., Hood, P., & McGonigle-Gibson, P. (1991). Predictors of decline in Alzheimer's disease. *Cortex, 27*, 9–17.

Borkowski, J., Benton, A., & Spreen, O. (1967). Word fluency and brain damage. *Neuropsychologia, 5*, 135–140.

Bourgeois, M. (1991). Communication treatment for adults with dementia. *Journal of Speech and Hearing Research, 34*, 831–844.

Bourgeois, M. S. (1992). Evaluating memory wallets in conversations with dementia. *Journal of Speech and Hearing Research, 35*, 13–44.

Bowles, N., Obler, L., & Albert, M. (1987). Naming errors in healthy aging and dementia of the Alzheimer type. *Cortex, 23*, 519–524.

Brookshire, R. (2003). *An introduction to neurogenic communication disorders* (6th ed.). St. Louis, MO: Mosby Yearbook.

Brush, J., & Camp, C. (1998). *A therapy technique for improving memory: Spaced retrieval*. Beachwood, OH: Mcnorah Park Center for the Aging.

Cappa, S. F., Binetti, G., Pezzini, A., Padovani, A., Rozzini, L., & Trabucchi, M. (1998). Object and action naming in Alzheimer's disease and frontotemporal dementia. *Neurology, 50*, 351 355.

Chapman, S. B. (1997). Discourse markers of Alzheimer's disease versus normal advanced aging. *Neurophysiology and Neurogenic Speech and Language Disorders, 7*(4). (Special Interest Division 2 Newsletter, 20–26). Rockville, MD: American Speech-Language-Hearing Association.

Chapman, S., Weiner, M., Rackley, A., Hynan, L., & Zientz, J. (2004). Effects of cognitive-communication stimulation for Alzheimer's disease patients treated with donopezil. *Journal of Speech, Language, and Hearing Research, 47*, 1149–1163.

Chenery, H. J., Murdoch, B. E., & Ingram, J. C. L. (1996). An investigation of confrontation naming performance in Alzheimer's dementia as a function of disease severity. *Aphasiology, 10*, 423–441.

Critchley, M. (1970). *Aphasiology and other aspects of language*. London, UK: Edward Arnold.

Cummings, J. (1990). Introduction. In J. Cummings (Ed.), *Subcortical dementia* (pp. 3–16). New York, NY: Oxford University Press.

Cummings, J., & Benson, D. (1992). *Dementia: A clinical approach* (2nd ed.). Stoneham, MA: Butterworth-Heinemann.

Cycyk, L. M., & Wright, H. H. (2008). Frontotemporal dementia: Its definition, differential diagnosis, and management. *Aphasiology, 22*, 422–444.

D'Hornicthun, P., & Pillon, A. (2008). Verb comprehension and naming in fronto-temporal degeneration: The role of the static depiction of actions. *Cortex, 44*, 834–847.

Dick, M., Kean, M., & Sands, D. (1989). Memory for internally generated words in Alzheimer-type dementia: Breakdown in encoding and semantic memory. *Brain and Cognition, 9*, 88–108.

Druks, J., Masterson, J., Kopelman, M., Clare, L., Rose, A., & Rai, G. (2006). Is action naming better preserved (than object naming) in Alzheimer's disease and why should we ask? *Brain and Language, 98*, 332–340.

Ehlhardt, L. A., Sohlberg, M. M., Kennedy, M., Coelho, C., Ylvisaker, M., Turkstra, L., & Yorkston, K. (2008). Evidence-based practice guidelines for instructing individuals with neurogenic memory impairments: What have we learned in the past 20 years? *Neuropsychological Rehabilitation, 1*, 1–43.

Eustache, F., Lambert, J., Cassier, C., Dary, M., Rossa, Y., Rioux, P., . . . Lechevalier, B. (1995). Disorders of auditory identification in dementia of the Alzheimer type. *Cortex, 31*, 119–127.

Folstein, M. F., Folstein, S. F., & McHugh, P. R. (1975). Mini-mental state: A practical guide for grading the cognitive state of patients for the clinician. *Journal of Psychiatric Research, 12,* 196–198.

Fromm, D., & Holland, A. (1989). Functional communication in Alzheimer's disease. *Journal of Speech and Hearing Disorders, 54,* 535–540.

Fromm, D., Holland, A., Nebes, R., & Oakley, M. (1991). A longitudinal study of word reading ability in Alzheimer's disease: Evidence from the National Adult Reading Test. *Cortex, 27,* 367–376.

Gewirth, L., Shindler, A., & Hier, D. (1984). Altered patterns of word associations in dementia and aphasia. *Brain and Language, 21,* 307–317.

Goldfarb, R., & Goldberg, E. (2004). Communicative responsibility and semantic task in the language of adults with dementia. *Perceptual and Motor Skills, 98,* 1177–1186.

Goldfarb, R., & Santo Pietro, M. J. (2004). Support systems: Older adults with neurogenic communication disorders. *Journal of Ambulatory Care Management, 27,* 376–385.

Granholm, E., & Butters, N. (1988). Associative encoding and retrieval in Alzheimer's and Huntington's disease. *Brain and Cognition, 7,* 335–347.

Grasby, P. M., Frith, C. D., Friston, K. J., Simpson, J., Fletcher, P. C., Frackowiak, R. S., & Dolan, R. J. (1994). A graded task approach to the functional mapping of brain areas implicated in auditory-verbal memory. *Brain, 117,* 1271–1282.

Grossman, M., D'Esposito, M., Hughes, E., Onishi, K., Biassou, N., White-Devine, T., & Robinson, K. (1996). Language comprehension profiles in Alzheimer's disease, multi-infarct dementia, and fronto-temporal degeneration. *Neurology, 48,* 183–189.

Halpern, H. (1986). Therapy for agnosia, apraxia, and dysarthria. In R. Chapey (Ed.), *Language intervention strategies in adult aphasia* (pp. 420–436). Baltimore, MD: Williams & Wilkins.

Halpern, H., Darley, F., & Brown, J. (1973). Differential language and neurologic characteristics in cerebral involvement. *Journal of Speech and Hearing Disorders, 38,* 162–173.

Haynes, W., & Pindzola, R. (2004). *Diagnosis and evaluation in speech pathology.* Boston, MA: Pearson Education.

Haynes, W., Pindzola, R., & Emerick, L. (1992). *Diagnosis and evaluation in speech pathology.* Englewood Cliffs, NJ: Prentice-Hall.

Hearst Business Communications, Inc., RAI Division (n.d.). *Improving your ability to recall information.* New York, NY: Author.

Henry, M. L., Beeson, P. M., & Rapcsak, S. Z. (2008). Treatment for anomia in semantic dementia. *Seminars in Speech and Language, 29,* 60–67.

Hier, D., Hagenlocker, K., & Shindler, A. (1985). Language disintegration in dementia: Effects of etiology and severity. *Brain and Language, 25,* 117–133.

Hodges, J. R., Martinos, M., Woolams, A. M., Patterson, K., & Adlam, A-L. (2008). Repeat and point: Differentiating semantic dementia from progressive non-fluent aphasia. *Cortex, 44,* 1265–1270.

Holland, A., McBurney, D., Moossy, J., & Reinmuth, O. (1985). The dissolution of language in Pick's disease with neurofibrillary tangles: A case study. *Brain and Language, 24,* 36–58.

Hopper, T., & Bayles, K. (2008). Management of neurogenic communication disorders associated with dementia. In R. Chapey (Ed.), *Language intervention strategies in aphasia and related neurogenic communication disorders* (pp. 988–1008). Baltimore, MD: Lippincott Williams & Wilkins.

Hopper, T., Bayles, K., Harris, F., & Holland, A. (2001). The relationship between minimum data set ratings and scores on measures of communication and hearing among nursing home residents with dementia. *American Journal of Speech-Language Pathology, 10,* 370–381.

Hopper, T., Mahendra, N., Kim, E., Azuma, T., Bayles, K., Cleary, S., & Tomoeda, C. (2005). Evidence-based practice recommendations for working with individuals with dementia: Spaced-retrieval training. *Journal of Medical Speech-Language Pathology, 13,* 27–34.

Horley, K., Reid, A., & Burnham, D. (2010). Emotional prosody perception and production in dementia of the Alzheimer's type. *Journal of Speech, Language, and Hearing Research, 53,* 1132–1146.

Horner, J., Dawson, D., Heyman, A., & Fish, A. (1992). The usefulness of the Western aphasia battery for differential diagnosis of Alzheimer dementia and focal stroke syndromes: Preliminary evidence. *Brain and Language, 42,* 77–88.

Homer, J., Heipman, A., Aker, C., Kanter, J., & Royall, J. (1982, October). *Misnamings of Alzheimer's dementia compared to misnaming associated with left and right hemisphere stroke.* Paper presented at the Academy of Aphasia, New Paltz, NY.

Huber, S., & Shuttleworth, E. (1990). Neuropsychological assessment of subcortical dementia. In J. Cummings (Ed.), *Subcortical dementia* (pp. 71–86). New York, NY: Oxford University Press.

Huff, F. J., Corkin, S., & Growden, J. H. (1986). Semantic impairment and anomia in Alzheimer's disease. *Brain and Language, 28,* 235–249.

Huff, F., Mack, L., Mahlmann, J., & Greenberg, S. (1988). A comparison of lexical-semantic impairments in left hemisphere stroke and Alzheimer's disease. *Brain and Language, 34,* 262–278.

Johnson, K., & Bourgeois, M. (1998). Language intervention for patients with dementia attending a respite program. *Neurophysiology and Neurogenic Speech and Language Disorders, 8*(4). (Special Interest Division 2 Newsletter, 11–16). Rockville, MD: American Speech-Language-Hearing Association.

Kavé, G., & Levy, Y (2003). Morphology in picture descriptions provided by persons with Alzheimer's disease. *Journal of Speech, Language, and Hearing Research, 46,* 341–352.

Kavé, G., & Levy, Y (2004). Preserved morphological decomposition in persons with Alzheimer's disease. *Journal of Speech, Language, and Hearing Research, 47,* 835–847.

Kempler, D., Curtiss, S., & Jackson, C. (1987). Syntactic preservation in Alzheimer's disease. *Journal of Speech and Hearing Research, 30,* 343–350.

Kertesz, A. (1982). *The Western aphasia battery.* New York, NY: Gruen & Stratton.

Kim, E. S., Cleary, S. J., Hopper, T., Bayles, K. A., Mahendra, N., Azuma, T., & Rackley, A. (2006). Evidence-based practice recommendations for working with individuals with dementia: Group reminiscence therapy. *Journal of Medical Speech-Language Pathology, 14,* 23–34.

Kontiola, P., Laaksonen, R., Sulkava, R., & Erkinjunnti, T. (1990). Pattern of language impairment is different in Alzeimer's disease and multi-infarct dementia. *Brain and Language, 38,* 364–383.

MacDonald, M. C., Almor, A., Henderson, V. W., Kempler, D., & Andersen, E. S. (2001). Assessing working memory and language comprehension in Alzheimer's disease. *Brain and Language, 78,* 17–42.

Mahendra, N., Bayles, K., & Harris, F. (2005). Effect of presentation modality on immediate and delayed recall in individuals with Alzheimer's disease. *American Journal of Speech-Language Pathology, 14,* 144–155.

Mahendra, N., Hopper, T., Bayles, K., Azuma, T., Cleary, S., & Kim, E. (2006). Evidence-based practice recommendations for working with individuals with dementia: Montessori-based interventions. *Journal of Medical Speech-Language Pathology, 14,* 15–25.

Mahendra, N., Kim, E. S., Bayles, K. A., Hopper, T., Cleary, S. J., & Azuma, T. (2005). Evidence-based practice recommendations for working with individuals with dementia: Computer-assisted cognitive interventions (CACIs). *Journal of Medical Speech-Language Pathology, 13,* 35–44.

Marcie, P., Roudier, M., Goldblum, M., & Boller, F. (1993). Principal component analysis of language performances in Alzheimer's disease. *Journal of Communication Disorders, 26,* 53–63.

Martin, A., & Fedio, P. (1983). Word production and comprehension in Alzheimer's disease: The breakdown of semantic knowledge. *Brain and Language, 19,* 124–141.

Masterson, J., Druks, J., Kopelman, M., Clare, L., Garley, C., & Hayes, M. (2007). Selective naming (and comprehension) deficits in Alzheimer's disease. *Cortex, 43,* 921–934.

Mateer, C., & Sohlberg, M. (1988). A paradigm shift in memory rehabilitation. In H. Whitaker (Ed.), *Neuropsychological studies of non-focal brain injury: Dementia and closed head injury.* New York, NY: Springer.

Mathews, P., Obler, L., & Albert, M. (1994). Wernicke and Alzheimer on the language disturbances of dementia and aphasia. *Brain and Language, 46,* 439–462.

Mattis, S. (1976). Mental status examination for organic mental syndrome in the elderly patient. In R. Black & B. Karasu (Eds.), *Geriatric psychiatry* (pp. 77–121). New York, NY: Gruen & Stratton.

Mayo Clinic Health Letter (1995, November). *Dementia—When you suspect a loved one's problem.* Retrieved October 24, 2011 from: http:// www.pspinformation.com /disease/dementia/dementiax.shtml

McCabe, P., Sheard, C., & Code, C. (2007). Pragmatic skills in people with HIV/AIDS. *Disability and Rehabilitation, 29,* 1251–1260.

McCabe, P., Sheard, C., & Code, C. (2008). Communication impairment in the AIDS dementia complex (ADC): A case report. *Journal of Communication Disorders, 41,* 203–222.

McKhann, G., Drachman, D., Folstein, M., Katzman, R., Price, D., & Stadlan, E. (1984). Clinical diagnosis of Alzheimer's disease: Report of the NINCDS-ADRDA work group under the auspices of the Dept. of Health and Human Services task force on Alzheimer's disease. *Neurology, 34*, 939–944.

McNamara, P., Obler, L., Au, R., Durso, R., & Albert, M. (1992). Speech monitoring skills in Alzheimer's disease, Parkinson's disease, and normal aging. *Brain and Language, 42*, 38–51.

Mentis, M., Briggs-Whitaker, J., & Gramigna, G. (1995). Discourse topic management in senile dementia of the Alzheimer's type. *Journal of Speech and Hearing Research, 38*, 1054–1066.

Morris, R. (1987). Articulatory rehearsal in Alzheimer type dementia. *Brain and Language, 30*, 351–362.

Murdoch, B., Chenery, H., Wilks, V., & Boyle, R. (1987). Language disorders in dementia of the Alzheimer type. *Brain and Language, 31*, 122–137.

Nebes, R., & Boller, F. (1987). The use of language structure by demented patients in a visual search task. *Cortex, 28*, 87–98.

Neils, J., Roeltgen, D., & Constantinidou, F. (1995). Decline in homophone spelling associated with loss of semantic influence on spelling in Alzheimer's disease. *Brain and Language, 49*, 27–49.

Neils-Strunjas, J., Groves-Wright, K., Mashima, P., & Harnish, S. (2006). Dysgraphia in Alzheimer's disease: A review for clinical and research purposes. *Journal of Speech, Language, and Hearing Research, 49*, 1313–1330.

Nicholas, M., Obler, L., Albert, M., & Helm-Estabrooks, N. (1985). Empty speech in Alzheimer's disease and fluent aphasia. *Journal of Speech and Hearing Research, 28*, 405–410.

Obler, L., & Albert, M. (1981). Language in the elderly aphasic and in the dementing patient. In M. Sarno (Ed.), *Acquired aphasia* (pp. 385–398). New York, NY: Academic Press.

Obler, L., Albert, M., Estabrooks, N., & Nicholas, M. (1982, October). *Noninformative speech in Alzheimer's dementia and in Wernicke's aphasia.* Paper presented at the Academy of Aphasia, New Paltz, NY.

Orange, J. B., & Colton-Hudson, A. (1998). A case study of spousal communication education and training program for Alzheimer's disease. *Neurophysiology and Neurogenic Speech and Language disorders, 8*(4). (Special Interest Division 2 Newsletter, 22–29). Rockville, MD: American Speech-Language-Hearing Association.

Orange, J., Lubinski, R., & Higginbotham, D. (1996). Conversational repair by individuals with dementia of the Alzheimer's type. *Journal of Speech and Hearing Research, 39*, 881–895.

Patterson, J., & Chapey, R. (2008). Assessment of language disorders in adults. In R. Chapey (Ed.), *Language intervention strategies in aphasia and related neurogenic communication disorders* (pp. 64–160). Baltimore, MD: Lippincott Williams & Wilkins.

Rabins, P., Mace, N., & Lucas, M. (1982). The impact of dementia on the family. *Journal of the American Medical Association, 248*, 333–336.

Reisberg, B., Ferris, S., DeLeon, M., & Crook, T. (1982). The global deterioration scale (GDS): An instrument for the assessment of primary degenerative dementia (PDD). *American Journal of Psychiatry, 139*, 1136–1139.

Ripich, D., & Horner, J. (2004, April 27). The neurodegenerative dementias: Diagnoses and interventions. *The ASHA Leader.*

Ripich, D., & Terrell, B. (1988). Patterns of discourse, cohesion, and coherence in Alzheimer's disease. *Journal of Speech and Hearing Disorders, 53*, 8–15.

Rochon, E., Waters, G., & Caplan, D. (1994). Sentence comprehension in patients with Alzheimer's disease. *Brain and Language, 46*, 329–349.

Rochon, E., Waters, G., & Caplan, D. (2000). The relationship between measures of working memory and sentence comprehension in patients with Alzheimer's disease. *Journal of Speech, Language, and Hearing Research, 43*, 395–413.

Sander, A., Nakase-Richardson, R., Constantinidou, F., Wertheimer, J., & Paul, D. (2007). Memory assessment on an interdisciplinary rehabilitation team: A theoretically based framework. *American Journal of Speech-Language Pathology, 16*, 316–330.

Santo Pietro, M. J., & Boczko, F. (1998). The Breakfast Club: Results of a study examining the effectiveness of a multi-modality group communication treatment. *American Journal of Alzheimer's Disease, 13*, 146–159.

Santo Pietro, M. J., & Goldfarb, R. (1995). *Techniques for aphasia rehabilitation: Generating effective treatment* (TARGET). Vero Beach, FL: The Speech Bin.

Santo Pietro, M. J., & Goldfarb, R. (1985). Characteristic patterns of word association responses in institutionalized elderly with and without senile dementia. *Brain and Language, 26,* 230–243.

Shuttleworth, E., & Huber, S. (1988). The naming disorder of dementia of Alzheimer type. *Brain and Language, 34,* 222–234.

Small, J., Gutman, G., Makela, S., & Hillhouse, B. (2003). Effectiveness of communication strategies used by caregivers of persons with Alzheimer's disease during activities of daily living. *Journal of Speech, Language, and Hearing Research, 46,* 353–367.

Small, J., & Perry, J. (2005). Do you remember? How caregivers question their spouses who have Alzheimer's disease and the impact on communication. *Journal of Speech, Language, and Hearing Research, 48,* 125–136.

Smith, S., Murdoch, B., & Chenery, H. (1989). Semantic abilities in dementia of the Alzheimer's type. *Brain and Language, 36,* 314–324.

Tomoeda, C., Bayles, K., & Boone, D. (1990). Speech rate and syntactic complexity effects in the auditory comprehension of Alzheimer patients. *Journal of Communication Disorders, 23,* 151–190.

Vanhalle, C., Van der Linden, M., Belleville, S., & Gilbert, B. (1998). Putting names on faces: Use of a spaced retrieval strategy in a patient with dementia of the Alzheimer type. *Neurophysiology and Neurogenic Speech and Language Disorders, 8*(4). (Special Interest Division 2 Newsletter, 22–29). Rockville, MD: American Speech-Language-Hearing Association.

Volin, R., Goldfarb, R., Raphael, L., & Weinstein, B. (1990). Language, speech and hearing in Pick's disease: A case study. *Clinical Gerontologist, 10,* 93–98.

Wechsler, D. (1981). *Wechsler adult intelligence scale—Revised manual.* New York, NY: Psychological Corp.

Weinstein, B., & Amsel, L. (1986). Hearing loss and senile dementia in the institutionalized elderly. *Clinical Gerontology, 4,* 3–15.

Welland, R., Lubinski, R., & Higginbotham, D. J. (2002). Discourse comprehension test performance of elders with dementia of the Alzheimer type. *Journal of Speech, Language, and Hearing Research, 45,* 1175–1187.

Wilson, R., Kazniak, A., Bacon, L., Fox, J., & Kelly, M. (1982). Facial recognition memory in dementia. *Cortex, 18,* 329–336.

Zientz, J., Rackley, A., Chapman, S. B., Hopper, T., Mahendra, N., Kim, E. S., & Cleary, S. (2007). Evidence-based practice recommendations for dementia: Educating caregivers on Alzheimer's disease and training communication strategies. *Journal of Medical Speech-Language Pathology, 15,* 53–64.

Communication Disorders Associated with Traumatic Brain Injury

Definition and Etiology

Traumatic brain injury (TBI) occurs when a swiftly moving object hits the head (e.g., bullet wounds), or when the moving head strikes a stationary object (e.g., falls). Coelho (1997) noted that the damage following TBI is the result of primary and secondary damage, along with physiologic changes that can affect brain function. Primary damage is caused by the actual impact to the brain. Secondary damage is a consequence of such factors as infection, hypoxia, edema, elevated intracranial pressure, infarction, and hematomas. Physiologic changes can result from a number of metabolic disturbances such as hyperthermia, electrolyte imbalances, and damage to the hypothalamus or pituitary gland.

Open head injury (or penetrating brain injury) is where the skull is fractured or perforated, and the meninges are torn or lacerated. In open head injuries, primary damage usually occurs along the path of the penetrating object (shrapnel, stones, bullets, blunt or sharp instruments). Secondary damage can result from the effects of swelling, bleeding, infections, increased intracranial pressure, and scarring.

Closed head injury (or nonpenetrating brain injury) is where the meninges (three layers of tissue that cover the brain) remain intact. Trauma at the point of impact is known as *coup*. Injuries to the brain on the opposite side from the point of impact are known as *contrecoup*. In closed head injuries, primary damage usually occurs because the brain is involved in high levels of acceleration and deceleration (e.g., automobile and motorcycle accidents, falls). The rapid twisting and rotation of the brain can result in a shearing, stretching, or tearing of nerve fibers and is identified as diffuse axonal injury. As mentioned previously, secondary damage can occur as a result of such factors as infection, hypoxia (lack of oxygen), edema (swelling), elevation of intracranial pressure, infarction (cell death due to lack of oxygen in the brain), and hematomas (accumulation of blood).

Deep coma is a state of profound unconsciousness where the person cannot be aroused and makes no response to external stimuli (e.g., pain, sound, touch, smell). The lightest stages of coma are where the person responds to external stimuli but in a general and nonspecific manner (e.g., whole body or nonspecific motor movements). Coma can occur through interference with the reticular system of the brain, which is responsible for attention and alertness. Coma is more prevalent in closed head injury than in open head injury because of the widespread damage caused by diffuse axonal injury.

Traumatic brain injury (Adamovich, 1992; Coelho, 1997; Netsell & Lefkowitz, 1992; Sarno, Buonaguro, & Levita, 1986) can also cause aphasia, the communication disorders associated with right hemisphere damage, dysarthria, and apraxia of speech, all of which are discussed elsewhere in this text. The symptoms described in the next section typically result from diffuse brain damage.

The State of the Skull

Any injury causing an opening of the skull is classified as an open head, or penetrating injury. It is a visible injury located at a specific point in the brain. This visible injury may involve penetration or fracture, and may be the result of an accident, gunshot wound, or a variety of external factors. Closed head injury (CHI) occurs when the head accelerates and then rapidly decelerates (an *inertial* type of injury), or when it collides with another object (a *contact* type of injury). CHI may be further subdivided into temporal-causal categories. A *primary injury* occurs instantaneously at the moment of initial impact or acceleration, and *secondary injury* occurs as a result of the primary injury. There may also be a third category, *delayed injury*, which is more delayed than secondary injury (Gennarelli, 1993). This results from the pathophysiology of the primary event, involving interruption or elimination of afferent nerve function, cell dysfunction, and cell death.

The primary pathologies associated with CHI fall into *focal* and *diffuse* categories. The term *focal* means that one hemisphere of the brain or any part of one hemisphere is involved. Focal lesions usually accompany contact types of injury. Inertial types of injury may disrupt neurons at their axons. Resultant diffuse axonal injury of the white matter is the major type of diffuse traumatic pathology (Katz, 1992). Axonal damage occurring throughout the nervous system can disturb the motor subsystems that serve speech production and swallowing. It is common for speakers who are dysarthric secondary to CHI to have a wide array of abnormal speech features as well as physiological deficits in the mechanisms for speech production and swallowing (Theodoros, Murdoch, & Stokes, 1995).

Neuropathology of TBI

The frontal lobes are particularly vulnerable to injury because of their location at the front of the cranium, their large size, and their proximity to the greater wings of the sphenoid bone. Frontal lobe damage is the most common site of damage in closed head injury. There is no other part of the brain where damage can cause such a variety of symptoms. The frontal lobes are involved with motor function, memory, language, and problem solving, as well as with spontaneity, social control, initiation, judgment, and impulse control. There are well-known asymmetrical differences in the frontal lobes, particularly that of language-related movement, controlled by the left frontal lobe in most speakers. However, other parts of the brain are affected in TBI as well.

Inertial forces involving acceleration and deceleration often result in *coup-contrecoup* types of lesions. At the site of direct contact, or in the initial stage of inertia injury, translational forces produce movement of the brain in a horizontal plane (the *coup* stage). Inertial or rotational injury may be followed by angular forces. For example, in a motor vehicle accident, the head may pitch forward into the steering wheel or the windshield. Movement of the skull (brain case) is suddenly stopped, but the brain continues to pitch forward, crushing against the internal brain case as a result of translational forces. The brain then pitches back or at an angle to the site of contact, as a result of angular forces, causing the brain to bounce around the rough and jagged inner surfaces of the skull (the *contrecoup* stage). Therefore, if the site of the coup is the frontal lobe, the site of the contrecoup may be the occipital lobe. According to Adamovich (1997), damage frequently occurs about the diencephalic-midbrain junction.

The diencephalon is composed of the epithalamus, the dorsal thalamus, the subthalamus, and the hypothalamus. The midbrain develops from the middle of the three primary cerebral vesicles of the embryo; prominent cell groups include the motor nuclei of the trochlear and oculomotor nerves, the red nucleus, and the substantia nigra (McDonough, 1994).

Strain injuries are associated with the unrestricted head movement seen in inertial types of brain injury. Strains cause deformation of brain tissue, and are characterized by the direction of the inertial force. The subtypes are *tensile* strain, which indicates pulling apart, *compressive* strain, which involves pushing together, and *shear* strain, which involves parallel deforming forces (Katz, 1992).

Three separate pairs of processes work to injure the brain. In the first pair, *bruising* or *bleeding*, the force of impact when the brain is propelled against the internal brain case may cause blood vessels to rupture. In the resultant hemorrhage, or uncontrolled release of blood, further damage occurs. As the hard and brittle brain case will not expand, pressure of the blood against the softer brain tissue may cause *necrosis* (cell death) in some areas and *stunning* in larger areas. Stunning occurs when neural connections are severed and areas of the brain that have not been destroyed cease to function. The purpose of rehabilitation will be to rewire the stunned portions of the brain to restore function. Clearly, our understanding of how to accomplish this is inexact.

Brain tissue, which is gelatinous in consistency, has a very small degree of rigidity, making it susceptible to damage from even slight distortions of shape. The second pair of processes, *tearing* or *shearing*, may occur in both contact and inertial types of brain injury. Translational acceleration occurs in a contact injury, say, a blow to the back of the head. The initial impact is similar to that which occurs from a poorly hammered nail, where energy transfer causes weblike cracks to appear in the wall. Next, because of different densities in the brain and skull, the brain will fail to keep up with the faster-moving skull, and will be dragged forward. The brain abrades against the rough internal surfaces of the brain case, is suddenly stopped (say, against the frontal calvarium), and the brain and skull undergo several more oscillations before reaching zero velocity.

The third pair of processes involves pressure injuries from *swelling* or *edema*, which occur on CHI but not in skull fractures, where pressure may be released. Brain swelling is caused by an increase in fluid content following the trauma. As with intracranial bleeding, the brain case will not expand to accommodate the extra volume, so pressure is exerted on the brain by its increased size. Intracranial pressure is elevated because of the increased mass of the swollen brain, which decreases the protective capacity of the cerebrospinal fluid within the finite intracranial space, and which, left unchecked, may lead to brain herniation (Coelho, 1997). One explanation for the survival of Rep. Gabrielle Giffords of Arizona, after she was shot in the head on January 8, 2011, is that surgeons removed (and later reattached) a portion of her skull, which allowed her swelling brain to avoid additional intracranial pressure.

Symptoms

The communication disorder discussed here is a condition that can fit into the category labeled by American Speech-Language-Hearing Association (ASHA, 1991) as cognitive-communicative disorders. Adamovich (1992), Brookshire (2007), Coelho (1997), Hartley (1994), and Ylvisaker, Szekeres, and Feeney (2008) have elaborated on the origin of this communication breakdown. Factors to consider are cognitive, executive, linguistic, and behavioral. TBI may also lead to dysphagia.

Swallowing Impairments

About one-fourth of TBI survivors exhibit some form of dysphagia, defined as pain or difficulty in the act of swallowing. Traumatic injury to the brain, brainstem, or cranial nerves (especially Cranial IX, the glossopharyngeal, which innervates the cricopharyngeal or upper esophageal sphincter) may result in oral-level, pharyngeal-level, or oropharyngeal dysphagia. Note that similar characteristics may be found in poststroke dysphagia. Videofluoroscopy remains the gold standard of evaluation, as the bedside examination may lack both specificity and sensitivity (Baylow et al., 2009). The most frequent swallowing impairments, in descending order, tend to be delayed triggering of the swallow response, reduced tongue control, and reduced pharyngeal transit (Logemann, 1997). After the acute onset of TBI, spontaneous recovery will vary, based on the degree and severity of brain damage, as well as coexisting or subsequent medical complications (Musson, 1998). In addition, coexisting cognitive impairments may interfere with intervention plans aimed at self-feeding, and respiratory impairments may interfere with the ability to produce reflexive, volitional, and effective coughing.

Cognitive Functioning

Cognitive functioning involves orientation, arousal, attention, speed of processing, memory (see the section on communication disorders associated with dementia for further discussion of memory), abstract reasoning, and visuospatial perception. Because attention and memory problems are so prevalent in patients with TBI, an expanded description is presented in the following paragraphs.

In seeking to provide guidance for treatment of impaired self-regulation after TBI, Kennedy and Coelho (2005) included an update of the concepts of executive functions, metacognition, and self-regulation. From the perspective of the "self," metacognition is the highest level in the cognitive system. The prefix "meta-" refers to the ability to view, observe, and assess other processes; the concept of metacognition can be defined as thinking about thinking. Subsystems would include metamemory, metalinguistics, and metacomprehension. Metacognition is also used for self-monitoring and self-control during an activity.

Executive functions give feedback up to the self and down to more basic processes, such as self-regulation. The cognitive processes that determine behavior that is purposeful and directed to goals are the foundations of executive functions, which may also be seen as fostering an orderly execution of functions of daily living (Kennedy & Coelho, 2005, p. 243). Specific examples are offered in the section on executive functioning below.

After traumatic brain injury, individuals may have difficulty starting (initiating) and stopping (inhibiting), as well as shifting and adjusting. In addition, these individuals may show impaired self-monitoring and self-control. A common goal of intervention is for the individual to gain strategies that generalize outside the therapy room. Interventions that focus on self-awareness and self-regulation often address problems in memory, learning, and problem solving.

A fundamental assumption of attention training is that individual aspects of cognition may be isolated and targeted with exercises (Sohlberg et al., 2003). These cognitive aspects include the following: vigilance, or ability to sustain attention over time; information capacity; shift of attention; speed of processing; and ability to screen distractions. A comprehensive search of attention remediation literature (Sohlberg et al., 2003) focused on participants, components of attention training, outcomes of intervention, methodologies, and clinically applicable trends. The six studies (three Class I and three Class II) that met criteria of contributing to evidence-based practice in TBI reported no improvements in attention training during the acute rehabilitation phase, although methodological concerns qualify this conclusion.

Confounding issues included presence of posttraumatic amnesia, level of agitation, confusion, and fatigue.

In reviewing databases for articles published more recently (after 1999), another 27 articles were identified and evaluated as Class II level of research (Sohlberg et al., 2003). A commercially available attention training program facilitated (re)learning of specific skills, but not improvement in attention functions. Interpreting the evidence is further confounded by heterogeneity and subject variability, varied settings and practitioners, and differences in operational definitions regarding meaningful change.

Overall, certain aspects of attention training may be helpful for some adults with TBI. Attention training may best be used in combination with self-reflective logs, anticipation/prediction activities, feedback, and strategy training (Sohlberg et al., 2003, p. 36).

Mateer (1996) reviewed the various models of attention that can be used to assess and treat disorders of the attentional system such as TBI. One of them is the clinical model of attention (Sohlberg & Mateer, 1989). The model is hierarchical, with each level viewed as more complex and requiring effective functioning at the previous level. Components of the model are as follows:

1. *Focused attention.* This is the ability to respond discretely to specific visual, auditory, or tactile stimuli (e.g., looking at a glass globe in which snow or confetti moves when the globe is turned upside down). This level does not imply purposefulness of response.
2. *Sustained attention.* This is the ability to maintain a consistent behavioral response during continuous and repetitive activity (e.g., matching playing cards correctly according to number, color, or suit). This level incorporates concepts of vigilance.
3. *Selective attention.* This is the ability to maintain a behavioral or cognitive set in the face of distracting or competing stimuli (e.g., paying attention to the clinician even though a television is playing or other people are in the background). This level incorporates the concept of "freedom from distractibility."
4. *Alternating attention.* This is the capacity for mental flexibility that allows one to shift his or her focus of attention and move between tasks that have different cognitive requirements or require different behavior responses (e.g., attending correctly to the clinician, then properly responding to a phone call or visitor who interrupts, and then correctly resuming with the clinician). This level controls which information will be selectively attended to and incorporates the concept of shifting an established set easily.
5. *Divided attention.* This is the ability to respond simultaneously to multiple tasks or multiple task demands (e.g., attending correctly to the clinician while keeping track of a child in the same room). At this level, two or more behavioral responses may be required, or two or more kinds of stimuli may need to be monitored.

Memory is an essential aspect of cognitive functioning. TBI patients are quite susceptible to pretraumatic and posttraumatic amnesia.

Pretraumatic amnesia is the loss of memory of events occurring before the trauma. Often the patient cannot remember the minutes, hours, or even days before the injury. The memory loss can last for up to a year, sometimes longer. As the patient begins to recover, the memory loss preceding the trauma gets shorter in terms of the time period mentioned. Pretraumatic amnesia may be caused by problems with the retrieval processes.

Posttraumatic amnesia refers to the loss of memory of events occuring after the trauma. The memory loss can last for several minutes, hours, days, months, and in some cases years. As the patient begins to recover, memory of day-to-day events slowly becomes better. Posttraumatic amnesia is the more serious problem of the two because it involves everyday activities and appears to be a problem involving storage of memory processes.

Executive Functioning

Executive functioning includes goal setting, awareness of self, initiation of goal-directed behavior, sequencing, planning, organizing, monitoring and controlling behavior, problem solving, and self-evaluation. Some examples of executive functioning would be planning one's daily activities (e.g., getting dressed); how one gets to the doctor; the steps used in preparing foods; arranging items from large to small or vice versa; arranging items from most to least important; putting theme cards in a logical sequence (e.g., supermarket shopping from start to finish; taking a cab from beginning to end of destination); looking at the success or failure in performing a particular task and knowing why it succeeded or failed and the steps needed to rectify the failure; and so forth. Douglas (2010) found a significant association between executive impairment and the pragmatic communication difficulties experienced by 43 individuals with severe TBI. (See the section on communication disorders associated with dementia for additional comments on executive dysfunction.)

Linguistic Functioning

A linguistic functioning problem can occur because of a lesion in a language area of the brain; this would be called *aphasia*. In aphasia, communication is impaired because the components of language (phonologic, morphologic, syntactic, and semantic) are directly interfered with.

Linguistic functioning problems also can be caused by a lesion or lesions in parts of the brain that control cognitive and executive functioning and behavior; this would be called a *cognitive-communicative disorder*. In a cognitive-communicative disorder, communication is impaired because the components of cognition (orientation, arousal, attention, speed of processing, memory, abstract reasoning, and visuospatial perception), executive functioning, and behavior are directly interfered with, and this in turn indirectly interferes with language. For example, a patient with aphasia will have an auditory comprehension problem due to a lesion in Wernicke's or other areas, and will respond erroneously because he did not understand the instruction (e.g., "Point to the window"). A patient with a cognitive-communicative disorder will have an auditory comprehension problem and give an erroneous response because from among several possibilities, her attention span for the auditory stimulus (e.g., "Point to the window") was limited or wandering.

Darley (1982), Halpern, Darley, and Brown (1973), and Wertz (1985) have called this condition the *language of confusion*, where, because of deficits in cognition, the patient usually manifests an inability to follow directions, bizarre and irrelevant responses (see Drummond, 1986), unawareness of the inappropriateness of his or her responses, and confabulations (a fictitious story reported through oral and/or written expression). Dalla Barba (1993) has reviewed the different patterns of confabulation and noted that confabulation is different from lying, where there is intention to deceive. (See the section on communication disorders associated with right hemisphere damage for additional discussion of confabulation.)

Geschwind (1967) described the syndrome of "nonaphasic misnaming," which typically occurs in disorders that diffusely involve the nervous system, especially when the disturbance comes on fairly rapidly. Characteristically the errors tend to "propagate." Thus the patient, if asked where he or she is, may say, "In a bus," and may continue by identifying the examiner as the bus driver, those around her as passengers, and her bed as one being used by the driver for resting.

It is usually obvious, once a sequence of questions is asked, that ordinary aphasic misnaming is readily ruled out. In aphasic misnaming there is no tendency to propagation, although perseveration (e.g., repetition of the same incorrect word) occurs frequently. The connected or propagated character of the errors may show up particularly in relation to the hospital and the patient's illness. The patient may call the hospital a "hotel," the doctors "bellboys," and the nurses "chambermaids," and will not accept correction.

Stengel (1964) stated that people in confusional states, when called upon to name objects, do not respond in the same way as adults with aphasia, who say, "I know what it is, but I can't find the word." Confused patients boldly and sometimes recklessly improvise and produce words on the spur of the moment. These words may show effects of perseveration, slang, and other associations.

Weinstein, Lyerly, Cole, and Ozer (1966) used the term "jargon aphasia" to describe subjects who had bilateral brain involvement and showed confabulation, particularly about the onset of the illness as the reason for coming to the hospital; disorientation for place and time; unawareness of errors; and lack of any catastrophic response.

From the studies cited, it is obvious that among the language skills, the factor of impairment of relevance is a key differentiating point (Halpern et al., 1973). In working with a patient after TBI, one of the authors found the following to be typical examples of irrelevant responses: "A measure of violence" was given as the definition for bargain. "Should watch out for mailboxes, should watch out for people, should watch out for papers" was a response to the question, "What three things should every good citizen do?" In response to this same question, another TBI patient said, "Have your tires checked, know a good auto shop, buy a Ford, and go to Sears."

Hartley (1994) and Ylvisaker et al. (2008) reviewed a number of studies about the language deficits that occur after TBI. These studies have revealed that (1) TBI can produce deficits in all four modalities and at all levels of severity, as does aphasia; (2) there are fewer cases of aphasia after TBI in acute care facilities than there are in rehabilitation centers; (3) the predominant kind of aphasia after TBI is fluent and anomic; (4) language therapy for aphasia caused by TBI is generally the same as for aphasia caused by cerebrovascular accident (CVA).

Behavioral Functioning

Behavioral functioning impairment can manifest itself as irritability and aggression, anxiety, depression, decreased initiation, disinhibition, and social inappropriateness. (See "Treatment for Mild Impairment" in this section.)

Diagnosis

Diagnostic procedures for determining the communication disorders associated with traumatic brain injury can involve (1) establishing background information, (2) giving a neurologic evaluation, (3) testing or assessing cognition and language, and (4) employing information about differential diagnosis.

In accordance with the World Health Organization's International Classification of Functioning categories (WHO, 2001), Coelho, Ylvisaker, and Turkstra (2005) proposed functional assessment of activities and contexts for planning and monitoring clinical intervention in TBI. Shortcomings of standardized testing primarily related to the disparity seen in patients' good performance on office-bound language testing, compared to the more severe dysfunction observed in daily living activities. The authors reported this dissociation as a feature of frontal lobe injury.

Among the 28 different nonstandardized tasks or procedures reported in a survey of speech-language pathologists (SLPs) working with individuals with TBI (Coelho et al., 2005), most used subtests from published assessment batteries. Results of aphasia batteries overestimated communicative performance, probably because of the limited scope and ceiling effect of these tests, which were not intended to assess subtle deficits demonstrated by many individuals with TBI. There were some consistent findings regarding impairments in:

1. Initiating and maintaining conversational topics; and
2. Conveying content during conversation, including word retrieval deficits, transfer of information, and response adequacy.

The nonstandardized tests most useful for identifying conversational impairments were those that measured content and topic management.

In establishing guidelines for clinical assessments of TBI, the Academy of Neurologic Communication Disorders and Sciences (ANCDS) committee (Turkstra et al., 2005, pp. 9–10) focused on two questions:

1. What tests can or should be used by SLPs for evaluating and assessing communication abilities in individuals with TBI?
2. What unique contribution does the SLP make in the process of interdisciplinary evaluation?

The committee gathered information by surveying SLPs engaged in clinical practice with individuals with TBI, surveying test publishers and distributors, reviewing test manuals, reviewing published literature appearing in four databases, and reviewing published expert opinion.

Most tests showed strengths in content and face validity, but weaknesses in other elements of reliability and validity. For example, a majority of tests did not meet strict criteria for interrater reliability, internal consistency, and test–retest reliability. They were also much more likely to show concurrent validity than predictive validity. Overall, despite some strengths in content validity, many of the tests designed for and administered to individuals with TBI were weak psychometrically, lacking established relationships between test scores and important measures of outcomes (Turkstra et al., 2005, p. 23).

Assessing cognitive-communication disorders in individuals after TBI is challenging for SLPs. The clinical population tends to be heterogeneous, showing complex constellations of strengths and limitations (Turkstra, Coelho, & Ylvisaker, 2005, p. 216). Evaluation addresses the following questions:

1. Does the individual with TBI have a cognitive-communication problem?
2. If there is such a problem, what are its characteristics?
3. What are the implications of the test results?
4. How do the test results inform treatment?

The ANCDS writing committee (Turkstra, Coelho, & Ylvisaker, 2005) reviewed 84 tests recommended by practicing SLPs and 40 tests recommended by publishers and distributors. After eliminating tests that did not mention TBI in the test manual, 31 tests for children, adolescents, and adults remained.

Most experts agreed that standardized tests constitute only one component of an evaluation, leading the committee (Turkstra, Coelho, & Ylvisaker, 2005, p. 220) to recommend the following:

1. Use caution when using existing standardized tests to evaluate individuals with TBI.
2. In addition to standardized testing, evaluate the individual's preinjury characteristics (based on a reliable informant), stage of development and recovery, and demands and contexts for communication in the individual's activities of daily living.
3. Collaborate with other professionals when considering how to interpret cognitive impairment level based on tests.

Establishing Background Information and Giving the Neurologic Evaluation

These procedures can be found at the beginning of the "Diagnosis" part of the section on aphasia.

Tests for Assessing Cognition and Language

Screening tools are evaluated according to two criteria: sensitivity, which refers to identification of mild through severe forms of the impairment; and specificity, which refers to identification of only the target population (e g., individuals with cognitive impairment), as opposed to related populations (e.g., individuals with language impairment). The most commonly used cognitive screening tool is the *Mini-Mental State Examination* (MMSE) (Folstein, Folstein, & McHugh, 1975), which assesses language and memory skills. It is convenient, but not sensitive to mild cognitive impairment, and it is influenced by age, socioeconomic status, and level of education.

The *Montreal Cognitive Assessment* (MoCA) (Aggarwal & Kean, 2010) shows promise as a more sensitive screening tool for mild–moderate cognitive impairment. However, it takes twice as long to administer as the MMSE, and is based on data from only 50 patients. It has been reported to have high sensitivity and specificity for the detection of mild cognitive impairment, with a score of less than 25 as the optimal cutoff point for a diagnosis for mild cognitive impairment. The authors' (Aggarwal & Kean, 2010) claim of high specificity is questionable, as patients who were medically unstable, had aphasia, refused, or were from a non-English-speaking background were excluded from the study.

Depending upon which stage of recovery the TBI patient is in, different diagnostic procedures can be used. If the patient is severely impaired, the *Glasgow Coma Scale* (Jennett & Teasdale, 1981) evaluates eye-opening abilities, motor responses, and verbal responses. Eye-opening items include: (1) opens eyes spontaneously (best score), (2) opens eyes to verbal command, (3) opens eyes in response to pain, and (4) no response (worst score). Motor response items include: (1) obeys verbal commands (best score), (2) attempts to pull examiner's hand away during painful stimulation, (3) moves limb away from painful stimulus, (4) flexes body in response to pain, (5) extends limbs, becomes rigid in response to pain, and (6) no response (worst score). Verbal response items include: (1) converses and is oriented (best score), (2) converses but is disoriented, (3) utters intelligible words but does not make sense, (4) produces unintelligible sounds, and (5) no response (worst score).

Another instrument is the *Rancho Los Amigos Scale of Cognitive Levels* (Hagen, 1984), which evaluates the patient's cognitive and behavioral course of recovery. The test measures the patient's responses to stimuli that range from Level I–No Response (no response to pain, touch, sound, or sight) to Level VIII–Purposeful and Appropriate (responds appropriately in most situations, can generalize new learning across situations, does not require daily supervision, may have poor tolerance for stress, and may exhibit some abstract reasoning disabilities).

Many patients with TBI suffer from posttraumatic amnesia. The *Galveston Orientation and Amnesia Test* (GOAT) (Levin, O'Donnell, & Grossman, 1979) can be used to assess the patient's memory, amnesia, and orientation. The memory portion evaluates short-term memory for words, the alphabet, and counting backward. The amnesia portion asks the patient to tell his or her name, place of birth, age, and where he or she lives. The orientation portion checks the patient's knowledge of time (year, month, day, hour) and place (present location).

Currently, there are two tests that can evaluate the TBI patient's cognitive and linguistic abilities. One is the *Brief Test of Head Injury* (BTHI) (Helm-Estabrooks & Hotz, 1990), which is designed to assess orientation and attention, following commands, linguistic organization, reading comprehension, naming, memory, and visuospatial skills. Items are scored by type of response (linguistic, gestural), and communicative quality of the response. The other is the *Scales of Cognitive Ability for Traumatic Brain Injury* (SCATBI) (Adamovich & Henderson, 1992), which is constructed to evaluate perception/discrimination, orientation, organization, recall, and reasoning.

Although most batteries that assess cognition are conceived by individuals in other professions, the two preceding tests were designed by speech-language pathologists. It is quite important to know not only for assessment, but for the treatment that follows, whether the problem in communication is due to a direct language impairment (aphasia) or an indirect language problem due to an impairment in cognition that impedes communication in a certain way.

Finally, the *Ross Information Processing Assessment* (RIPA-2) (Ross-Swain, 1996) can be used to test communicative and cognitive functioning (for additional description see the section on communication disorders associated with right hemisphere damage), and the *Discourse Comprehension Test* (Brookshire and Nicholas, 1997) assesses both listening and reading comprehension (see "Diagnosis" in the section on aphasia).

Differential Diagnosis

The findings of the following studies can be used to aid in the language diagnosis. The language findings of the study by Halpern et al. (1973) indicated that the group with confused language was differentiated from the other groups (aphasia, generalized intellectual impairment, and apraxia of speech) by impairment in reading comprehension, writing words to dictation, and relevance.

Groher (1977) studied the memory and language skills of 14 patients who had suffered closed head trauma. He noted that initially his subjects manifested both aphasia (a reduced capacity to interpret and formulate language symbols) and confused language skills (faulty short-term memory, mistaken reasoning, inappropriate behavior, poor understanding of the environment, and disorientation). After a period of 1 month, both language and memory skills improved significantly. Continued improvement was made after 1 month and for up to 4 months in both language and memory abilities, although deficits were still present in both areas at 4 months.

Comparing a single patient with the language of confusion with 10 aphasic patients, Mills and Drummond (1980) found that naming ability could be used as a discriminating factor between the two disorders. The factors of error rate and response time in naming tasks were more variable in the patient with the language of confusion than in the aphasic patients. The greatest error rate and the longest response time took place in the early stages of recovery in the patient with confused language. In the latter stages of recovery, error rate and response time were close to normal. The aphasic patients were consistent throughout this time period. A greater percentage of semantically unrelated responses was found in the patient with confused language than in the aphasia group.

In another study of a single patient with the language of confusion, Drummond (1986) noted that a monologue context ("Tell me how you would fry an egg") was more effective for observing linguistic irrelevancy than was picture description. The monologue context provides a topic and requires the speaker to introduce different referents, expand on each of these referents, and then arrange them in a temporal hierarchy utilizing the past, present, and future. She also found that total utterance and impaired topic-focus organization were probably the most valid variables for describing linguistic irrelevancy. Both of these factors diminish progressively with physiological recovery.

Ehrlich (1988) found that in picture description tasks, adults with head injury were more verbose and slower than normal subjects in imparting information. Liles, Coelho, Duffy, and Zalagens (1989) observed that adults with closed head injury were differentiated from normal subjects by story generation and story retelling tasks. Tompkins et al. (1990) found that injury severity and existence and severity of previous psychological, physical, or cognitive disorders were the best predictors of recovery for adults with closed head injury. In children with closed head injury, parental marital status was the best predictor.

Gruen, Frankle, and Schwartz (1990) measured the word-fluency generation tasks (animal naming and single-letter–based word generation) of 218 closed head injury subjects, and noted significant differences in response quality and quantity relative to normal subjects. Peach (1992) found that perceptual functioning, general language abilities, and mental efficiency were the major factors underlying neuropsychological test performance in chronic severe TBI.

Campbell and Dollaghan (1990, 1995) conducted two studies to examine the speaking rate following TBI in nine children and adolescents. Study I (1990) showed that the average speaking rate of the group with TBI was slower than that of the age-matched control subjects. Study II (1995) showed that articulatory speed and linguistic processing speed may contribute independently to slowed speaking rates more than one year after TBI.

Turkstra (2005) found that there were no significant differences between participants in the TBI group and their typically developing peer group in eye-to-face gaze while listening or speaking, in average gaze times, but the within-group variability was significantly greater in the TBI group. Le, Coelho, Mozeiko, and Grafman (2011) evaluated a new measure of story narrative performance. They combined organizational (story grammar) and completeness measures and tested 24 adults with acquired brain injuries and 46 typically developing adults, and found significant group differences on both story grammar and story completeness. They concluded that the combination of measures provided a more accurate depiction of discourse performance than either measure alone, and suggested that this measure is sensitive, is reliable, and has potential utility for investigating discourse deficits in clinical populations.

Therapy

Kennedy and Turkstra (2006) admonished SLPs to study the role of good judgment in clinical practice as rigorously as we do in clinical trials (p. 158). Both require logic, knowledge, and experience to make good decisions.

A recent review (Kennedy et al., 2008) focused on intervention for improving everyday problem solving, planning, organizing, and multitasking. Using several databases, more than 2500 published articles were identified in these areas. Most were excluded because they were not intervention studies with objective outcomes, leaving 15 quantitative intervention studies. The strength of evidence was evaluated as Class I for five studies, Class II for three, and Class III for seven. Treatment dosage varied from two 15-minute sessions to 48 hours, with therapy provided individually in most cases (87%). Treatment outcomes were classified according to the International Classification Framework for Enablement (WHO, 2001) at the impairment level and at the activity/participation level.

Goals of intervention varied according to the aspect of executive function targeted. All studies focused on some aspect of problem solving, planning, organizing, and multitasking, but some specifically addressed social or behavioral problem solving; time management; goal management; decision making; self-regulation; verbal reasoning; complex activities with cues; organization strategies during functional activities; or dual-task training. Intervention approaches tended to include metacognitive strategy instruction, including self-monitoring, self-recording of performance, basing strategy decisions on goals, and adjusting or modifying plans based on self-assessment or external feedback (Kennedy et al., 2008, p. 35).

Nearly all studies reported positive treatment outcomes immediately following the experimental interventions. Positive activity/participation treatment effects were also reported in most studies. A majority of studies (60%) also reported positive maintenance effects, that is, generalization to untrained tasks and contexts. In other words, there was strong evidence of efficacy of treatment.

The first goal of therapy is to inform the patient and the caretaker(s) about the nature and the consequences of the disorder.

The TBI patient will show cognitive impairment directly related to the mild (or late), moderate (or middle), and severe (or early) stages of the condition. The language components are affected according to the stage of the disorder.

Ylvisaker et al. (2008) noted the stages of recovery for the CHI patient, which falls under the heading of TBI. These stages are based on the *Rancho Los Amigos Scale of Cognitive Levels* (Hagen, 1984), an eight-stage recovery scale. The early stage (severe impairment) starts with the first generalized responses to the environment (inconsistent responses to pain, touch, sound, or sight) and ends with stimulus-specific responses (e.g., visual tracking, localizing to sound), recognition of some common objects, and comprehension of some simple commands. The middle stage (moderate impairment) starts with heightened alertness and increased activity, along with confusion and agitation, and ends with improved orientation and behavior that is generally goal-directed and can consistently follow simple directions. The late stage (mild impairment) starts with adequate orientation (although insight, judgment, and problem solving may be poor) and performance of daily routine tasks in a highly familiar environment (usually done in an automatic, robot-like manner) and ends with the patient responding appropriately in most situations and generalizing new learning across most situations (some abstract reasoning abilities may still be impaired). Patients do not require daily supervision but may have poor tolerance for stress.

The second goal of therapy is to provide the appropriate treatment approaches and techniques.

Efficacy of Therapy for the Communication Disorders Associated with Traumatic Brain Injury

Coelho, DeRuyter, and Stein (1996) reviewed several treatment efficacy studies of cognitive rehabilitation. In their review, they found that there are a number of treatment techniques that have been successfully applied to deficits of attention, memory, and executive function in various TBI patients. Patients with more severe cognitive-communicative deficits can receive treatment directed toward the development of compensatory strategies, such as the use of memory aids (e.g., appointment book, alarm watch, or a detailed daily schedule).

For patients with profound deficits, the treatment may best be focused on environmental modifications or the arrangement of permanent support systems (e.g., training caretakers to prompt the patient during daily living activities). Single-subject, multiple baseline designs are well suited for studying the efficacy of these treatment approaches to cognitive rehabilitation. Social skills retraining, timing of treatment during recovery, treatment location and its effectiveness (e.g., hospital, home, school, work), and the benefits of early intervention were also stressed.

Coelho et al. (1996) noted that functional gains were realized in receptive and expressive language, speech production, reading, writing, and cognition for TBI patients receiving speech-language treatment. Inpatients receiving cognitive rehabilitation returned to productive living at the same rate as a less severely impaired group who had not received treatment. When patients with similar severity were compared, those who had received cognitive rehabilitation had better average cost outcomes than those not receiving rehabilitation services.

Fraas and Calvert (2009) investigated the factors leading to successful recovery and productive lifestyles after acquired brain injury (ABI). After interviews of 31 survivors of ABI, the following four major themes emerged: (1) development of social support networks (e.g., support of friends/family, initial loss of friends), (2) grief and coping (e.g., denial, frustration, anger), (3) acceptance of injury and redefinition of self (e.g., vocational adjustment, productivity), and (4) empowerment (e.g., motivation, making own decisions and setting goals). The authors stated that stories of inspiration such as these may serve to provide hope and motivation to others as they progress through the recovery process.

Cognitive Rehabilitation

When the ANCDS writing committee for TBI searched the literature for evidence-based practice recommendations (Sohlberg, Ehlhardt, & Kennedy, 2005), they included the fields of special education and neuropsychology. They specifically addressed instruction of individuals with cognitive-communication disorders. Several models were subjected to experimental scrutiny. *Direct instruction* explicitly addressed teaching such subjects as reading, mathematics, and social skills. *Strategy-based instruction* emphasized self-monitoring and monitoring one's own thinking. A *combined model* included both of the above, and *nondirect* or *nonstrategy instruction* did not specify methods, but addressed reinforcement and modeling.

A review of instructional literature over 12 years identified errorless learning as the focus of more than 30 relevant studies. In errorless learning, errors are eliminated, or at least substantially reduced, during the acquisition phase of learning. Components of errorless learning tend to include the following: breaking down tasks into small steps; modeling before asking for the target response or task; discouraging guessing; correcting errors immediately; and fading prompts. In contrast, errorful learning is based on trial and error or discovery, which may include guessing. Some techniques that facilitate errorless learning follow.

Frequent practice of correct responses, repeated until accurate performance is achieved, sounds like drill work, because it is. This may also be called *massed practice*. In distributed practice, or spaced retrieval, individuals with severe memory loss practice successful recall of information over expanded time intervals. Perhaps surprisingly, distributed rather than massed practice has been shown to be better for individuals with dementia or aphasia to remember specifically, personally relevant information (for a review see Sohlberg et al., 2005). In chaining, new steps are linked sequentially with a previous step. Chaining may go forward and backward. For example, in the method of vanishing cues, a form of backward chaining, targeted information is presented right away, and then faded, one cue at a time, after each successful recall trial.

Coelho (1997) stated that the treatment of cognitive-communicative disorders that arises from TBI is known as *cognitive rehabilitation*. Cognitive rehabilitation embodies a treatment program directed at raising functional abilities in everyday activities. This is done primarily by improving the patient's ability to process and interpret incoming information. The two approaches to cognitive rehabilitation are restorative and compensatory.

The restorative approach is based on neuronal growth through repetitive exercises and drilling of neuronal circuits. The compensatory approach is based on circumventing the impaired functions. Usually, the restorative approach is used first, and if that does not work, the compensatory approach is implemented. After a while, these approaches can be used simultaneously in therapy to achieve functional abilities in everyday life.

Treatment for Severe Impairment (Early Stage)

It is not within the scope of practice for the SLP to treat the personality changes common after severe traumatic brain injury. However, behavior and social changes that accompany communication problems may need to be addressed. This becomes even more complicated because risky and impulsive behavior, which may predispose an individual to traumatic brain injury, may be a preexisting problem (Ylivsaker, Turkstra, & Coelho, 2005).

The ANCDS committee (Ylvisaker et al., 2005, 2007), in reviewing 59 nonpharmacological studies of behavioral intervention for individuals with behavior problems following TBI, concluded that there is a reasonably strong evidence base for efficacy of treatment. They recommended that SLPs should consider behavioral interventions as a practice guideline (Ylvisaker et al., 2005, p. 260).

The two approaches to treatment are applied behavior analysis (ABA) and positive behavior supports (PBS). Both approaches use the operant conditioning paradigm, where $S^D \rightarrow R \rightarrow S^{r+}$ or$^-$. S^D, the antecedent event, sets the occasion for the occurrence of a performance (R), which leads to a consequent event (S^r), which may be positive or aversive. In a behavioral chain, the first consequent event (S^{r1}) can be seen as being identical to the second antecedent event (S^{D2}), so that more complex behaviors can be structured, with behavioral approaches focused on both immediate and more remote supports (see, for example, Goldfarb, 1981). Traditional ABA, focusing on the last part of the operant conditioning paradigm, manages maladaptive behaviors through deliberate manipulation of consequent events (sometimes called "reinforcement" or "payoffs"). Behaviors should increase or decrease based on positive or aversive payoffs. The PBS approach, which emphasizes the first part of the operant conditioning paradigm, manages and modifies immediate and remote antecedent events. The goal is for the individual with TBI to acquire repertoires of behavior leading to success in social contexts (Ylvisaker et al., 2005, 2007).

Because of problems primarily in arousal, attention, orientation, and pretraumatic and posttraumatic amnesia, communicative functioning can be very limited. Treatment is geared, on a basic functional level, toward stimulating those problem areas. For early stage or slow-to-recover patients, Ansell (1991) suggested the following sensory stimulation examples (with some adaptation):

1. Present visual stimuli (e.g., a glass globe with "snow" or confetti that moves when the globe is turned upside down, or a colorful pinwheel) to engage the patient's attention and facilitate visual tracking.
2. Give orientation information to patients, including greeting them by name; identifying the clinician by name and title; and telling patient the day, date, name of facility in which the patient resides, the length of time the patient has been there, and the reason for his or her placement at the facility.
3. Present multisensory stimulation to facilitate auditory comprehension (e.g., put a soft ball in the patient's hand and aid in squeezing the ball while saying "Squeeze the ball").
4. Present tactile/gustatory stimulation to the lips via flavored popsicles, to facilitate purposeful oral movement and awareness/recognition of flavors and temperature. Olfactory stimuli (e.g., extracts, perfumes, colognes, spices, soaps, vinegar) and additional

gustatory stimuli (e.g., extracts, lemon, vinegar) have also been recommended to see if the patient consistently reacts and to assess the nature of that reaction.

If the patient is progressing in recovery, the clinician can begin the early application of environmental modification. Ylvisaker et al. (2008) suggested some forms of environmental modification. These activities include developing and practicing routines to structure the patient's day (e.g., time to get up, shower, dress, eat breakfast, therapy appointments). Visual cues such as pictures of personnel, calendars, datebooks, signs, and posters of upcoming events will help the patient acquire and maintain control of his or her environment.

Treatment for Moderate Impairment (Middle Stage)

Treatment in this stage consists of continuing and elaborating on environmental modification and ameliorating the patient's cognitive impairment. Adamovich (1992) suggested the following activities for bolstering cognition. They are presented here with some adaptation.

1. *Perception.* Visual and auditory perceptual tasks involve tracking and scanning; perception of sounds, words, and objects (e.g., use large print, use finger or card to maintain place, place items in best visual field, request repetition through auditory mode, request slowing down through auditory mode, request breakdown of smaller units of information through auditory mode); tracing or copying; following simple commands; and naming objects.

2. *Discrimination.* Activities begin with the visual discrimination of colors, shapes, and sizes followed by the discrimination of pictures, words, sentences, and situations (e.g., matching of colors; classifying light to dark; classifying round or long shapes; classifying small to large; putting words, sentences, and situations into categories function) and seeing how many stimulus items the patient can handle at once. This is progression from one to two, three, four, and more items at the same time.

3. *Organization.* Organizational skills include the categorization or grouping of items by physical attributes, meaningful units, function, likenesses, and differences (e.g., grouping objects according to round or long shapes, or small or large items; grouping words according to fruits or vegetables, or cities). Closure activities include the identification of missing elements of pictures, letters, words, sentences, stories, conversations, and situations. Sequencing activities include the sequencing of visual information (e.g., smallest to largest, lightest to darkest); sequencing of letters (e.g., from A to Z), words, and sentences (e.g., putting parts of a letter—date, Dear Sir, body of letter, Sincerely Yours, signature, and postscript—in their proper order); and sequencing functional activities (e.g., taking a shower, making coffee, frying an egg, shopping).

4. *Recall/Memory.* Treatment of memory disturbances includes internal retrieval strategies and external memory aids. Internal strategies include rehearsal, associations, and mnemonic devices. External memory aids include calendars, appointment books, notepads, daily logs/diaries, memo pads, lists, structured routines, reminder alarms, tape recorders, and watch alarms. For additional items that improve the ability to recall information, see the section on communication disorders associated with dementia.

5. *Reasoning/Problem Solving.* Several types of reasoning should be addressed, beginning with the most concrete (e.g., Will your car fit into the parking space?) and extending to more abstract reasoning (e.g., You forgot where you parked your car at a large shopping mall; figure out where it is by thinking through which mall entrance you came into, which store you shopped at first, which section of the department store you entered first, etc.). Additional activities can include simple arithmetic problems, simple maze designs, analogies, same and different aspects (e.g., doctor-lawyer), and so forth.

Treatment for Mild Impairment (Late Stage)

Executive and Behavior Problems

Due to frontal lobe damage, the patient with TBI will quite often have problems in executive function and behavior. Lezak (1982) described executive functioning as the ability to think about goals (e.g., a graduate student thinks about a topic for a term paper as part of a course requirement that will lead to a graduate degree), develop a plan (e.g., the same graduate student thinks about whether the format of the paper should be an experimental design, a case study, a review and analysis of the literature, and so on, and whether symptoms, etiology, diagnosis, therapy, or any combination of these areas will be covered), and successfully execute the plan (e.g., the same graduate student goes to the library, tests subjects if applicable, gathers and analyzes data, types it up, and completes it in time to hand in to the instructor).

Jacobs (1992) noted that the behavioral problems of the patient with TBI include anxiety, depression, withdrawal, aggressive behavior, temperament, decreased initiation, poor self-control, and attention seeking. These behavior problems can be caused directly by a lesion in particular areas of the brain that govern behavior (e.g., frontal and temporal lobes), or indirectly by a lesion in areas that govern cognition (e.g., attention, perception, memory, orientation), an impairment that can produce aberrant behavior when the patient tries to cope.

Behavior problems can also occur when the patient is trying to cope with associated injuries (e.g., amputation of limbs), or because of environmental factors that cause the patient to react or cope erratically (e.g., adjusting to a noisy or stuffy room, getting used to personnel). Many times, the behavior problems decrease as the patient regains cognitive abilities, executive function, and language abilities, and adjusts to the environment. Some patients may need additional treatment (e.g., counseling, medication).

Problems in executive function and behavior may have been present in the first two stages of recovery, but become most apparent in the last stage. It is during this stage that the TBI patient plans to re-enter society. Taking on and completing everyday activities (e.g., dressing, eating breakfast, preparing to go to school or work) are interwoven with a good deal of social interaction, which, of course, involves the use of language.

Executive Function Deficits

As suggested by Brookshire (2007), and Ylvisaker et al. (2008), treatment for executive function problems might include the following:

1. Break complex and demanding tasks into smaller segments.
2. Ask others to write down complex instructions and schedules.
3. Establish consistent routines and regular schedules for daily activities.
4. Get help from family members, friends, and associates in how to successfully ease the patient into daily life activities.
5. Keep possessions in designated places.
6. Organize the work space and set aside specific times for work at difficult tasks (i.e., when patient is rested and alert).
7. Set time limits (using alarms, timers) for working at difficult tasks.
8. Use a written daily schedule of events and appointments, with a place to check them off when completed.
9. Use an alarm watch or timer to signal appointments or other scheduled duties or events.
10. Use a daily log in which the day's activities can be recorded by the patient and/or others.
11. Place signs or notes in strategic locations as reminders for certain activities (e.g., Do you have your keys?).

Cazzato (1998) reported on the use of functionally based rehabilitation with a mild TBI patient. Complex attention skills, organizational activities, and memory strategies were worked on in the clinical setting and then in the actual work setting (the patient's home office). The patient's job required a great deal of travel and phone contact, and the need to structure and organize time and schedules. Referring to spreadsheets on the computer, making phone calls, collecting mailings, and sending or receiving faxes, all occurring in rapid succession or simultaneously, were at first simulated in the clinic. These activities were then shifted into the patient's home office, where the functional setting allowed for treatment gains to be generalized more effectively than in the clinical setting.

Kennedy (2004), in her preliminary study, found that when working with patients with TBI, the clinician should continue to directly train self-regulation (self-monitoring and self-control) for each learning activity. Kennedy cited Detterman (1993), who wrote, "The lesson learned from studies of transfer is that, if you want people to learn something, teach it to them. Don't teach something else and expect them to figure out what you really want them to do."

Language and Discourse Problems

Hartley (1994) noted that the area of language most likely affected during social interaction is discourse. Social interaction requires the blending of cognitive, social-behavioral, executive, and language skills. The discourse of TBI patients has been described as tangential, confused, and inappropriate in content and length. Hartley reviewed several studies dealing with narrative discourse after TBI; problems included decreased use of cohesive ties, decreased amount of information conveyed, use of ambiguous pronouns, slowed rate of production, excessive disfluencies, and use of shorter sentences.

Nicholas and Brookshire (1995) reviewed several studies and concluded that impaired listening comprehension is a frequent problem with TBI. Using an earlier version of their *Discourse Comprehension Test* (see the section on aphasia), they found that in the comprehension of spoken narrative discourse, 20 TBI subjects had more correct responses when questions assessed main ideas than when they assessed details, and more correct responses when questions assessed stated information than when they assessed implied information. In addition, stated information had stronger effects on their comprehension of details than on their comprehension of main ideas.

Coelho (2002) found that adults with CHI produced fewer words and clauses than non-brain-injured (NBI) adults on all discourse measures, and this was attributed to content organization. It was concluded that story generation was a more challenging task than story retelling for both groups. Concerning socioeconomic status, unskilled workers demonstrated poorer cohesive adequacy than either the skilled workers or professionals, regardless of group or story task. Kennedy and Nawrocki (2003) found that adults with TBI recalled narratives less well than 15 adults without TBI, regardless of question type. All participants recalled main ideas and implied information better than details and stated information.

Some treatment suggestions by Brookshire (2007) and Ylvisaker et al. (2008) for problems in language, specifically discourse, include the following:

1. Use scripts (e.g., going to a restaurant, shopping in the supermarket) to generate real or imagined descriptions of experiences.
2. Note topic of any conversation.
3. Self-examine regarding the main point.
4. Alert others before shifting topics.
5. Rehearse important comments and self-examine.

6. Ask for clarification or repetition when confused about what others are saying.
7. Watch others for feedback as to whether your comments are clear.
8. Watch facial expression of listener or ask about clarity of your remarks.
9. Practice retelling a story (e.g., view a picture story and then express it verbally).
10. Practice generating a story (e.g., view a single action picture and create a narrative for it).

The third goal of therapy is to encourage the patient and the caretaker(s) to continue the rehabilitative process outside of the clinical setting.

Treatment for Attention Deficit

Mateer (1996) suggested several attention-compensation techniques for use with TBI patients. These techniques to enhance concentration include the following:

1. Reduce distractions (e.g., turn off radio, TV, or loud machinery, close curtains, close eyes, use earplugs).
2. Avoid crowds (e.g., shop and drive during off-hours in small stores and streets, visit with people in small numbers, if a crowd is unavoidable take someone who can assist or act as a guide if necessary).
3. Watch out for fatigue (e.g., take frequent breaks when starting to get overwhelmed or nearing information overload).
4. Avoid interruptions (e.g., unplug phone or use answering machine, use a "Do Not Disturb" sign, ask others not to interrupt, do only one thing at a time).
5. Get enough sleep and exercise (e.g., naps and physical exercise help both sleep and attention).
6. Ask for help (e.g., tell trusted ones about your problems and ask for assistance, if needed, for items mentioned above).

Treatment for Confabulations

Sohlberg and Ehlhardt (1998) reported on assisting a caretaker in data collection and analysis of the confabulations uttered by a patient who also exhibited memory loss and personality change. The caretaker was provided with some education about the nature of confabulations (e.g., accompanying memory loss, no intent to deceive, due to brain damage).

The hope was that the caretaker (the mental health counselor) and the staff would develop strategies for managing and decreasing the confabulations, which indeed they did. The most interesting result was that the patient became more accepting and less argumentative when given correct information following a confabulation. The authors presented a summary of the seven-step therapy process used in their study.

Treatment for Executive Function and Behavior Deficits

Ylvisaker and Feeney (1998) reported on the use of a well-trained paraprofessional staff to help a TBI patient with a history of alcohol and drug abuse in defining goals, planning, decision making, and interpreting others' behavior during daily routine activities. Along with waking and eating times, the daily routine involved practice using memory aids, vocational activities for help in getting a job, and group therapy for understanding drug and alcohol abuse. What was once a source of negativism in the patient's daily routine turned into a more positive situation with the help of the staff.

The authors gave examples of negative daily encounters (e.g., waking the patient up and ordering him to participate in the day's activities, which resulted in cursing from the patient and agitation in the staff member) and positive daily encounters (e.g., pleasantly waking the patient who, after dressing and eating breakfast, reviews his goals and, with the aid of a staff member, his plans for accomplishing them). Because of this positive interaction with the staff, the once very negative patient increasingly asked for guidance in making a plan and for feedback regarding his perceptions and decisions.

Advanced Study

It is well known that children, because of greater brain plasticity, may recover more completely from brain traumas than adults who suffer the same kinds of injuries. One observation is that the homologous centers in an unaffected cerebral hemisphere may compensate better for brain damage in children than in adults. For example, a child who suffers a traumatic injury to the third frontal convolution in the left hemisphere may show subsequent growth of brain tissue in the third frontal convolution in the right hemisphere, with resultant improvement in naming and word retrieval.

Native or primary language also relates to lateralization of function. For example, functional magnetic resonance imaging (fMRI) studies of English-speaking neurotypical participants listening to English sentences (Schlosser, Aoyagi, Fulbright, Gore, & McCarthy, 1998) revealed a stronger activation of the left superior temporal sulcus compared to the right homologous region. When the same participants listened to Turkish sentences, none had similar cerebral activations. Although studies confirm a left hemisphere specialization for receptive language processing, there is controversy regarding the specific involvement of different brain regions at each level of processing. Accordingly, we may ask:

How is language processed by individuals with TBI who were bilingual premorbidly?

Does processing of sentences with canonical subject-verb-object structure involve a pathway that includes the frontal inferior gyrus, the supplementary motor area, and the temporal inferior gyrus (as suggested by Ikuta et al., 2006)? How is this process affected by TBI?

There are no studies of the effect of episodic memory and mental imagery on brain activation in receptive language processing, either for neurotypical adults or for those with TBI. Paquette et al. (2010) suggest presenting a known story compared to an unknown one to address this issue.

Is fMRI, which requires the patient to remain as still as possible for an extended period of time, the best way to measure language lateralization of individuals with TBI? Might techniques shown to be more tolerant to motion artifacts, such as near-infrared spectroscopy (NIRS) (Paquette et al., 2010), be better?

Website

The Brain Injury Association of America is a nonprofit organization dedicated to people with brain injury and their families. The association offers research, education, and advocacy programs through a national office, network of state affiliates, support groups, and a helpline. The website is *http://www.ninds.nih.gov/find_people/voluntary_orgs/volorg226.htm*.

CASE DESCRIPTION

We met CB when she entered the graduate program in speech-language pathology, having received an undergraduate degree from a university for deaf and hard-of-hearing students.

She presented with a moderate right hemiparesis, flaccid dysarthria, impaired naming and word retrieval, difficulty with both procedural and lexical/semantic memory, and impaired organizational skills. Writing with the nondominant (left) hand was characterized by tremulous letter and number formation, but overall legibility was fair. She reported chronic and constant pain in her right foot.

Etiology was traumatic brain injury, secondary to a violent sexual assault, where CB was dragged down a flight of concrete steps. She was reportedly taken to the hospital, where she was initially noted to be DOA (dead on arrival), and remained comatose for several weeks. She initially suffered from severe nonfluent aphasia, but recovered to the extent that comprehension was minimally impaired. Language production was moderately nonfluent with poor intelligibility, so CB undertook to learn American Sign Language, using her left hand primarily, and enrolled in the undergraduate program. Here are her words (actually a synopsis of several individuals with TBI):

"After the craniotomy and the first CT scan were done, five hours after I arrived at the hospital, the neurosurgeon met with B [CB's husband], saying that the surgery had been a success. B commented, 'Thank God she's all right.' The doctor told him that was not what he said; he said the surgery, which was to remove the blood, was a success. They wouldn't know for five days, and more tests, whether I would be all right. I was not aware of any of it. Not even that the hair had been shaved from half of my head.

"I spent the first two days following surgery in the recovery room attached to tubes and console machines. I recognized B from the first day. I responded with one squeeze of B's hand for yes and two for no. I indicated pain from the mouthpiece, where I was receiving oxygen; sometimes that my head hurt; and sometimes that the pain was from the needles in my arms.

"As I became aware of the situation I discovered my speech was extremely slow and lobored. I didn't use the proper words to describe things. I tried to write things down, but my motor control was very sluggish. I found I was sleeping a great deal. Someone had come in and asked if I was sleeping, and I replied that, "No, I was just douching," instead of "dozing." Word retrieval, speech motor control, all were difficult. I tried reading. My eyes would scan from left to right, but stop just slightly past the middle of the line. I was frightened. There was a ticking in my head, like a time bomb. My ears felt clogged, although I seemed to hear well enough. I was not allowed to lie flat, but had to stay at a 45-degree angle. There were a number of medications being given to me. There were steroids and some other things I don't remember. Tagamet was given to prevent the other medications from causing stomach problems. I was allowed Tylenol, but no aspirin.

"I tried to record my progress and feelings [one of the authors gave her a tape recorder to use at her bedside], but I couldn't put into words or sequence what I wanted to say. There was still a lot of medication, causing me to feel very lax and uncaring. I mostly wanted to sleep and I did a great deal of that. For several weeks my moving around was slow, my muscles wouldn't respond quickly. My vision was still distorted and things looked reduced in size. I was not seeing colors properly, particularly reds. There was also a difference in my hearing. I was aware of the sounds, but they sounded like I was in a cavern. There was still a great deal of ticking inside of my head. When I tried to walk for a few minutes, my head began to feel twice its normal size. It ached most of the time, and the area of incision was still draining."

About 10 years later, CB was graduated with the Master of Arts degree in speech-language pathology, passed the Praxis examination, and received ASHA CCC and state licensure. She began her professional career working with deaf children. Twenty years after the assault, she wrote to indicate that she was finally ready to work with a TBI population. She reports continuing lexical/semantic, working memory, word retrieval, and organizational problems. The experience of rehabilitation, according to CB, was not one of adapting to her damaged brain, but rather of learning how to use her new brain. After numerous surgical procedures, the pain in her right foot persists. She has also changed her name.

Discussion Questions: Theory

1. What is the difference between closed head injury and open head injury?

2. What is the difference between primary damage and secondary damage?

3. What are the effects of different points of contact (e.g., coup-contrecoup, rotational injuries)?

4. What is meant by the term "executive functioning?" What are the subtypes?

5. Why are deficits in TBI revealed in divided attention tasks?

Discussion Questions: Therapy

1. What language deficits are associated with TBI?

2. Describe one of the test batteries for TBI.

3. Should SLPs limit their focus of treatment to language deficits, or is it within the SLP's scope of practice to address cognitive deficits?

4. What are some criteria for differential diagnosis (say, between language deficits in TBI versus the language of confusion)?

5. What is the efficacy of language therapy after TBI (i.e., does it work)?

Assignment: Write a multiple-choice question with five options. Explain why the key option is correct, and why the distractors or decoys are incorrect. Avoid using forms such as, "All of the following are (in)correct *except*" in the stem, and "All (or none) of the above" in the options.

Example: Although language impairments are common in people with traumatic brain injury (TBI), not all language disturbances are aphasic, or even aphasic-like. Which of the following language impairments occur in TBI, but not in aphasia?

a. Impairments in word retrieval
b. Reading and writing impairments
c. Semantic and phonemic paraphasias
d. Circumlocutions
e. Disproportionately impaired pragmatic skills

The correct answer is *e*: It is said that people with TBI speak better than they communicate, while the reverse is true for people with aphasia. *a* is incorrect because it is the principal language deficit in both aphasia and TBI; *b* is incorrect because alexia (or deep dyslexia) and agraphia can occur when a lesion in Wernicke's area extends into the angular gyrus; *c* is incorrect because semantic and phonemic (also called verbal and literal) paraphasias occur in both conditions; and *d* is incorrect because circumlocutions (talking around a subject) occur in both conditions in the presence of a word retrieval deficit.

References

Adamovich, B. (1992). The role of the speech-language pathologist in the evaluation and treatment of adolescents and adults with traumatic brain injury. *Neurophysiology and Neurogenic Speech and Language Disorders, 2*(1). (Special Interest Division 2 Newsletter). Rockville, MD: American Speech-Language-Hearing Association.

Adamovich, B. (1997). Traumatic brain injury. In L. L. LaPointe (Ed.), *Aphasia and related neurogenic language disorders* (2nd ed.) (pp. 226–237). New York, NY: Thieme.

Adamovich, B. B., & Henderson, J. (1992). *Scales of cognitive ability traumatic brain injury*. Chicago, IL: Riverside Publishing Company.

Aggarwal, A., & Kean, E. (2010). Comparison of the Folstein mini mental state examination (MMSE) to the Montreal cognitive assessment (MoCA) as a cognitive screening tool in an inpatient rehabilitation setting. *Neuroscience and Medicine, 1,* 39–42.

American Speech-Language-Hearing Association (1991). Guidelines for speech-language pathologists serving persons with socio-communicative and/or cognitive impairments. *ASHA, 33* (Suppl 5), 21–28.

Ansell, B. (1991). Slow-to-recover brain-injured patients: Rationale for treatment. *Journal of Speech and Hearing Research, 34,* 1017–1022.

Baylow, H. E., Goldfarb, R., Taveira, C., & Steinberg, R. (2009). Accuracy of clinical judgment of the chin-down posture for dysphagia during the clinical/bedside assessment as corroborated by videofluoroscopy in adults with acute stroke. *Dysphagia, 24,* 423–433.

Boyle, M., Golper, L. A. C., & Cherney, L. (1999). Back to basics: Assessment practices with neurogenic communication disorders. *Neurophysiology and Neurogenic Speech and Language Disorders, 9*(3). (Special Interest Division 2 Newsletter, 3–8). Rockville, MD: American Speech-Language-Hearing Association.

Brookshire, R. (2007). *An introduction to neurogenic communication disorders* (6th ed.). St. Louis, MO: Mosby Elsevier.

Brookshire, R., & Nicholas, L. (1997). *Discourse comprehension test*. Bloomington, MN: BRK Publishers.

Campbell, T., & Dollaghan, C. (1990). Expressive language recovery in severely brain-injured children and adolescents. *Journal of Speech and Hearing Disorders, 55,* 567–581.

Campbell, T., & Dollaghan, C. (1995). Speaking rate, articulatory speed, and linguistic processing in children and adolescents with severe traumatic brain injury. *Journal of Speech and Hearing Research, 38,* 864–875.

Cazzato, K. R. (1998). A case of functionally based rehabilitation following a mild traumatic brain injury. *Neurophysiology and Neurogenic Speech and Language Disorders, 8*(2). (Special Interest Division 2 Newsletter, 3–8). Rockville, MD: American Speech-Language-Hearing Association.

Coelho, C. A. (1997). Cognitive-communicative disorders following traumatic brain injury. In C. T. Ferrand & R. L. Bloom (Eds.), *Introduction to organic and neurogenic disorders of communication* (pp. 110–138). Needham Heights, MA: Allyn & Bacon.

Coelho, C. (2002). Story narratives of adults with closed head injury and non-brain-injured adults: Influence of socioeconomic status, elicitation task, and executive functioning. *Journal of Speech and Hearing Research, 45,* 1232–1248.

Coelho, C., DeRuyter, F., & Stein, M. (1996). Treatment efficacy: Cognitive-communicative disorders resulting from traumatic brain injury in adults. *Journal of Speech and Hearing Research, 39,* S5–S17.

Coelho, C., Ylvisaker, M., and Turkstra, L. (2005). Nonstandardized assessment approaches for individuals with traumatic brain injuries. *Seminars in Speech and Language, 26,* 223–241.

Dalla Barba, G. (1993). Different patterns of confabulation. *Cortex, 29*, 567–581.

Darley, F. (1982). *Aphasia*. Philadelphia, PA: Saunders.

Douglas, J. (2010). Relation of executive functioning to pragmatic outcome following severe traumatic brain injury. *Journal of Speech and Hearing Research, 53*, 365–382.

Drummond, S. (1986). Characterization of irrelevant speech. *Journal of Communication Disorders, 19*, 175–183.

Ehrlich, J. (1988). Selective characteristics of narrative discourse in head-injured and normal adults. *Journal of Communication Disorders, 21*, 1–9.

Folstein, M. F., Folstein, S. F., & McHugh, P. R. (1975). Mini-mental state: A practical method for grading the cognitive state of patients for the clinician. *Journal of Psychiatric Research, 12*, 196–198.

Fraas, M., & Calvert, M. (2008). The use of narratives to identify characteristics leading to a productive life following acquired brain injury. *American Journal of Speech-Language Pathology, 18*, 315–328.

Gennarelli, T. A. (1993). Mechanisms of brain injury. *The Journal of Emergency Medicine, 11*, 5–11.

Geschwind, N. (1967) The varieties of naming errors. *Cortex, 3*, 97–112.

Goldfarb, R. (1981). Operant conditioning and programmed instruction in aphasia rehabilitation. In R. Chapey (Ed.), *Language intervention strategies in adult aphasia* (pp. 249–264). Baltimore, MD: Williams & Wilkins.

Groher, M. (1977). Language and memory disorders following closed head trauma. *Journal of Speech and Hearing Research, 20*, 212–223.

Gruen, A., Frankle, B., & Schwartz, R. (1990). Word fluency generation skills of head-injured patients in an acute trauma center. *Journal of Communication Disorders, 23*, 163–170

Hagen, C., 1984. Language disorders in head trauma. In A. Holland (Ed.), *Language disorders in adults: Recent advances* (pp. 245–282). San Diego, CA: College-Hill.

Halpern, H., Darley, F., & Brown, J. (1973). Differential language and neurologic characteristics in cerebral involvement. *Journal of Speech and Hearing Disorders, 38*, 162–173.

Hartley, L. (1994). Linguistic deficits after traumatic brain injury. *Neurophysiology and Neurogenic Speech and Language Disorders, 4*(1). (Special Interest Division 2 Newsletter). Rockville, MD: American Speech-Language-Hearing Association.

Helm-Estabrooks, N., & Hotz, G. (1990). *The brief test of head injury* (BTHI). Austin, TX: Pro-Ed.

Ikuta, N., Sugiura, M., Sassa, Y., Watanabe, J., Akitsuki, Y., Iwata, K., . . . Kawashima, R. (2006). Brain activation during the course of sentence comprehension. *Brain and Language, 97*, 154–161.

Jacobs, H. (1992). Behavior disorders and traumatic brain injury. *Neurophysiology and Neurogenic Speech and Language Disorders, 2*(1). (Special Interest Division 2 Newsletter). Rockville, MD: American Speech-Language-Hearing Association.

Jennett, B., & Teasdale, G. (1981). *Management of head injuries*. Philadelphia, PA: Davis.

Katz, D. I. (1992). Neuropathology and neurobehavioral recovery from closed head injury. *Journal of Head Trauma Rehabilitation, 7*, 1–15.

Kennedy, M. (2004). Self-monitoring recall during two tasks after traumatic brain injury: A preliminary study. *American Journal of Speech-Language Pathology, 13*, 142–154.

Kennedy, M., & Coelho, C. (2005). Self-regulation after traumatic brain injury: A framework for intervention of memory and problem solving. *Seminars in Speech and Language, 25*, 242–255.

Kennedy, M., Coelho, C., Turkstra, L., Ylvisaker, M., Sohlberg, M., Yorkston, K., . . . Kan, P-F. (2008). Intervention for executive functions after traumatic brain injury: A systematic review, meta-analysis and clinical recommendations. *Neuropsychological Rehabilitation, 1*, 1–43.

Kennedy, M., & Nawrocki, M. (2003). Delayed predictive accuracy of narrative recall after traumatic brain injury: Salience and effectiveness. *Journal of Speech and Hearing Research, 46*, 98–112.

Kennedy, M., & Turkstra, L. (2006). Group intervention studies in the cognitive rehabilitation of individuals with traumatic brain injury: Challenges faced by researchers. *Neuropsychology Review, 16*, 151–159.

Le, K., Coelho, C., Mazeiko, J., & Grafman, J. (2011). Measuring goodness of story narratives. *Journal of Speech and Hearing Research, 54*, 118–126.

Levin, H., O'Donnell, V., & Grossman, R. (1979). The Galveston orientation and amnesia test: A practice scale to assess cognition after head injury. *Journal of Nervous and Mental Disease, 167*, 675–684.

Lezak, M. (1982). The problem of assessing executive functions. *International Journal of Psychology, 17,* 281–297.

Liles, B., Coelho, C., Duffy, R., & Zalagens, M. (1989). Effects of elicitation procedures on the narratives of normal and closed head injured adults. *Journal of Speech and Hearing Disorders, 54,* 356–366.

Logemann, J. (1997). Structural and functional aspects of normal and disordered swallowing. In C. T. Ferrand & R. L. Bloom (Eds.), *Introduction to organic and neurogenic disorders of communication* (pp. 229–246). Boston, MA: Allyn & Bacon.

Mateer, C. (1996). Managing impairments in attention following traumatic brain injury. *Neurophysiology and Neurogenic Speech and Language Disorders, 6*(3). (Special Interest Division 2 Newsletter). Rockville, MD: American Speech-Language-Hearing Association.

McDonough, J. T. (1994). *Stedman's concise medical dictionary* (2nd ed.). Philadelphia, PA: Williams & Wilkins.

Mills, R., & Drummond, S. (1980, November). *Analysis of impaired naming in language of confusion.* Paper presented at the American Speech-Language-Hearing Association, Detroit, MI.

Musson, N. D. (1998). An introduction to neurogenic swallowing disorders. In A. F. Johnson & B. H. Jacobson (Eds.), *Medical speech-language pathology: A practitioner's guide* (pp. 354–389). New York, NY: Thieme.

Netsell, R., & Lefkowitz, D. (1992). Speech production following traumatic brain injury: Clinical and research implications. *Neurophysiology and Neurogenic Speech and Language Disorders, 2*(4). Special Interest Division 2 Newsletter). Rockville, MD: American Speech-Language-Hearing Association.

Nicholas, L., & Brookshire, R. (1995). Comprehension of spoken narrative discourse by adults with aphasia, right-hemisphere brain damage, or traumatic brain injury. *American Journal of Speech-Language Pathology, 4,* 69–81.

Paquette, N., Gonzalez-Frankenberger, B., Vannasing, P., Tremblay, J., Florea, O., Beland, R., . . . Lassonde, M. (2010). Lateralization of receptive language function using near infrared spectroscopy. *Neuroscience and Medicine, 1,* 64–70.

Patterson, J., & Chapey, R. (2008). Assessment of language disorders in adults. In R. Chapey (Ed.), *Language intervention strategies in aphasia and related neurogenic communication disorders* (pp. 64–160). Baltimore, MD: Lippincott Williams & Wilkins.

Peach, R. (1992). Factors underlying neuropsychological test performance in chronic severe traumatic brain injury. *Journal of Speech and Hearing Research, 35,* 810–818.

Ross-Swain, D. (1996). *Ross information processing assessment* (2nd ed.). Austin, TX: Pro-Ed.

Sarno, M. T., Buonaguro, A., & Levita, E. (1986). Characteristics of verbal impairment in closed head injury. *Archives of Physical Medicine and Rehabilitation, 67,* 400–405.

Schlosser, M. J., Aoyagi, N., Fulbright, R. K., Gore, J. C., & McCarthy, G. (1998). Functional MRI studies of auditory comprehension. *Human Brain Mapping, 6,* 1–13.

Sohlberg, M., Avery, J., Kennedy, M., Ylvisaker, M., Coelho, C., Turkstra, L., & Yorkston, K. (2003). Practice guidelines for direct attention training. *Journal of Medical Speech-Language Pathology, 11,* 19–39.

Sohlberg, M. M., & Ehlhardt, L. (1998). Case report: Management of confabulation after subarachnoid hemorrhage. *Neurophysiology and Neurogenic Speech and Language Disorders, 8*(2). (Special Interest Division 2 Newsletter, 9–13). Rockville, MD: American Speech-Language-Hearing Association.

Sohlberg, M., Ehlhardt, L., & Kennedy, M. (2005). Instructional techniques in cognitive rehabilitation: A preliminary report. *Seminars in Speech and Language, 26,* 268–279.

Sohlberg, M. M., & Mateer, C. A. (1989). *Introduction to cognitive rehabilitation theory and practice.* New York, NY: Guilford Press.

Stengel, E. (1964). Speech disorders and mental disorders. In A. DeReuck & M. O'Connor (Eds.), *Disorders of language* (pp. 285–292). London, UK: Churchill.

Theodoros, D. G., Murdoch, B. E., & Stokes, P. D. (1995). Variability in the perceptual and physiological features of dysarthria following severe closed head injury: An examination of five cases. *Brain Injury, 9,* 671–696.

Tompkins, C., Holland, A., Ratcliff, G., Costello, A., Leahy, L., & Cowell, V. (1990). Predicting cognitive recovery from closed head injury in children and adolescents. *Brain and Cognition, 13,* 86–97.

Turkstra, L. (2005). Looking while listening and speaking: Eye-to-face gaze in adolescents with and without traumatic brain injury. *Journal of Speech and Hearing Research, 48*, 1429–1441.

Turkstra, L., Coelho, C., & Ylvisaker, M. (2005). The use of standardized tests for individuals with cognitive-communicative disorders. *Seminars in Speech and Language, 26*, 215–222.

Turkstra, L., Ylvisaker, M., Coelho, C., Kennedy, M., Sohlberg, M., Avery, J., & Yorkston, K. (2005). Practice guidelines for standardized assessment for persons with traumatic brain injury. *Journal of Medical Speech-Language Pathology, 13*, 9–38.

Weinstein, E., Lyerly, O., Cole, M., & Ozer, M. (1966). Meaning in jargon aphasia. *Cortex, 2*, 165–187.

Wertz, R. (1985). Neuropathologies of speech and language: An introduction to patient management. In D. F. Johns (Ed.), *Clinical management of neurogenic communicative disorders* (pp. 1–96). Boston, MA: Little, Brown.

World Health Organization. (2001). *International classification of functioning, disability and health*. Geneva, Switzerland: Author.

Ylvisaker, M., & Feeney, T. (1998). A Vygotskyan approach to rehabilitation after TBI: A case illustration. *Neurophysiology and Neurogenic Speech and Language Disorders, 8*(2). (Special Interest Division 2 Newsletter, 14–19). Rockville, MD: American Speech-Hearing-Language Association.

Ylvisaker, M., & Szekeres, S. (1994). Communication disorders associated with closed head injury. In R. Chapey (Ed.), *Language intervention strategies in adult aphasia* (pp. 546–567). Baltimore, MD: Williams & Wilkins.

Ylvisaker, M., Szekeres, S., & Feeney, T. (2008). Communicative disorders associated with traumatic brain injury. In R. Chapey (Ed.), *Language intervention strategies in aphasia and related neurogenic communication disorders* (pp. 879–962). Baltimore, MD: Lippincott Williams & Wilkins.

Ylvisaker, M., Turkstra, L., & Coelho, C. (2005). Behavioral and social interventions for individuals with traumatic brain injury: A summary of the research with clinical implications. *Seminars in Speech and Language, 26*, 256–267.

Ylvisaker, M., Turkstra, L., Coelho, C., Yorkston, K., Kennedy, M., Sohlberg, M., & Avery, J. (2007). Behavioural interventions for children and adults with behaviour disorders after TBI: A systematic review of the evidence. *Brain Injury, 21*, 769–805.

Communication Disorders Associated with Schizophrenia

Definition

There is general agreement that schizophrenia is a disorder that affects the total personality in all aspects of its functioning. Not all patients show the same range in magnitude of disturbance, and even the same individual's symptoms will vary from time to time, but the striking feature of this disorder is that it permeates every aspect of the individual's functioning (Bemporad & Pinsker, 1974). Day and Semrad (1978, pp. 199–241) pointed out that most schizophrenia begins in the mid-teens and continues at a high level of incidence until the mid-fifties. More women than men develop schizophrenia. Married people are less susceptible than those who are single, separated, or divorced. Schizophrenia may affect the patients' perceptions, thoughts, mood, will, speech, motor control, and social behavior.

According to the *Diagnostic and Statistical Manual of Mental Disorders* (DSM-IV) (American Psychiatric Association, 2000), schizophrenia is diagnosed if at least two of the following symptoms are present for at least a one-month period: delusions, hallucinations, disorganized speech, grossly disorganized or catatonic behavior, and negative symptoms of affective flattening, alogia, or avolition. Catatonic behavior is defined as marked motor abnormality, either immobility or nongoal-directed excitement, resistance to being moved, posturing, echopraxia, and stereotypical movements. Examples of catatonic speech are mutism and echolalia. For diagnosis of schizophrenia to be confirmed, symptoms of schizophrenia have to cause significant social or occupational dysfunction for at least six months (American Psychiatric Association, 2000).

Symptoms and Etiology

Language Abilities

Neurology and psychiatry in Germany, particularly at the Breslau school during the late nineteenth and early twentieth centuries, related the disordered language in schizophrenia and aphasia (Geschwind, 1966). The language of schizophrenia, as aphasia, may be viewed as a neurogenic disorder, that is, its characteristic cognitive symptoms may be organic in origin. Different clinical pictures may result from differences in pathoanatomy. One subtype, according to the German school, was *schizophasia*, a form of schizophrenia characterized primarily by disorganized language.

That there is not universal agreement among professionals studying schizophrenic language becomes apparent when reading articles in a single journal. Such language has been seen as no different from normal slips of the tongue (Fromkin, 1975), as an episodical form of pathologically deviant language behavior (Lecours & Vanier-Clement, 1976), or as resulting from an intermittent aphasia (Chaika, 1974). Part of the confusion probably relates to the semantic behaviors produced in aphasia and the language of schizophrenia. Clinical intervention, which follows diagnosis, would be different if individuals were thought to have aphasia. Except in rare cases where symptoms progress to more severe forms, aphasia is characterized by spontaneous recovery and responsiveness to clinical speech-language intervention. The language of schizophrenia is not characterized by spontaneous recovery and the disorder is resistant to speech-language therapy.

The behavior of schizophrenia has been given more attention than the language of adults with this condition. Linguistic output, as opposed to extreme behavioral symptoms, has been examined in a relatively smaller number of studies. Whereas the patterns of language of adults with aphasia have been long framed and mapped, the same rigor of focus has not been devoted to the verbal behavior of adults with schizophrenia.

In the present section, we aim to illustrate neurolinguistic patterns associated with chronic undifferentiated schizophrenia, and to focus on issues concerning the relationship between the language of schizophrenia and aphasia. In particular, we seek to address the following questions:

1. Is there a "schizophrenic language?"
2. Does the language of schizophrenia differ qualitatively as well as quantitatively from the language of neurotypical adults? If so, how?
3. Does it differ from the language of aphasia? If so, how?
4. Is the abnormality observed in the language of schizophrenia due to an underlying abnormality in thought (as the true cause of the abnormality in language), or is the adult with schizophrenia somehow deficient in linguistic competence?
5. If the adult with schizophrenia lacks linguistic competence, is the abnormality syntactic, semantic, or pragmatic?
6. Are the linguistic abnormalities observed in schizophrenia under conscious control?

Speech Abilities

The treatment for psychotic symptoms, such as delusions and hallucinations, are medications, which block dopamine receptors in the mesolimbic pathway. The side effects of pure dopamine antagonists, such as Haldol and Thorazine, are tremor, rigidity, dystonia, and *tardive dyskinesia*. Such neurological side effects are caused by the general and indiscriminate blockade of dopamine in the brain. The *nigrostriatal* area of the brain, which is rich in dopamine receptors, is inadvertently affected by pure dopamine antagonists. Due to the neurological side effects, first-generation antipsychotic medications were called *neuroleptics*. An early sign of impending tardive dyskinesia is hyperkinetic dysarthria, when symptoms might be reversed by cessation of neuroleptic medications (Portnoy, 1979). Speech-language pathologists treating individuals with psychiatric disorders need to be sensitive to changes in speech and voice, in order to make appropriate referrals.

Dopamine blockade in an already dopamine-deficient prefrontal cortex may further worsen cognitive symptoms. Second-generation antipsychotic medications minimize neurological side effects by blocking both serotonin and dopamine in the brain (Sprague, Loewen, & Raymond, 2004). Since serotonin and dopamine are in a state of reciprocal inhibition, the blockade of serotonin reverses the blockade of dopamine in the nigrostriatal area, causing fewer movement disorders. For that reason, second-generation antipsychotic medications, such as Clozaril, Risperdal, Zyprexa, Abilify, Seroquel, and Geoden, are called *atypical neuroleptics*. Atypical neuroleptics have been shown to improve cognitive functioning in schizophrenia by reducing dopamine deficiency (Bilder et al., 2002).

Frequently, speech and communication problems such as dysarthria and dysprosody are observed in schizophrenia, and often precede the onset of psychosis (Nasrallah & Smeltzer, 2002). A communication disorder in schizophrenia is often described by clinicians as a thought disorder. Loosening of associations, which is the loss of logical associations between antecedents and subsequent associations, is a common feature in schizophrenia language. It may be helpful to view the disorders of associations as disorders of the word and disorders of the sentence. Disorders of word range from loss of symbolic meaning of a word or making up new words (*neologisms*) to approximate use of words, where disorders of sentence include associative failures. Words combined based on sounds rather than meaning are referred to as clang associations. Neologisms as well as *echolalia* and verbigeration (use of words in a repetitive manner) are often observed in the language of schizophrenia. Difficulty in maintaining a specific topic, which is often referred to as tangential and disorganized speech, is a pragmatic characteristic common to schizophrenia. There may be different thought disorder subtypes, which may be differentially related to different language production problem subtypes (Barach & Berenbaum, 1996).

Halpern, McCartin-Clark, and Wallack (1989) evaluated the nonfluencies of eight adults with psychiatric problems (seven of the eight participants were diagnosed with schizophrenia, and one with atypical brain syndrome). Results indicated that 12% of total participant output were nonfluencies. Most nonfluencies were on tasks involving verbal formulation, picture description, spontaneous speech, and reading aloud of sentences and paragraphs, and least in automatic speech and repetitions of phrases and sentences.

The nonfluencies were mostly repetitions, followed by hesitations, and then prolongations. The nonfluencies appeared mostly on sounds, with words and phrases the next frequent, and sentences and syllables the least frequent. Finally, the most nonfluencies occurred on words in the middle or beginning of sentences, with the least occurring in words at the end of sentences.

DiSimoni, Darley, and Aronson (1977) tested 27 patients with schizophrenia, who were free of any known neurological deficit, with an aphasia test battery. Results showed that participants with schizophrenia were most deviant with regard to the relevance of their responses and in reading comprehension, while naming, syntax, and the adequacy of their responses were essentially normal. Participants with aphasia given similar tests typically have far less difficulty with reading comprehension and relevance, and have the most difficulty with adequacy. These authors used the term "adequacy" to signify the semantic component of language.

Goldfarb, Eisenson, Stocker, and DeSanti (1994) in their study of aphasia and "schizophasia" found differences in responses to semantic (divergent and convergent) and pragmatic (communicative responsibility) tasks. These language patterns were also different from those adults with Alzheimer and frontotemporal dementia (Goldfarb & Goldberg, 2004). Semantic behaviors in the language of schizophrenia are also characterized by a unique pattern of word association (Halpern, Goldfarb, Brandon, & McCartin-Clark, 1985). Andreasen (1979a, 1979b) reported what has been seminal research in describing language and thought in chronic undifferentiated schizophrenia. Her definitions of schizophrenic linguistic symptoms (Andreasen, 1979b) follow:

1. *Poverty of speech*: restriction in the amount of spontaneous speech.
2. *Poverty of content of speech*: speech that is adequate in amount, but conveys little information.

3. *Pressured speech*: an increase in the amount of speech. The patient speaks rapidly and is difficult to interrupt. Speech tends to be loud and emphatic.
4. *Distractible speech*: a tendency to change topic inappropriately in response to extraneous stimuli present in the environment, an object in the room, etc.
5. *Tangentiality*: replying in a tangential, irrelevant manner. Tangentiality refers only to immediate replies to questions (stimulus-response mode) and not to transitions in spontaneous speech.
6. *Derailment (loss of goal)*: a pattern of spontaneous speech in which ideas slip off the track in an obliquely related manner or in an unrelated manner. Errors are similar to tangentiality, but occur in the spontaneous conversational mode.
7. *Incoherence*: speech that is essentially incomprehensible; at times includes paragrammatism (syntactic confusions, random word choice). This disorder is rare.
8. *Illogicality*: speech in which conclusions reached do not follow logically. Includes *non sequiturs*, faulty inductive references. Does not include delusions.
9. *Clanging*: speech in which sounds govern word choice, so that intelligibility is impaired. Includes rhyming and puns.
10. *Neologisms*: new word formations that render language unintelligible.
11. *Word approximations*: words used in a new and unconventional way or actual new words that are developed by conventional rules of word formation, e.g., gloves = *handshoes*; pen = *paperskate*. (Authors' comment: While the example of *paperskate* seems fine as an illustration of a word approximation, *handschuh* is actually the Yiddish and German word for "glove.")
12. *Circumstantiality*: speech that is very indirect and delayed in reaching its goal. Includes the intrusion of many tedious details. It differs from poverty of content and derailment in that the goal of the communication is eventually reached by the speaker.
13. *Perseveration*: persistent repetition of words, phrases, ideas.
14. *Echolalia*: speech in which the patient echoes the words or phrases of the interviewer.
15. *Blocking*: interruption of a train of thought (speech) before completion of the thought or idea. After a period of silence, the patient indicates an inability to recall what he meant to say.
16. *Stilted speech*: speech with an excessively formal quality, overly pompous. The authors remember one patient who said, "To the knowledge of historians," before he gave an answer to any question that was presented to him.
17. *Self-reference (egocentric speech)*: the patient repeatedly refers the topic back to himself and refers neutral topics to himself (personalizes).

Speech and language characteristics of individuals with schizophrenia may be summarized as follows.

Prosody

Affective prosodic deficits are observed on an aprosodia battery, which uses stimuli having incrementally reduced verbal-articulatory demands. A study of 45 chronic, medication-stabilized adults with schizophrenia revealed that their performance on the aprosodia battery was statistically identical to patients with right hemisphere brain damage (RHD), but very different from those with left hemisphere brain damage (LBD) (Ross et al., 2001).

Suprasegmental features of rate, stress, and melodic intonation are not characteristically impaired. However, there are some individuals with schizophrenia who have a flat affect and, as a result, will produce a monotone voice.

Phonology

Phonological rules appear to be preserved. There is no evidence of characteristic phonological processes (e.g., final consonant or weak syllable deletion, cluster reduction) among individuals with schizophrenic language.

Syntax

Sentences are usually well-formed syntactically (Andreasen, 1979a). However, word association responses (Halpern et al., 1985) are often syntactically inappropriate, with significant numbers of responses scored as repetitious, anomalous, or unclassifiable. Several word-association studies (Chapman, 1958; Downing, Elbert, & Shubrooks, 1963; Faibish, 1961; Johnson, Weiss, & Zelhart, 1964) have shown that adults with schizophrenia produce fewer associations and more idiosyncratic associations, and are distracted by associatively linked words. Another study (Richman, 1968), found that emotionally tinged words caused participants with schizophrenia to distort and confuse the meanings of words, and that often they followed verbal and sound associations rather than referential ones. On the other hand, Wynne (1964) found that the pattern of popular word-association responses is similar for adults with schizophrenia and neurotypical controls.

Some researchers have attempted to categorize the word-association responses of participants with schizophrenia. Raven (1958) devised categories of "verbal dysfunction" based on vocabulary responses to 17 words. These categories included disordered syntax, perseveration, bizarre content, rigidity of expression, poverty of expression, circumstantial talk, vagueness of structure, distractions due to intrusions of psychological or geographic origin, chain associations, telescoped ideas, dissipated and echo responses, stylized language, and negativistic responses.

Semantics (Examples from Andreasen, 1979a, 1979b)

1. Adjectives attribute qualities to nouns they cannot ordinarily have (e.g., equipment is described as *stale*; a rug as *full of sandpaper*).
2. Pronouns and adverbs are used as if they have referents when in fact they do not ("Any kind of fruit has to disappear *there*." "So, if the equipment is stale plus *that*, what does *he* earn?").
3. Occasional true *word salad*: "Because of rodents, see, and as for being an explorer, any kind of fruit has to disappear there."
4. Semantic errors are similar to semantic paraphasias. Words are related semantically or topically to an earlier portion of the discourse, but they make no sense as they are used in a particular sentence. This may also be seen as an example of perseveration.

Semantic confusions (paraphasias) by participants with aphasia were more like than unlike word associations, although word associations were less specific than semantic confusions (Rinnert & Whitaker, 1973). Production of paradigmatic word-association responses varied inversely with the abstractness of words in samples from adults with both aphasia (Goldfarb & Halpern, 1981) and schizophrenia (Halpern et al., 1985). No clear pattern regarding abstractness emerged in associations produced by younger or older neurotypical controls (Goldfarb & Halpern, 1981, 1984). The unique pattern of word associations of adults with chronic undifferentiated schizophrenia was characterized by a marked reduction in paradigmatic responses and an increase in anomalous responses. Thus, the first and third of the generalizations cited above may be specific to the language of schizophrenia, while the second and fourth may be evidenced in both populations, those with schizophrenia and those with aphasia.

Research data both support and refute the existence of "schizophasia." One major focus of the study by Goldfarb et al. (1994) was the effect of certain semantic tasks on the language of adults with aphasia and those with schizophrenia. We hoped that these tasks would help us answer questions about the existence of "schizophasia" and to identify patterns of semantic behavior in three (aphasic, schizophrenic, and neurotypical) populations. Semantic behavior in schizophrenia sometimes resembles aphasia and sometimes does not. Some researchers consider the language of schizophrenia to be a form of aphasia, while others do not. Although we are inclined to reject the term "schizophasia" because it produces more confusion than clarification, we are chastened by Tachibana's (1980) citation of frequent negligence of the *Type II error* in behavioral studies. Failure to find a difference between categories does not mean there is no difference between them, particularly when the categories are diagnostic entities that may have criteria beyond those tested in a given study.

Pragmatics

1. Language violates the rule of discourse that a topic must be adhered to or switched only after giving the listener some warning. There are no transitions, and there is evidence of presupposition.
2. The speaker may appear to show awareness that there is a listener. An example is the use of the word *see* in the word salad (#3, above) as a discourse marker. However, the speaker is often not aware of any difficulty in communicating (much the same as an individual with Wernicke's aphasia).
3. There is frequent self-reference (similar to the language of dementia).
4. There is evidence of confabulation (also seen in confused language and TBI).
5. There is evidence of propagation (also seen in confused language and TBI).

Level of demand for creativity, a pragmatic measure of communicative responsibility on the *Stocker Probe for Fluency and Language, 3rd Edition* (Stocker & Goldfarb, 1995), may be useful in discriminating the language of schizophrenia from aphasia. Adults with aphasia are said to communicate better than they speak. Those with traumatic brain injury are said to speak better than they communicate, an observation that may also be true for adults with schizophrenia. A Level IV request on the *Stocker Probe*, which follows presentation of a common object stimulus, is, "Tell me everything you know about it," a task that requires the participant to identify semantic features of form and function. The question posed in Level V is, "What does this make you think of," a request that provides no contextual support. Adults with schizophrenia provided better responses to Level IV than to V, while the reverse occurred for adults with aphasia.

To conclude, the language of schizophrenia often tends to consist of incoherent monologues delivered as if the speaker were unaware that dialogue is even possible. Language disorder in schizophrenia may be exacerbated by institutional neurosis. This condition, which is characterized mostly by apathy and sometimes a stereotyped posture and gait, may affect individuals who are institutionalized for two years or longer (Goldfarb & Halpern, 1989). The probable causes of this condition are (1) loss of contact with the outside world; (2) enforced idleness and loss of responsibility; (3) bossiness of medical and nursing staff; (4) loss of friends, possessions, and personal effects; (5) drugs; (6) ward atmosphere; and (7) loss of prospects outside the institution.

Temporal lobe overactivation has been demonstrated in a number of studies (e.g., Frith et al., 1995; Kubicki et al., 2003). Temporal lobe volume reduction is a very consistent finding in schizophrenia. In addition, although there is a debate about the findings, a facilitated semantic priming effect has also been found repeatedly in schizophrenia and could be interpreted as lexical overactivation in temporal regions (e.g., Moritz, Woodward, Kuppers, Lausen, & Schickel, 2001). Many of the "frontal" findings in schizophrenia could stem from abnormalities in processing at an earlier stage in posterior regions such as the temporal and inferior parietal cortex.

The functional frontal deficit model does not address the decreased right ear (left hemisphere) advantage of adults with schizophrenia, compared to depressed and typical participants in dichotic listening tasks (Bruder et al., 1995). There was no difference in hemispheric advantage while on or off medication, and those schizophrenic participants with greater hallucinatory behaviors were found to have a lower right ear advantage. The temporal cortical language areas of individuals with schizophrenia may be abnormally lateralized, with less auditory language strength in the left hemisphere compared to the same language areas of typical individuals (Woodruff et al., 1997).

A recent theory of the evolutionary and genetic origins of schizophrenia (Crow, 2008) posits that the disease can be attributed to failure in hemispheric specialization for language. A particular speciation event in humans led to the formation of a dominant hemisphere for language, but this process of dominance has failed to occur in individuals with schizophrenia, at least for some key aspects of their language. A means of testing this theory may be found in a model of continuous phonological processing (Strelnikov, 2008). There are two streams of processing: a sequential stream, which is strictly modular and unidirectional; and a parallel stream, which is highly interactive and capable of forming predictions based on perceived linguistic information. Each hemisphere of the brain houses both processing streams, but one stream is dominant in each hemisphere. Inability of adults with schizophrenia to detect deviant stimuli in phonological processing might underlie failed hemispheric specialization, supporting Crow's theory. The paradigm of mismatch negativity (a type of deviance detection), which has been fruitful in event-related potential electroencephalographic (EEG) studies of aphasia, might also be worthwhile in research on the language of schizophrenia.

Diagnosis

Diagnostic procedures for determining the communication disorders associated with schizophrenia can involve (1) establishing background information, (2) giving a neurologic evaluation, (3) employing informal tests, and (4) employing formal tests.

The relationship between working memory and frontal lobe function is not clear or straightforward. An extensive review of the literature with regard to frontal lobe function did not find evidence that unilateral damage to the frontal lobe resulted in working memory impairment (D'Esposito & Postle, 1999). We conclude by affirming that, in many studies, temporal versus frontal lobe functioning in people with schizophrenia is not all that clear. It is possible that frontal lobe functioning was not significantly impaired relative to temporal lobe functioning on the tasks assessed, or that temporal lobe functioning was better than frontal lobe functioning. Finally, schizophrenia is thought to be a neurodegenerative disorder, which is frequently associated with the worsening of cognitive symptoms over time.

It can also be argued that a preference for nouns (associated with temporal lobe function) over verbs (a frontal lobe function) in adults with schizophrenia (Goldfarb & Bekker, 2009) may stem from an overactivation of temporal regions, not functional damage to prefrontal regions. In word-association tests (Halpern, Goldfarb, Brandon, & McCartin-Clark, 1985), adults with schizophrenia gave the most paradigmatic (same grammatical class) responses to nouns, followed by adjectives, and then verbs, regardless of speed or modality of presentation of stimuli. This appeared to be an exclusively schizophrenic response, as adults with aphasia, as well as neurotypical control participants (Goldfarb & Halpern, 1981), showed that the greatest-to-least numbers of paradigmatic associates were to adjectives, nouns, and verbs. Verbs may also elicit a significantly stronger emotional reaction than nouns in adults with schizophrenia, since anticipation of being harmed through some action is part of paranoid ideation that patients may experience.

Meilijson, Kasher, and Elizur (2004) found that 43 participants with chronic schizophrenia showed a high degree of inappropriate pragmatic abilities compared to participants with mixed anxiety-emotion disorder and participants with hemispheric damage. The pragmatic abilities were analyzed according to the pragmatic protocols of Prutting and Kirchner (1987) and consisted of the following:

1. Speech acts (e.g., using natural language in communicating assertions, commands, requests);
2. Topic (e.g., maintenance, change);
3. Turn-taking (e.g., eye gaze, repair/revision, feedback);
4. Lexical (e.g., cohesion, specificity/accuracy, prosody); and
5. Nonverbal communication (e.g., gestures, body posture, facial expressions).

With an eye toward differential diagnosis, Halpern and McCartin-Clark (1984) compared language data from adults with schizophrenia to the language data of participants with a generalized intellectual impairment (dementia), confused language (TBI), and apraxia of speech (Halpern et al., 1973). This comparison revealed the following: (1) participants with a generalized intellectual impairment (dementia) showed more impairment in auditory retention span, naming, and syntax, than participants with the language of schizophrenia; (2) participants with confused language (TBI) tended to be more impaired in reading comprehension, syntax, naming, relevance, writing words to dictation, and general overall language ability than individuals with the language of schizophrenia; and (3) individuals with apraxia of speech were more impaired in syntax, more nonfluent, and less impaired in relevance than those with the language of schizophrenia. It seems that the more preserved naming and syntactic abilities of individuals with schizophrenia differentiate them from the above cerebrally involved groups, except for those with apraxia of speech, where only syntactic ability differentiated them.

For individuals with schizophrenia, length of institutionalization and speaking (especially adequacy, a semantic ability, and naming) were positively correlated, indicating that the longer the institutionalization, the more errors in speaking (especially adequacy and naming) are produced (Halpern & McCartin-Clark, 1984). This finding agrees with Wynne (1963), who stated that schizophrenic language can be influenced by long-term institutionalization.

Many utterances of the adult with schizophrenia resemble the adequacy (semantic) errors of the adult with aphasia. Although the end product, an adequacy error, is the same, in the patient with aphasia it seems to be part of a word-finding disturbance (a linguistic inaccessibility), whereas in the patient with schizophrenia it seems to be due to the underlying thought disorder, a lack of stimulation or socialization, and not caring. It seems that if the thought disorder component takes control, a bizarre response will be produced. If the lack of stimulation or socialization and the not-caring components take over, an adequacy (semantic) error is produced. The results of the Halpern et al. (1973) and Halpern and McCartin-Clark (1984) studies show that adequacy (semantic) problems were the most common or least differentiating language symptoms of all the groups tested.

As a final note, the speech-language pathologist (SLP) must always consider the specific work environment. For example, working in a typical elementary school is quite different than working in a hospital. Typically, the differences can be seen in the age of the patient, the etiology of the communication disorder, the severity of the communication disorder, and the physical setting.

In light of this, the authors remember a screening evaluation of all patients in a specific ward of a psychiatric center. One individual who was on the list was nowhere to be found. Suddenly, one of the aides in the center spotted that missing individual at the other end of this large open ward room and motioned for him to come over to where we were standing. The patient who was summoned weighed about 200 pounds, was built like Mike Tyson (former heavyweight boxing champion) or Arnold Schwartznegger (when he was a champion weightlifter), and could sprint like a cornerback in the National Football League. He started running toward us at about 100 miles per hour, causing the author either to stay put or move to one side or the other. The author stayed put (and alive), and the patient came to a screeching halt about 2 feet in front of him. By the way, the screening evaluation that followed found that the patient did not need speech or language therapy (whew!).

In a psychiatric center, the SLP should be alerted to the possible sudden temporary bizarre changes in speech, language, cognition, mood, and behavior. With this knowledge, the formal and informal speech and language evaluation materials and procedures used in other settings and environments can be used with the individuals in a psychiatric center.

Therapy

Speech Disorders Related to Tardive Dyskinesia

Uncontrolled movement of the oral structures, particularly the tongue and the mandible, may be associated with tardive dyskinesia (TD). The condition, as noted above, may occur as a consequence of long-term ingestion of antipsychotic medications. Treatments for voice and speech disorders characteristic of hyperkinetic dysarthria, described in Portnoy (1979), are discussed elsewhere in this text (see the section on dysarthria).

A shaping and fading procedure may be effective in reducing or eliminating the adventitious movements of the mandible associated with TD, as well as ritualistic behaviors, such as tongue protrusions, associated with schizophrenia. In a case study (Aaron, DeSanti, & Goldfarb, 1984), therapy bands of differing tension, borrowed from the physical therapy department, were wrapped from below the patient's mandible to the top of her head. As maladaptive behaviors of jaw jerks and tongue protrusions decreased, therapy bands with lower tension were introduced. The patient was also instructed to assume the pose made famous by Rodin's sculpture of "The Thinker" when she was listening to her communicative partner. Having her balled right fist below her mandible served as a paired stimulus to maintain head stability when use of the therapy bands was faded. Ward personnel remarked that the patient seemed to be more involved as a listener, based on her use of the "Thinker" pose.

Language Disorders

Therapy tends to follow the same format as that prescribed for both the patient with communication problems associated with traumatic brain injury and, to a lesser extent, the patient with dementia. Initially, keep the questions and responses as succinct as possible so as not to tax the patient. The next step would be short, simple conversations. Accomplish this task by gradually increasing the complexity of the verbalizations. Each time the patient demonstrates understanding of the particular level of syntactic structure, move to a higher level and observe the patient's responses.

Kondel et al. (2006) reported results of a 4-week lexical training program for nine adults with chronic schizophrenia. The authors claimed that a storage size problem, rather than word retrieval impairment (characteristic of aphasia), was the source of the anomia displayed by these individuals. While the authors reported a linear improvement in the partcipants' ability to identify 64 line drawings over the 4-week period of retraining, the follow-up test 1 month after completion revealed results similar to those observed in the first retraining session. Accordingly, it may not be beneficial to incorporate lexical retraining tasks into a speech-language intervention program for individuals with chronic undifferentiated schizophrenia.

To prevent or at least to limit the irrelevant verbiage by the patient when a given stimulus requires a specific response, one has several options. Initially, request the patient to stop talking. Use a time-out procedure with the patient each time his response becomes irrelevant and wordy. If a positive consequent event has been established (e.g., 5 minutes playing a computer game), use a grid with 10 boxes across and 10 down. Write a check mark in each of the 10 boxes across for an appropriate response, and erase a check for a disinhibited response. Write a star after each set of 10 checked boxes, and proceed to the next lower set of 10 boxes. When 10 stars are earned (100 correct responses), the patient is given computer time.

Speech and language therapy for the adult with chronic undifferentiated schizophrenia can focus on any coexisting aphasia, dysarthria, stuttering, or voice problem. In addition, therapy can focus on overcoming institutional neurosis by strengthening unimpaired communication skills, educating the communication partner, and addressing atherapeutic aspects of the environment (see the set theory model in the section on aphasia).

Halpern (1990) noted that traditional methods of speech therapy might not work for individuals with schizophrenia who stutter. Such factors as poor attention span, an inability to follow directions, memory deficits, compulsive behavior, or additional language problems are the reasons. However, with some tailor-made modifications, such techniques as relaxation, slowed speech, easy onset, choral speaking, and the *Stocker Probe* (Stocker & Goldfarb, 1995) have been demonstrated to be successful. Even if all objectives of therapy for stuttering are not met, the rapport created between patient and clinician, the individual knowledge that a patient will have a set time twice a week for self-expression, improvement of skills, feedback of accomplishments, and special attention often makes therapy very worthwhile.

Advanced Study: Neurobiology and Psychopharmacology of Schizophrenia

Adults with *chronic undifferentiated schizophrenia* commonly exhibit one or more neurological "soft signs," such as attention deficit, speech problems, right–left confusion, perseveration, abnormal gait, dysdiadochokinesia (inability to perform rapidly alternating movements), hypotonia, and nystagmus (abnormal eye movements) (Nasrallah & Smeltzer, 2002). Soft neurological signs are common not only in patients with schizophrenia, but also in their first-order relatives, supporting a biological and genetic etiology of this illness. Schizophrenia is never diagnosed on the basis of neurological signs, but rather on the basis of psychiatric symptoms. In a recent study (Goldfarb & Bekker, 2009), the 30 participants with chronic undifferentiated schizophrenia scored between 30 and 40 on the *Global Assessment of Functioning Scale* (GAF) in the DSM-IV (American Psychiatric Association, 2004, p. 34). This level indicates some impairment in reality testing or communication. For example, speech is at times illogical, obscure, or irrelevant. The neurotypical range on the GAF is 80–100. Another useful assessment tool for level of pathology associated with psychosis is the *Positive and Negative Syndrome Scale* (PANSS) (Geddes, Freemantle, Harrison, & Bebbington, 2000).

The proposed basic neurocircuit abnormality in schizophrenia, which causes delusions and hallucinations, is excessive *dopamine* activity in the *mesolimbic* pathway (Cohen &

Servan-Schreiber, 1992). Cognitive dysfunction and disorganization of schizophrenia may be related to a functional deficit in the dorsolateral prefrontal cortex (Brodmann's area 46/9). Deficient dopamine activity in this area may be responsible for reduced *working memory* and language disorder associated with schizophrenia (Perlstein, Carter, Noll, & Cohen, 2001). However, a recent meta-analysis of working memory experiments concluded that it is only the very early portion of working memory, the encoding phase, that is primarily deficient in schizophrenia. This may call into question the importance of frontal lobe function in producing the deficit. Prefrontal abnormalities have not been consistently demonstrated in postmortem, volumetric, or functional imaging studies of schizophrenia (see Van Snellenberg, Thornton, & Torres, 2006; Zuffante et al., 2001, for a review of these studies). In addition, working memory deficits were not found to be associated with the volume of area 46 (one presumed dorsolateral prefrontal working memory region) in participants with schizophrenia (Zuffante et al., 2001).

CASE DESCRIPTION 1

Note the remarkable coincidence in the decision of the attending neurologist to lower the patient's medication dosage, as well as her discovery of new symptoms in the patient, immediately after the consulting SLP filed his report.

I. *Report by consulting speech-language pathologist:*

This 39-year-old inpatient presented with a history of schizophrenia, chronic undifferentiated type, resulting in treatment at C. Psychiatric Center for the past 20 years, with continuous treatment for the past 15 years. During that time he has been treated with neuroleptic medications, primarily of the phenothiazine class.

Speech and language evaluation indicated evidence of tardive dyskinesia, characterized by frequent tongue protrusions and occasional random movement of the right upper limb. These behaviors can be controlled volitionally by the patient. A ward assistant reported noting these behaviors at least as early as 11 months ago.

During the evaluation the patient demonstrated fleeting periods of lucidity, accompanied by eye contact and relevant, propositional language. For example, the patient, who claims to be a professional baseball player (Johnny Logan), was engaged in a conversation about baseball. He responded quickly and appropriately to questions involving defensive and offensive plays and statistics. During this interchange, the predominant communication impairment was the patient's imprecise consonant formation and rapid-fire delivery, characteristic of a cluttering disorder.

Most of the patient's communicative behavior is typical of those with schizophrenic language. The following verbal and nonverbal communicative behaviors were noted: echolalia, or the tendency to repeat verbatim the examiner's questions or previous statements; perseveration, or the tendency to repeat an utterance made previously by the patient or examiner, although not an elicited or direct imitation; stereotypic utterances, or frequent repetitions of an idiosyncratic statement, such as, "My name is Dr. S. Johnny Logan Protector"; self-stimulatory behavior, exemplified by the patient's tendency to ball his right fist and rotate it across his right temple; rejection of attempts at interaction, characterized by the patient positioning his body away from the speaker and averting his eyes.

The following is recommended:

1. *A trial period of clinical intervention in speech-language pathology to determine which of the patient's maladaptive communicative behaviors are alterable;*

2. *A complete audiological evaluation; and*

3. *A neuropsychiatric evaluation to determine the extent of tardive dyskinesia, and to determine if any of these symptoms are reversible through titration of dosage of antipsychotic medications.*

II. *Report by the attending neurologist (later that same day):*

Pertinent Clinical History and Reason for Referral: 39-year-old white male who has been hospitalized for 15 years. He has been in our service for 2 years, 4 months. He has continued to have ritualistic behavior sticking his tongue out, patting his stomach, and putting his hand above his head in a peculiar way. He has been examined by me several times in the past for tardive dyskinesia. He was also examined by Dr. W. of TD group from H. Hospital 18 months ago. According to him he was not having TD at that time. At that time he was receiving 1000 milligrams of thorazine a day, which has been reduced. On [same date as SLP evaluation] it was further reduced to 600 milligrams/day. He was examined by [author] who felt patient has TD. I examined him today and found new movements in toes bilaterally and left elbow and some in wrist. Please examine him and give your recommendation and opinion. SK, M.D.

III. *Report by Tardive Dyskinesia Group (4 days later):*

Adventitious movements recorded by Dr. K., and found today, are compatible with possible tardive dyskinesia, spontaneous psychotic movement disorder, and Huntington disease. Patient's age is younger than what would ordinarily be expected for Jakob-Creutzfeldt disease.

Substantiation of diagnosis would depend on factors such as family history and relation of time of onset of movements to time of onset of mental illness and start of neuroleptic therapy.

Substantiation of the reported opinion excluding TD may possibly have been related to some of these factors; also the fact that the ritualistic movements are abolished with certain maneuvers, viz, the athetoid limb postures on assumption of the Romberg stance; bucco-lingual dyskinesia on wide opening of the mouth; and adventitious hand movements abolished by praxis (unlacing and lacing shoes).

Treatment for TD has been generally unsatisfactory. Currently there are research efforts attempting amelioration with alpha and beta adrenergic blockers but reported results have not been such as to encourage adoption. JS, M.D.

CASE DESCRIPTION 2

Following is a portion of an unedited e-mail response from a 36-year-old male with chronic undifferentiated schizophrenia to an invitation to lunch. He was living in a car, and reported that he was taking his medications, which were of the atypical neuroleptic class. Identifying information has been abbreviated or deleted.

I left a voice mail, thanks again for thinking of me, C. is a bit thoughtless or reacting too, just in case there is any miscommunication because of rumor or assumption. This creates more work and needed effort for me in my busy and difficult days with new financial responsibility and industry understanding beyond simple market "investments." I wish this was funny, but F. wouldn't stop, it became un-intended slander towards me from a couple of others also. It wound up reversing with my patience and accurate understanding, not his. I go on in this email to say I am worried about him, not just saying that. Also, C. is not supposed to be speaking for me, even on something as simple as a ride, this would also be false. No one is supposed to be speaking for me, that is dangerous at this level, especially with my added and corresponded "Security and Concerns Update" relevant to the "socially" concerned Network Radio invention. I should be there Saturday, I will call you if I'm not coming.

Beyond the wordiness of this email, please understand the presence of irrational conclusion from others, stemming from those close to me, you are clearly different. That irrational conclusion has and can be easily used to wedge a discomfort in something as simple as a lunch invitation, usually for fearful self-protection that is based on untruth. This does not come from me or you but is a program of sorts, if you have heard that "talk," and not a game or evaluative circumstance to disagree, maybe to understand fully—yes!

Further in this email, I explain that I work very, very hard, avoiding laziness and encouragement of harmful things that would end up in your home or on your table. For example, like C. telling you that I am not going after I told her a few times I would. She is doing her best, but it is unfair to her and not enough. We spoke about that conversation with you. It has only made more difficulty by slandering, self-protective conclusions that are understandable, but completely unwhole and irrational. I understand your difference in perspective, easily not being the same quick, unwhole, or inaccurate conclusion—the same for this long email, detail relevant. These conclusions written, too easily deniable by those others are what is difusing correctly. This is only about these small personal things, not much else. The rest of the email introduces the topic of a whole understanding, the appropriate note I am copying for you explains details, otherwise I am hurt further.

. . . on a positive note, that less-negative or progressive skill is developed too, non-encouraging to end in the same healing result.

Discussion Questions: Theory

1. Neurological "soft signs" are common in adults with schizophrenia, but are not used as the basis for a diagnosis. What are some of these soft signs? What are some of the psychiatric signs?

2. Why is the notion of reduced working memory in individuals with schizophrenia controversial?

3. Andreasen has identified 17 linguistic symptoms associated with schizophrenia. Which of these symptoms might also be characteristic of aphasia?

4. What are some potential effects of reciprocal inhibition of neurotransmitters on the patient receiving antipsychotic medications?

5. The apparent preference for nouns over verbs may indicate functional frontal lobe deficit or temporal lobe overactivation. Explain.

Discussion Questions: Therapy

1. Regarding the case description, why did the neurologist (Dr. K.) lower the dosage of medication, and why did she choose this particular time to do so?

2. What speech and voice symptoms might prompt an SLP to refer an individual with schizophrenia for an evaluation of tardive dyskinesia?

3. Should treatment of the language of schizophrenia by an SLP be reimbursed by third-party payers (health insurance)? Why or why not?

4. How are semantic and pragmatic language deficits in schizophrenia similar to and different from those deficits in aphasia?

5. How does treatment of speech and language disorders in chronic undifferentiated schizophrenia differ from speech-language intervention for aphasia?

Assignment: Write a multiple-choice question with five options. Explain why the key option is correct, and why the distractors or decoys are incorrect. Avoid using forms such as, "All of the following are (in)correct *except*" in the stem, and "All (or none) of the above" in the options.

Example: Differentiating between diagnostically related groups may be facilitated by errors in language comprehension, production, and use. When adjectives attribute qualities to nouns they do not typically have (equipment is described as "stale"), the underlying disorder is more likely to be:

a. Broca's aphasia than Wernicke's aphasia
b. Nonfluent aphasia than fluent aphasia
c. The language of schizophrenia than fluent aphasia
d. The language of Alzheimer dementia than the language of frontotemporal dementia
e. Dysarthria than apraxia of speech

The correct answer is *c*: Semantic paraphasias in fluent aphasia affect nouns and verbs more than adjectives, while the thought disorder in schizophrenia can result in semantic errors of the type noted in the example above. *a* is incorrect because semantic paraphasias are more typical of Wernicke's than of Broca's aphasia; *b* is incorrect because semantic paraphasias are more typical of fluent than of nonfluent aphasia; *d* is incorrect because language in Alzheimer disease becomes empty with an increasing loss of substantives, while in vascular dementia, language becomes more concise because of preservation of substantive words; *e* is incorrect because both dysarthria and apraxia of speech affect articulation, not semantics.

References

Aaron, I., DeSanti, S., & Goldfarb, R. (1984, April). *Tardive dyskinesia: Assessment and intervention*. Presentation to the New York State Speech-Language-Hearing Association.

American Psychiatric Association. (2000). *Diagnostic and statistical manual of mental disorders* (4th ed.). Washington, DC: Author.

Andreasen, N. C. (1979a). The clinical assessment of thought, language, and communication disorders: I. Diagnostic significance. *Archives of General Psychiatry, 36*, 1325–1330.

Andreasen, N. C. (1979b). Thought, language, and communication disorders: I. Clinical assessment, definition of terms, and evaluation of their reliability. *Archives of General Psychiatry, 36*, 1315–1321.

Barach, D., & Berenbaum, H. (1996). Language production and thought disorder in schizophrenia. *Journal of Abnormal Psychology, 105*, 81–88.

Bemporad, J., & Pinsker, H. (1974). Schizophrenia: The manifest symptomatology. In S. Arieti & E. Brody (Eds.), *American handbook of psychiatry* (Vol. 3, pp. 524–550). New York, NY: Basic Books.

Bilder, R. M., Goldman, R. S., Volavka, J., Czobor, P., Hoptman, M., Sheitman, B., . . . Lieberman, J. (2002). Neurocognitive effects of clozapine, olanzapine, risperidone, and haloperidol in patients with chronic schizophrenia or schizoaffective disorder. *American Journal of Psychiatry, 159,* 1018–1028.

Bruder, G., Rabinowitz, E., Towey, J., Brown, A., Kaufmann, C. A., Amador, X., . . . Gorman, J. M. (1995). Smaller right ear (left hemisphere) advantage for dichotic fused words in patients with schizophrenia. *The American Journal of Psychiatry, 152,* 932–935.

Chaika, E. (1974). A linguist looks at "schizophrenic" language. *Brain and Language, 1,* 257–276.

Chapman, L. J. (1958). Intrusion of associative responses into schizophrenic conceptual performance. *Journal of Abnormal and Social Psychology, 56,* 373–379.

Cohen, J., & Servan-Schreiber, D. (1992). Context, cortex, and dopamine: A connectionist approach to behavior and biology in schizophrenia. *Psychological Review, 99,* 45–77.

Crow, T. J. (2008). The "big bang" theory of the origin of psychosis and the faculty of language. *Schizophrenia Research, 102,* 31–52.

Day, M., & Semrad, E. (1978). Schizophrenic reactions. In A. Nicholi (Ed.), *The Harvard guide to modern psychiatry* (pp. 191–241). Cambridge, MA: Harvard University Press.

D'Esposito, M., & Postle, B. R. (1999). The dependence of span and delayed-response performance on prefrontal cortex. *Neuropsychologia, 37,* 1303–1315.

DiSimoni, F., Darley, F., & Aronson, A. (1977). Patterns of dysfunction in schizophrenic subjects on an aphasia test battery. *Journal of Speech and Hearing Disorders, 42,* 498–513.

Downing, R., Ebert, J., & Shubrooks, S. (1963). Effects of three types of verbal distractors on thinking in acute schizophrenia. *Perceptual and Motor Skills, 17,* 881–882.

Faibish, G. (1961). Schizophrenic responses to words of multiple meaning. *Journal of Personality, 29,* 414–427.

Frith, C. D., Friston, K. J., Herold, S., Silbersweig, D., Fletcher, P., Cahill, C., . . . Liddle, P. F. (1995). Regional brain activity in chronic schizophrenic patients during the performance of a verbal fluency task. *British Journal of Psychiatry, 167,* 343–349.

Fromkin, V. (1975). A linguist looks at "A linguist looks at 'schizophrenic' language." *Brain and Language, 2,* 498–503.

Geddes, J., Freemantle, N., Harrison, P., & Bebbington, P. (2000). Atypical antipsychotics in the treatment of schizophrenia: Systematic overview and meta-regression analysis. *British Medical Journal, 321,* 1371–1376.

Geschwind, N. (1966). Carl Wernicke, the Breslau school, and the history of aphasia. In E. C. Carterette (Ed.), *Brain function: Speech, language, and communication* (Vol. III, pp. 1–17). Berkeley, CA: University of California Press.

Goldfarb, R., & Bekker, N. (2009). Noun-verb ambiguity in chronic undifferentiated schizophrenia. *Journal of Communication Disorders, 42,* 74–88.

Goldfarb, R., Eisenson, J., Stocker, B., & DeSanti, S. (1994). Communicative responsibility and semantic class in aphasia and "schizophasia." *Perceptual and Motor Skills, 79,* 1027–1039.

Goldfarb, R., & Goldberg, E. (2004). Communicative responsibility and semantic class in the language of dementia. *Perceptual and Motor Skills, 98,* 1177–1186.

Goldfarb, R., & Halpern, H. (1981). Word association of time-altered auditory and visual stimuli in aphasia. *Journal of Speech and Hearing Research, 24,* 233–246.

Goldfarb, R., & Halpern, H. (1984). Word association responses in normal adult subjects. *Journal of Psycholinguistic Research, 13,* 37–55.

Goldfarb, R., & Halpern, H. (1989). Impairments of naming and word finding. In C. Code (Ed.), *The characteristics of aphasia* (pp. 33–52). London, UK: Taylor & Francis.

Halpern, H. (1990). Stuttering therapy for nonfluent psychiatric adults. *Perceptual and Motor Skills, 71,* 914.

Halpern, H., Darley, F. L., & Brown, J. (1973). Differential language and neurologic characteristics in cerebral involvement. *Journal of Speech and Hearing Disorders, 38,* 162–173.

Halpern, H., Goldfarb, R., Brandon, J., & McCartin-Clark, M. (1985). Word-association responses to time-altered stimuli by schizophrenic adults. *Perceptual and Motor Skills, 61,* 239–253.

Halpern, H., & McCartin-Clark, M. (1984). Differential language patterns in aphasic and schizophrenic subjects. *Journal of Communication Disorders, 17,* 289–307.

Halpern, H., McCartin-Clark, M., & Wallack, W. (1989). The non-fluencies of eight psychiatric adults. *Journal of Communication Disorders, 22,* 233–241.

Johnson, R., Weiss, R., & Zelhart, P. (1964). Similarities and differences between normal-psychotic subjects in response to verbal stimuli. *Journal of Abnormal and Social Psychology, 63,* 422–427.

Kondel, T. K., Hirsch, S. R., & Laws, K. R. (2006). Name relearning in elderly patients with schizophrenia: Episodic and temporary, not semantic and permanent. *Cognitive Neuropsychiatry, 11,* 1–12.

Kubicki, M., Westin, C. F., Nestor, P. G., Wible, C. G., Frumin, M., Maier, S. E., . . . Shenton, M. E. (2003). Cingulate fasciculus integrity disruption in schizophrenia: A magnetic resonance diffusion tensor imaging study. *Biological Psychiatry, 54,* 1171–1180.

Lecours, A. R., & Vanier-Clement, M. (1976). Schizophasia and jargonaphasia: A comparative description with comments on Chaika's and Fromkin's respective looks at "schizophrenic" language. *Brain and Language, 3,* 516–565.

Meilijson, S., Kasher, A., & Elizur, A. (2004). Language performance in chronic schizophrenia: A pragmatic approach. *Journal of Speech, Language, and Hearing Research, 47,* 695–713.

Moritz, S., Woodward, T. S., Kuppers, D., Lausen, A., & Schickel, M. (2001). Increased automatic spreading of activation in thought-disordered schizophrenic patients. *Schizophrenia Research, 59,* 181–186.

Nasrallah, H. A., & Smeltzer, D. J. (2002). *Contemporary diagnosis and management of the patient with schizophrenia.* Newtown, PA: Handbooks in Healthcare.

Perlstein, W., Carter, C., Noll, D., & Cohen, J. (2001). Relation of prefrontal cortex dysfunction to working memory and symptoms of schizophrenia. *American Journal of Psychiatry, 158,* 1105–1113.

Portnoy, R. A. (1979). Hyperkinetic dysarthria as an early indicator of impending tardive dyskinesia. *Journal of Speech and Hearing Disorders, 44,* 214–219.

Prutting, C., & Kirchner, D. (1987). A clinical appraisal of the pragmatic aspects of language. *Journal of Speech and Hearing Disorders, 52,* 105–119.

Raven, J. (1958). Verbal dysfunction in mental illness. *Language and Speech, 1,* 218–225.

Richman, J. (1968). Symbolic distortion in the vocabulary definitions of schizophrenics. In H. J. Vetter (Ed.), *Language behavior in schizophrenia.* Springfield, IL: Thomas.

Rinnert, C., & Whitaker, H. (1973). Semantic confusions by aphasic patients. *Cortex, 9,* 56–81.

Ross, E. D., Orbelo, D. M., Cartwright, J., Hansel, S., Burgard, M., Testa, J. A., & Buck, R. (2001). Affective-prosodic deficits in schizophrenia: Comparison to patients with brain damage and relation to schizophrenic symptoms. *Journal of Neurology, Neurosurgery, and Psychiatry, 70,* 597–604.

Sprague, D. A., Loewen, P. S., & Raymond, C. B. (2004). Selection of atypical anti-psychotics for the management of schizophrenia. *Annals of Pharmacotherapy, 38,* 313–319.

Stocker, B., & Goldfarb, R. (1995). *The Stocker probe for fluency and language* (3rd ed.). Vero Beach, FL: The Speech Bin.

Strelnikov, K. (2008). Activation-verification in continuous speech processing: Interaction of cognitive strategies as a possible theoretical approach. *Journal of Neurolinguistics, 21,* 1–17.

Tachibana, T. (1980). Persistent erroneous interpretation of negative data and assessment of statistical power. *Perceptual and Motor Skills, 51,* 37–38.

Van Snellenberg, J. X., Thornton, A. E., & Torres, I. J. (2006). Functional neuroimaging of working memory in schizophrenia: Task performance as a moderating variable. *Neuropsychology, 20,* 497–510.

Woodruff, P. W. R., Wright, I. C., Bullmore, E. T., Brammer, M., Howard, R. J., Williams, S. C. R., . . . Murray, R. M. (1997). Auditory hallucinations and the temporal cortical response to speech in schizophrenia: A functional magnetic resonance imaging study. *The American Journal of Psychiatry, 154,* 1676–1682.

Wynne, R. D. (1963). The influence of hospitalization on the verbal behavior of chronic schizophrenics. *British Journal of Psychiatry, 109,* 380–389.

Wynne, R. D. (1964). Are verbal word association norms suitable for schizophrenia? *Psychological Reports, 61,* 121–122.

Zuffante, P., Leonard, C. M., Kuldau, J. M., Bauer, R. M., Doty, E. G., & Bilder, R. M. (2001). Working memory deficits in schizophrenia are not necessarily specific or associated with MRI-based estimates of area 46 volumes. *Psychiatry Research: Neuroimaging Section, 108,* 187–209.

Dysarthria

Definition

The condition known as dysarthria can occur alone or can accompany other speech and language disorders. In a seminal study, Darley, Aronson, and Brown (1969a, 1969b, 1975) stated that dysarthria is a collective name for a group of speech disorders that result from disturbances in muscular control over the speech mechanism due to damage of the central or peripheral nervous system.

Dysarthria designates an impairment in oral communication due to paralysis, which is a weakness, slowness, or incoordination of the speech musculature. This is in contrast to impairments due to damage in higher centers related to the faulty programming of movement and sequences of movements (apraxia of speech), and to the inefficient processing of linguistic units (aphasia).

Darley et al. (1969a, 1969b, 1975) delineated the various types of dysarthria, each with its own neurologic and speech characteristics. Prior to this perceptual method for delineating the various types of dysarthria, professionals would just use the term *dysarthria* and provide a description of the speech symptom(s) (see Halpern, Hochberg, & Rees, 1967). The Darley et al. (1969a, 1969b) study showed that because speech production follows particular neuroanatomical and neurophysiological pathways, a reference to a specific type of dysarthria can be useful in localizing a lesion. This has clinical value, because it serves as a diagnostic tool and can lead to further investigation of the condition.

Darley et al. (1969a, 1969b, 1975) identified 36 different dimensions (symptoms) and 2 overall dimensions (intelligibility and bizarreness) in their dysarthria study (Darley et al., 1969a, 1969b). So as not to be overwhelmed by an avalanche of symptoms, the reader is advised to look primarily at those speech symptoms that distinguish one dysarthria from the others. It must be noted that some of the same symptoms may be ranked as most prominent in several dysarthrias and are therefore not considered as reliable differential signs. For example, imprecise consonants were found in all or practically all of the participants with dysarthria in all groups.

In later parts of this section, the terms *alternating motion rates* (AMRs) or *diadochokinetic rates* will be used. Both terms refer to checking the speed and consistency of alternating movements of the lips, tongue, and jaw during repetitive articulation.

The contributions of Darley, Aronson, and Brown (1969a, 1969b) remain crucial, but they are more than 40 years old. Kent et al. (2001) found that 30 years after the Darley, Aronson, and Brown (1969a) study that described 7 types of dysarthria, new information that relates the lesion to the speech disturbance can be applied to the pyramidal pathway, extrapyramidal pathway, and the cerebellum. More recently, the speech science laboratory has been a fruitful source of information about dysarthria, particularly in quantifying characteristics of the somewhat amorphous term *imprecise consonants*. A second concern is that the Mayo Clinic view may have motivated oromotor, nonverbal tasks for individuals with dysarthria.

Weismer (2006) reviewed literature that both supported and refuted the Mayo Clinic view of motor speech disorders. He concluded that there is weak theoretical and experimental support for the Mayo view. In another study (Bunton et al., 2007), the authors looked at interrater and intrarater agreement for the auditory-perceptual rating system developed by Darley, Aronson, and Brown (1969a, 1969b). Inexperienced and experienced listeners who evaluated 47 speakers with various types of dysarthria showed no significant differences in agreement on the perceptual features. The authors concluded that these auditory-perceptual ratings may be useful in identifying salient features of dysarthria. However, the scoring paradigm that clinicians use (e.g., phonetic, lexical, or semantic) to measure speech intelligibility does not seem to matter, as long as it is used consistently (Hustad, 2006a).

Weismer (2006) also indicated that using oromotor, nonverbal tasks for treatment of dysarthria is unwarranted. In fact, decreased tongue strength may not affect speech intelligibility (Neel et al., 2006). The present authors agree that physical therapy for the face (oromotor, nonverbal tasks) will not address the speech and voice problems associated with dysarthria, but note that (1) oromotor, nonverbal tasks are within the scope of practice of speech-language pathologists; and (2) improving facial symmetry through these tasks may address psychosocial concomitants of dysarthria, because individuals with facial droop may avoid social and communicative interactions.

Bunton-Weismer (2001) found that with dysarthric speakers the acoustic characteristics of tongue-height errors were not clearly differentiated from the acoustic characteristics of targets. The acoustic characteristics of errors often looked like noisy (nonprototypical) versions of the targets. Chen and Stevens (2001) found that in individuals with dysarthria, acoustic parameters are related to deviations in the temporal pattern of control of the articulators in providing fricative-vowel sequences and to lack of fine control of the tongue blade in achieving an appropriate target configuration for the fricative.

Yorkston (2007) reviewed 148 studies from 1997–2006 of degenerative dysarthrias associated with Parkinson disease, multiple sclerosis, and amyotrophic lateral sclerosis. The largest category by far was of studies that focused on neurophysiologic, acoustic, or perceptual aspects of speech production. For example, deep brain stimulation of the subthalamic nucleus does not seem to improve speech intelligibility in individuals with Parkinson disease (PD) (D'Alatri et al., 2008); and acoustic analysis alone, without perceptual analysis, does not adequately illuminate voice problems in dysarthria following stroke (Wang et al., 2009). The other large research issues were management, including assessment and treatment, and psychosocial aspects of dysarthria.

Some studies focused on peaks of resonance in the vocal tract, called *formants*, in the speech of individuals with dysarthria. The second formant (F2) has been known for more than 50 years to be important to intelligibility; it is also affected by various types of dysarthria. In a study by Rosen et al. (2008), 12 adults with multiple sclerosis and 16 neurotypical controls read the Grandfather Passage aloud, and F2 slopes were calculated. The mean and maximum F2 observations were used as examples of typical and extreme productions. The greatest differences between the two groups occurred for their best productions, that is, their maximum F2 slopes. This maximum F2 measure was shown to estimate the effects of mild to moderate dysarthria better than their typical productions did.

The second formant has also been used as a measure of treatment effects in dysarthria secondary to Parkinson disease (Sapir et al., 2007, 2010). Following treatment with the Lee Silverman Voice Treatment (LSVT) program, 14 individuals with idiopathic Parkinson disease were compared to 15 individuals with PD who did not receive LSVT and 15 age-matched neurotypical controls (Sapir et al., 2007). F2 differences for the vowels /i/, /u/, and /a/ between controls and the group that received LSVT were significant only for F2u and the ratio F2i/F2u. In a follow-up study (Sapir et al., 2010), the F2i/F2u ratio differentiated adults with dysarthria secondary to PD from healthy controls, and was not gender-sensitive. Kim et al. (2009) examined 40 speakers with dysarthria (20 with PD and 20 with stroke), and 5 neurotypical speakers, who were asked to repeat 6 words. Responses were examined according to the F2 slope. The authors concluded that acoustic variables such as F2 slope could be used in a quantitative metric of severity of speech deficits in dysarthria, but that further research was needed. Finally, Patel and Campellone (2009) noted that the acoustic cues commonly associated with prosody involve fundamental frequency (F_0), intensity, and duration, and found that their speakers with dysarthria relied more heavily on duration.

Kent, Vorperian, and Duffy (1999) reported on the robust reliability of the multidimensional voice program (MDVP), a computer program that can calculate as many as 33 acoustic parameters from a voice sample. In addition, the MDVP has potential as a tool for the semiautomatic analysis of voice samples in dysarthria. Tjaden (2003) found that anticipatory coarticulation for speakers with multiple sclerosis and speakers with Parkinson disease is preserved. Tjaden and Wilding (2005) found few group differences in coarticulation, suggesting that the organizational coherence of phonetic events is generally preserved for speakers with mild to moderate dysarthria. The finding that speech mode similarly affected acoustic measures of anticipatory coarticulation for speaker groups further suggests the feasibility of applying theories and models of neurologically typical speech production to the study of dysarthria. Tjaden, Rivera, Wilding, and Turner (2005) found that even those vowels characterized by relatively reduced vocal tract shapes, such as /I/ (as in "been"), /ɛ/ ("went"), and /U/ ("wood") are not free from the effects of dysarthria, although it was unclear whether dysarthria severity or neurologic disease has a primary role in determining the extent to which lax vowels are affected in speakers with dysarthria.

Rosen, Kent, Delaney, and Duffy (2006) found that hypokinetic dysarthria (HKD) can be consistently distinguished from healthy controls (HCs) on the basis of intensity, variation, and spectral range, when speech is in both sentence repetition and conversational modes. Although speakers with HKD were effectively able to produce higher contrastivity levels in sentence-repetition tasks, they habitually performed closer to the lower end of their production ranges. Caviness, Liss, Adler, and Evidente (2006) found that corticomuscular electroencephalographic-electromyographic (EEG and EMG) coherence existed for both healthy participants and those with Parkinson disease in all speech and nonspeech oromotor tasks, but to varying degrees in primary sensorimotor cortex and supplementary motor areas.

Technological advances have permitted nontraditional evaluation and treatment of dysarthria. Participants with long-standing dysarthria showed equivalent improvement in speech when treatment was either traditional or computer-based (Palmer, Enderby, & Hawley, 2007). The Munich Intelligibility Profile, a computer-based assessment of intelligibility of speakers with dysarthria, has been useful for standard diagnosis and for research (Ziegler & Zierdt, 2008). Last, an Internet-based assessment protocol shows promise, but needs further refinement (Hill, 2006).

Symptoms and Etiology

Flaccid Dysarthria

The first type of dysarthria is described as flaccid dysarthria and is, for example, found in the neurologic disorder called *bulbar palsy* (multiple cranial nerve damage, which can be caused by many of the conditions listed below). All patients in this group displayed evidence of a lower motor neuron lesion, implicating motor units of the cranial nerves involved in speech (V, VII, IX, X, XII). Lesions to lower motor neurons that innervate the respiratory musculature or to the cranial nerves that innervate the speech musculature can result in a flaccid dysarthria.

Weakness of muscle contraction and hypotonia (flaccidity) are the salient features of flaccid dysarthria. It is the only motor speech disorder in which a rapid breakdown of speech can occur after a short period of continuous speaking. Patients with myasthenia gravis can show this deterioration.

Duffy (2005) noted that the etiologies of 107 cases of flaccid dysarthria seen at the Mayo Clinic were as follows: traumatic (34%), composed of surgical trauma (29%) and nonsurgical trauma (5%); neuropathies of undetermined origin (27%); muscle disease (8%); tumor (6%); myasthenia gravis (6%); degenerative (6%); vascular (5%); infectious (3%); anatomic malformation (3%); demyelinating (1%); and other (1%).

Speech Symptoms

Following is a sampling of some of the studies and reports related to the speech symptoms found in flaccid dysarthria. Additional references are noted in the "Diagnosis" and "Therapy" parts of this section.

Darley et al. (1969a, 1969b, 1975), in their study of 30 patients with bulbar palsy, found that the most prominent speech deviations (from most to least severe) were hypernasality, imprecise consonants, breathiness (continuous), monopitch, nasal emission, audible inspiration, harsh voice quality, short phrases, and monoloudness.

The speech deviations that best distinguish flaccid dysarthria from the other dysarthrias are described by Darley et al. (1969a, 1969b, 1975), and by Duffy (2005) in his review of supportive studies in the literature, as hypernasality, often coupled with nasal emission of air (resulting from incomplete palatopharyngeal closure); breathiness that is continuous during phonation (resulting from poor adduction of the vocal folds); audible inspiration or stridor on inhalation (resulting from inadequate abduction of the vocal folds); and short phrases (resulting from the effect of air wastage through the nose and the need to replenish it frequently).

Respiration Symptoms

Hixon, Putnam, and Sharp (1983) described speech production in a case of flaccid paralysis of the rib cage, diaphragm, and abdomen. The patient was able to combine compensatory neck breathing and glossopharyngeal breathing with other biomechanical and linguistic adaptations into still another functional system for speech production. The authors described the kinematic analysis that took place with this patient.

Hoit, Banzett, Brown, and Loring (1990) used magnetometers to record surface motions of the chest wall in 10 men with traumatic cervical spinal cord injury. The speech characteristics of the subjects showed 3 with reduced loudness, 2 with breathiness, 1 with hypernasality, 1 with rough voice, 1 with imprecise articulation, 2 with short phrases, 1 with long phrases, 1 with long inspiration, and 3 who were normal. Abnormal chest wall activity was attributed mostly to loss of abdominal muscle function. The authors concluded that speech breathing in persons with cervical spinal cord injury may be improved by the use of abdominal binders.

Phonation Symptoms

Aronson (1990) noted that in the flaccid dysarthria of myasthenia gravis, the perceptual laryngeal-phonatory characteristics include the following: a breathy voice quality with weak intensity, a deterioration of phonation during stressful counting or other prolonged speaking activities, and a reduced sharpness of cough after stressful speaking.

The physical appearance of the vocal folds in milder cases may seem normal in structure and function, despite a dysphonia. Absence of findings does exclude presence of milder degrees of bilateral adductor weakness of the vocal folds. In more severe cases, the vocal folds bilaterally may fail to adduct and abduct completely. Bowing of the vocal folds may be present.

Murry (1978) studied 20 subjects with unilateral vocal fold paralysis and found that they had a reduced ability to reach upper pitch ranges. The affected fold becomes flaccid and sluggish, which accounts for the reduced speaking fundamental frequency range. This reduced vocal frequency range may produce a monotone, which is quite often perceived in flaccid dysarthria.

Hammarberg, Fritzell, and Schiratski (1984) analyzed the voice quality of 16 subjects with unilateral paralysis before and after a Teflon injection. A perceptual evaluation made after the injection showed that 11 of the 16 participants made improvement in their voices due to a reduction of breathiness and dysphonia, and in maintaining proper pitch functions. The acoustic measurement of LTAS (long term average spectrum) provided an objective measure of this improvement. Reich and Lerman (1978) found that after a Teflon injection in a patient with unilateral vocal fold paralysis there was a general reduction in perceived hoarseness and an enhancement of perceived pleasantness.

Watterson, McFarlane, and Menicucci (1990) studied 9 participants who had unilateral vocal fold paralysis. Of the 9 participants, 4 were injected with Teflon, 4 were not injected, and 1 was injected but served as a participant in both groups. An additional 3 participants without vocal fold pathology served as a typical control group. Results showed that participants in both groups with unilateral vocal fold paralysis (injected and not injected) showed abnormal vibratory characteristics of the vocal folds, whereas the typical participants showed a more normal picture. Teflon injections with the participants used in this study proved unsuccessful.

Duffy (2005), in his summary of respiratory and phonatory findings in flaccid dysarthria (based on the literature), confirmed the presence of the respiratory-phonatory symptom of short phrases, and the phonatory symptoms of breathiness and audible inspiration as distinguishing features.

Resonation Symptoms

Garcia and Cannito (1996) reported on a patient with severe flaccid dysarthria whose symptoms were primarily characterized by hypernasality, imprecise consonants, short phrases, and breathiness. The study demonstrated that for this speaker with dysarthria, speech produced with accompanying communication gestures, with highly predictive sentence content, or with situationally related contexts was more intelligible than speech lacking those characteristics.

Duffy (2005), in his summary of resonatory findings in flaccid dysarthria (based on the literature), confirmed the presence of hypernasality and nasal emission as distinguishing features.

Spastic Dysarthria

The second type of dysarthria is described as spastic dysarthria and is, for example, found in the neurologic disorder called *pseudobulbar palsy* (bilateral spastic paralysis affecting the bulbar musculature and most commonly caused by multiple or bilateral strokes, and head trauma). The patients in the pseudobulbar group present an upper motor neuron disorder, presumed to involve combined damage to the pyramidal system and a portion of the extrapyramidal system, both of which arise from the same motor cortex areas. Lesions to upper motor neurons produce spastic muscles that are stiff, move sluggishly through a limited range, and tend to be weak.

Duffy (2005) noted that the etiologies of 107 cases of spastic dysarthria seen at the Mayo Clinic were as follows: vascular (31%); degenerative (30%); traumatic (12%), composed of traumatic brain injury (10%) and surgical trauma (2%); undetermined (12%); demyelinating (6%); tumor (4%); multiple causes (3%); inflammatory (2%); and infectious (1%).

Speech Symptoms

Following is a sampling of some of the studies and reports related to the speech symptoms found in spastic dysarthria. Additional references are noted in the "Diagnosis" and "Therapy" parts of this section.

Darley et al. (1969a, 1969b, 1975), in their study of 30 patients with pseudobulbar palsy, found that the most prominent speech deviations (from most to least severe) were imprecise consonants, monopitch, reduced stress, harsh voice quality, monoloudness, low pitch, slow rate, hypernasality, strained-strangled quality, short phrases, distorted vowels, pitch breaks, breathy voice (continuous), and excess and equal stress.

The speech deviations that best distinguish spastic dysarthria from the other dysarthrias are described by Darley et al. (1969a, 1969b, 1975), and by Duffy (2005) in his review of supportive studies in the literature, as a strained-strangled voice quality (resulting from the increased tone of the laryngeal muscles, which causes narrowing of the glottis and increases the resistance to the flow of breath at that level), slow speech rate, and slow and regular alternating motion rates (AMRs), the latter two resulting from articulators that move sluggishly with a reduction of range, as well as weakness.

More recently, Nishio and Niimi (2006) used acoustic analysis to examine speaking rate, articulation rate, and AMR in 62 individuals with dysarthria and 34 neurotypical controls. All three parameters were much lower in speakers with dysarthria than in controls. AMR was notable because variation was more limited in controls, and, unlike in controls, AMR in speakers with dysarthria was markedly lower than their articulation rate. Accordingly, AMR may be used more easily and reliably to detect abnormal articulation than speaking rate and articulation rate.

Phonation and Resonation Symptoms

Aronson (1990) noted that in spastic dysarthria, the perceptual laryngeal-phonatory characteristics include the following: a hoarseness or harshness that has a strained-strangled quality, abnormally low pitch accompanied by monopitch, and reduced loudness accompanied by monoloudness. The strained-strangled, harsh voice quality is caused by hyperadduction of the true and false vocal folds, which produces glottic restriction and resistance to the exhalatory airflow.

At rest, the physical appearance of the vocal folds is normal. During speech, the vocal folds can range from looking normal to showing bilateral hyperadduction of the true and false vocal folds.

Duffy (2005), in his summary of phonatory findings in spastic dysarthria (based on the literature), confirmed the presence of strained-strangled voice quality as a distinguishing feature.

Articulation and Prosody Symptoms

Hirose, Kiritani, and Sawashima (1982) found a reduced range of articulatory movement in pseudobulbar palsy speech. Ziegler and von Cramon (1986) reported that speakers with spastic dysarthria showed a reduction of sound pressure level contrasts in the production of consonants, which may account for imprecise consonants.

Dworkin and Aronson (1986) found that speakers with spastic dysarthria had significantly slower rates than typical speakers. Hirose (1986) reported a reduced range of tongue movements and a slowed overall speech rate in spastic dysarthria. Hirose et al. (1982) found a slow rate of speaking in pseudobulbar palsy speech.

Linebaugh and Wolfe (1984) found that speakers with spastic dysarthria had significantly longer mean syllable duration than did typical speakers. Portnoy and Aronson (1982) confirmed that speakers with spastic dysarthria had a significantly slower and more variable rate in repetition tasks than did typical speakers. Ziegler and von Cramon (1986) reported that speakers with spastic dysarthria showed an increase in syllable and word duration, which might account for the slow rate.

Duffy (2005), in his summary of articulatory and prosody findings in spastic dysarthria (based on the literature), confirmed the presence of slow speech rate and slow and regular AMRs as distinguishing features.

Hypokinetic Dysarthria

The third type of dysarthria is described as hypokinetic dysarthria and is, for example, found in the neurologic disorder called *Parkinsonism*. The extrapyramidal system is responsible for regulating the muscle tone required for posture and for changing position. One of the symptoms of extrapyramidal disease is the reduction of movements, called *hypokinesia*. The characteristic symptoms of hypokinesia include slowness of movement, limited range of movement, immobility and paucity of movement, rigidity, loss of automatic aspects of movement, and rest tremor.

Parkinsonism is an example of hypokinesia and comes about through damage to the basal ganglia, cortex, and other structures. In particular, the substantia nigra, located in the brainstem, produces a chemical substance called dopamine and sends it to the corpus striatum in the basal ganglia. The corpus striatum turns it into a neural transmitter responsible for its inhibiting influence over muscle tone and movement. Damage to that mechanism is a major cause of Parkinsonism.

In relation to speech, the important feature of hypokinetic disorders is a marked limitation of range of movement. Individualized movements are slow and lack vigor, and often there are hesitations and false starts. Repetitive movements are sometimes slow and at other times very fast and of limited range. It is the only dysarthria in which rapid rate can occur and in which repeated phonemes and palilalia (the involuntary repetition of words and phrases with increasing rate and decreasing loudness) are often found.

Kim, Kent, and Weismer (2011) examined speech recordings from 107 speakers with dysarthria due to Parkinson disease, stroke, traumatic brain injury, and multiple system atrophy. This was used for acoustic analysis and for perceptual judgment of speech intelligibility. Results showed that (1) acoustic predictors of speech intelligibility differed slightly across diseases, and (2) classification accuracy by dysarthria type was typically worse than by disease type or severity.

Duffy (2005) noted that the etiologies of 107 cases of hypokinetic dysarthria seen at the Mayo Clinic were as follows: degenerative (75%), where Parkinson disease (31%) and Parkinsonism (26%) made up 57% of that total; vascular (10%); undetermined (6%); toxic/metabolic (3%); traumatic (2%); multiple (2%); infectious (1%); and other (1%).

Speech Symptoms

Following is a sampling of some of the studies and reports related to the speech symptoms found in hypokinetic dysarthria. Additional references are noted in the "Diagnosis" and "Therapy" parts of this section.

Darley et al. (1969a, 1969b, 1975), in their study of 32 patients with Parkinsonism, found that the most prominent speech deviations (from most to least severe) were monopitch, reduced stress, monoloudness, imprecise consonants, inappropriate silences, short rushes of speech, harsh voice quality, breathy voice (continuous), pitch level, and variable rate.

The speech deviations that best distinguish hypokinetic dysarthria from the other dysarthrias are described by Darley et al. (1969a, 1969b, 1975), and by Duffy (2005) in his review of supportive studies in the literature, as monopitch, monoloudness, decreased loudness, reduced stress, variable rate, short rushes of speech, overall increases in rate, increased rate within segments, rapid speech AMRs, repeated phonemes, and inappropriate silences (all deviations resulting from a limited range of movement of the musculature, and the rapid rate deviations resulting from the very fast, repetitive movements of a very reduced range that are seen only in Parkinsonism). Tjaden (2000) conducted a preliminary study of factors influencing listener perception of articulatory rate in nine men with mild to moderate idiopathic Parkinson disease. According to the author, the results hint at the possibility that perceptual impression of articulatory rate in PD may overestimate the actual physical rate.

Respiration Symptoms

Solomon and Hixon (1993) found that during speech breathing in Parkinson disease, the rib cage and abdominal activities were not as efficient as in normal adults. Duffy (2005), in his summary of respiratory-phonatory findings in hypokinetic dysarthria (based on the literature), confirmed the presence of decreased loudness as a distinguishing feature.

Recently, Huber and Darling (2011) evaluated 5 women with PD, 9 men with PD, and 14 age- and sex-matched control participants, who read a passage and spoke extemporaneously on a topic of their choice at comfortable loudness. The authors concluded that both respiratory-physiologic and cognitive-linguistic issues affected speech production by individuals with PD. Overall, individuals with PD had difficulty planning or coordinating language formulation and respiratory support, particularly during extemporaneous speech.

Phonation Symptoms

Aronson (1990) noted that in hypokinetic dysarthria of Parkinsonism, the perceptual laryngeal-phonatory characteristics include monopitch, reduced stress, monoloudness, reduced loudness, harsh voice quality, and breathy voice quality. Pitch changes require an elevating and lowering of the larynx, a stretching and loosening by contraction and relaxation of the vocal folds, and increase and decrease of infraglottal air pressure. The monopitch voice arises from the rigidity and reduced range of motion of the intrinsic and extrinsic laryngeal muscles needed for these movements.

Necessary for stress and emphasis in normal prosody are the controlled changes of infraglottal air pressure. Because of a reduced range of motion of the abdominal and thoracic muscles used in respiration, the controlled changes in respiration appear diminished in patients with Parkinson disease. This loss in emphasis and stress leads to an overall flattening of prosody.

The physical appearance of the vocal folds is normal. Adductor and abductor movements are bilaterally symmetric, but there may be incomplete closure of the vocal folds, which accounts for a breathy voice quality. Reduced loudness and breathiness in the absence of other neurologic signs can indicate early Parkinsonism.

With many Parkinson patients, the administration of the drug L-dopa has caused a lessening of the deviant voice and speech symptoms. Baker, Ramig, Johnson, and Freed (1997) found that fetal cell transplant (FCT) of dopamine into five individuals with Parkinson disease did not systemically influence their voice and speech production.

Gallena et al. (2001) found significant differences between idiopathic Parkinson disease (IPD) participants in the nonmedicated state. Those with higher levels of muscle activation had vocal fold bowing and greater impairment in voice onset and offset control for speech. Similarly, following levodopa administration, those with thyroarytenoid muscle activity reductions had greater improvements in voice onset and offset control for speech. Voice onset and offset control difficulties and vocal fold bowing were associated with increased levels of laryngeal muscle activity in the absence of medication.

Fox and Ramig (1997) observed in 40 patients with idiopathic Parkinson disease that vocal sound pressure level was significantly lower than in normal subjects, and that they rated themselves as significantly more impaired than normal subjects.

Kiran and Larson (2001) found that basal ganglia dysfunction may affect mechanisms relating to the execution and termination of the pitch-shift reflex for brief stimulus durations. The results also support hypotheses of impaired sensory integration of auditory feedback in patients with Parkinson disease.

Logemann, Fisher, Boshes, and Blonsky (1978) described the frequency of occurrence and the co-occurrence of speech and voice symptoms in 200 Parkinson patients. Of the 200 patients, 178 (89%) had laryngeal dysfunction symptoms, described in descending order of frequency as hoarseness, roughness, breathiness, and tremulousness.

Neel (2009) found that, in PD, both loud speech and amplification significantly improved intelligibility for sentences and words. Loud speech resulted in greater intelligibility improvement than amplification.

Resonation Symptoms

Hoodin and Gilbert (1989) found that as Parkinsonism deteriorates, the nasal airflow in speakers gets worse. Logemann et al. (1978) found that out of 200 Parkinson patients, 10% were hypernasal.

Articulation and Prosody Symptoms

Logemann et al. (1978) found that out of 200 Parkinson patients, 45% had articulation problems. In a follow-up study, Logemann and Fisher (1981) found a high rate of error on stops and affricates (both due to inadequate tongue elevation to achieve complete closure), and on fricatives (due to inadequate constriction of the airway).

Caligiuri (1989) studied the influence of speaking rate on articulation in Parkinsonian dysarthria and found decreased amplitude, movement time, and speed of labial movements during conversational speech rates, and a reduction of these abnormalities at slower rates. Canter and Van Lancker (1985), in studying a single Parkinson case, found that the rapid rate of this patient's speech was due to a decrease in syllable durations, which resulted from an abnormal shortening of vowels.

Darby, Simmons, and Berger (1984) found that 13 depressed subjects showed reduced stress, monopitch, and monoloudness, which are characteristic symptoms of hypokinetic dysarthria. They compared their results to the Parkinson subjects in the Darley et al. (1975) study. The depressed subjects showed significant improvement after antidepressant medication treatment. The authors suggested that on the basis of the speech signs, a hypokinetic disturbance of the extrapyramidal system exists in depression.

Darkins, Fromkin, and Benson (1988) found that the prosodic loss in Parkinson disease is due to motor control and not to a loss of linguistic knowledge. On the other hand, Natsopoulos et al. (1991), while acknowledging that dysarthria occurs in Parkinson patients, found that a language comprehension disturbance similar to aphasia existed when compared to neurotypical control subjects.

Walsh and Smith (2011) analyzed speech response latency, interarticulatory coordinative consistency, accuracy of speech production, and response latency and accuracy on a receptive language task in 16 individuals with Parkinson disease and 16 matched control participants. Results showed that individuals with PD had a higher oral motor coordination variability, took a longer time to initiate speech, and made more errors on the speaking task compared with the control group. They also received lower scores on the two complex conditions of the receptive language task. Increased length and syntactic complexity negatively affected performance in both groups of speakers.

Forrest and Weismer (1995) found that relative to normal geriatic speakers, Parkinsonian speakers produced stressed syllables with reduced movement, amplitude, and velocity. Hammen, Yorkston, and Minifie (1994) observed that synthetic alterations in rate did not increase intelligibility in Parkinsonian dysarthria. Logemann et al. (1978) found that out of 200 Parkinson patients, 20% had rate problems described as syllable repetitions, shortened syllables, lengthened syllables, and excessive pauses. Solomon, Robin, and Luschei (2000) assessed tongue strength, endurance, and stability in 16 persons with mild to severe Parkinson disease and a perceptible speech disorder. The same measures were taken from one hand for comparison. Only tongue endurance was found to be significantly lower in the participants with Parkinson disease than in 16 neurotypical control participants.

Ma, Whitehill, and So (2010) found that 14 speakers with hypokinetic dysarthria associated with Parkinson disease used acoustic cues similar to those of nondysarthric Cantonese speakers to mark the question–statement contrast. Listeners mainly used F_0 cues at final syllable for intonation identification. The authors concluded that these data add to understanding the production and perception of intonation in a lexical tone language.

Van Lancker Sidtis et al. (2010) found that participants with Parkinson disease who were being treated with bilateral deep brain stimulation (DBS) of the subthalamic nuclei with stimulators on and off improved in a voice measure, harmonic to voice ratio, in a repetition task and in the DBS-on condition. Disfluencies were more plentiful in conversation, with little or variable influence of DBS condition. The authors concluded that voice and fluency are differently affected by DBS treatment, and that task conditions, interacting with subcortical functionality, influence motor speech performance.

MacPherson, Huber, and Snow (2011) evaluated 8 women and 8 men with Parkinson disease (PD) and 16 age- and sex-matched control participants, and concluded that impaired intonational marking of syntactic boundaries likely contributes to dysprosody and reduced communicative effectiveness in PD. The effect of PD on intonation was sex-specific.

Duffy (2005), in his summary of articulatory and prosody findings in hypokinetic dysarthria (based on the literature), confirmed the presence of the articulatory symptoms of rapid speech AMRs and repeated phonemes, and the prosody symptoms of monopitch, monoloudness, reduced stress, variable rate, short rushes of speech, overall increase in rate, increased rate within segments, and inappropriate silences as distinguishing features.

Hyperkinetic Dysarthria

The fourth type of dysarthria is described as hyperkinetic dysarthria and is, for example, found in the neurologic disorders called *chorea* and *dystonia*. Basically, the hyperkinesias are abnormal involuntary movements, usually due to damage in the basal ganglia control circuit, or occasionally in the cerebellar control circuit or other parts of the extrapyramidal system.

Many involuntary movements are normal (e.g., blinking when the eye is in jeopardy, instantaneous removal of a hand from hot water). Abnormal movements occur in a setting that normally is typified by steady motor movements. The hyperkinesias arise from the failure of the inhibitory functions of the basal ganglia control circuit or the cerebellar control circuit upon the excitatory functions of the motor cortex.

These abnormal involuntary movements are excessive, and their speed can be fast, slow, or both. As a result, some hyperkinesias are called fast (e.g., chorea) and some are called slow (e.g., dystonia). Hyperkinetic dysarthria is a result of the abnormal involuntary muscular movements acting upon the respiratory, phonatory, resonatory, articulatory, and prosody components of speech production. Involuntary movements of the jaw, face, and tongue present during both speech and nonspeech situations are also associated with hyperkinetic dysarthria.

Duffy (2005) noted that the etiologies of 86 cases of hyperkinetic dysarthria seen at the Mayo Clinic were as follows: unknown (59%), where chorea and dystonia were part of that total; toxic/metabolic (17%); degenerative (9%), where Huntington chorea (5%) and dystonia (1%) were part of that total; multiple (5%), where chorea was part of that total; other (3%); infectious (2%), where Sydenham chorea made up all of that total; trauma (1%); and vascular (1%).

Huntington disease, whose onset occurs in adulthood, is an inherited, progressive, and fatal disease. Sydenham chorea, whose onset most frequently occurs in childhood, is a noninherited, nonprogressive, and curable disease.

Within the toxic /metabolic etiologic grouping is a condition called *tardive dyskinesia*. It is quite common for psychiatric patients to undergo long-term ingestion of neuroleptic or antipsychotic medication. These drugs can produce tardive dyskinesia, a potentially irreversible disturbance of the central nervous system. The characteristics of this condition are abnormal movements within the oral musculature such as sucking and smacking noises, sudden protrusions and retractions of the tongue, rhythmic opening and closing of the mouth, and lateral jaw movements. Portnoy (1979) noted that tardive dyskinesia is manifested in motor speech production as hyperkinetic dysarthria.

Murray and Stout (1999) found that patients with Huntington disease (HD) and patients with Parkinson disease showed a strong relationship in their general cognitive decline and in the discourse comprehensive difficulties. Although hyperkinetic dysarthria is a motor speech disorder, Murray (2000) investigated the presence and nature of spoken language abilities in Huntington disease and Parkinson disease. Regarding syntax, patients with HD produced shorter utterances, a smaller proportion of grammatical utterances, a larger production of simple sentences, and fewer embeddings per utterance than their non-brain-damaged peers. The HD group also produced utterances that were shorter and syntactically simpler than those of the PD group, despite similar performances in the cognitive and motor speech tasks. The only syntactic difference between the PD group and their control group was that patients with PD produced a smaller proportion of grammatical sentences. Although the patient and control participants tended to produce similar amounts of verbal output, less of what the patients said was informative. Correlations between language measures and test battery results suggested that the spoken language abilities of patients with HD or PD are related to a variety of neuropsychological and motor speech changes.

Chorea

Speech Symptoms

Following is a sampling of some of the studies and reports related to the speech symptoms found in the hyperkinetic dysarthria of chorea. Additional references are noted in the "Diagnosis" and "Therapy" portions of this section.

Darley et al. (1969a, 1969b, 1975), in their study of 30 patients with chorea, found that the most prominent speech deviations (from most to least severe) were imprecise consonants, prolonged intervals, variable rate, monopitch, harsh voice quality, inappropriate silences, distorted vowels, excess loudness variation, prolonged phonemes, monoloudness, short phrases, irregular articulatory breakdown, excess and equal stress, hypernasality, reduced stress, and strained-strangled quality.

The speech deviations that best distinguish the hyperkinetic dysarthria of chorea from the other dysarthrias are described by Darley et al. (1969a, 1969b, 1975) and by Duffy (2005), in his review of supportive studies in the literature, as hypernasality, strained harshness, transient breathing, articulatory distortions and irregular articulatory breakdowns, loudness variations, and sudden forced inspiration or expiration (all due to the variable and transient pattern of unpredictable movements).

Those speech deviations, along with the speaker's apparent attempt to avoid the interruptions or to compensate for them, result in prolonged intervals, prolonged phonemes, variable rate, inappropriate silences, voice stoppages, and excessive or insufficient stress patterns.

Respiration, Phonation, and Resonation Symptoms

Duffy (2005), in his summary of respiratory findings in the hyperkinetic dysarthria of chorea (based on the literature), confirmed the presence of loudness variations as a distinguishing feature.

Aronson (1990) noted that in the hyperkinetic dysarthria of chorea, the perceptual laryngeal-phonatory characteristics include the following: slow continuous changes in strained hoarse quality, breathiness, excess loudness variations, voice arrests, monopitch, monoloudness, reduced stress, and excess and equal stress on ordinarily unstressed syllables and words. Sudden uncontrolled movements of the respiratory and laryngeal musculature are responsible for irregular pitch fluctuations and voice arrests, thus producing speech that has a jerky quality. The physical appearance of the vocal folds is normal in structure and function, although there can be intermittent hyperadduction.

Duffy (2005), in his summary of phonatory and resonatory findings in the hyperkinetic dysarthria of chorea (based on the literature), confirmed the presence of the phonatory symptoms of strained harshness, transient breathiness, sudden forced inspiration or expiration, and voice stoppages, and the resonatory symptom of hypernasality as distinguishing features.

Articulation and Prosody Symptoms

Duffy (2005), in his summary of articulatory and prosody findings in the hyperkinetic dysarthria of chorea (based on the literature), confirmed the presence of the articulatory symptoms of articulatory distortions and irregular articulatory breakdowns, and the prosody symptoms of prolonged intervals and phonemes, variable rate, inappropriate silences, and excessive or insufficient stress patterns as distinguishing features.

Dystonia

Speech Symptoms

Following is a sampling of some of the studies and reports related to the speech symptoms found in the hyperkinetic dysarthria of dystonia. Additional references are noted in the "Diagnosis" and "Therapy" parts of this section.

Darley et al. (1969a, 1969b, 1975), in their study of 30 patients with dystonia, found that the most prominent speech deviations (from most to least severe) were imprecise consonants, distorted vowels, harsh voice quality, irregular articulatory breakdown, strained-strangled quality, monopitch, monoloudness, inappropriate silences, short phrases, prolonged intervals, prolonged phonemes, excess loudness variation, reduced stress, voice stoppages, and slow rate. Although below their mean scale value cutoff point of most prominent features, audible inspiration, voice tremor, and alternating loudness occurred with greater frequency than in the other dysarthrias.

The speech deviations that best distinguish the hyperkinetic dysarthria of dystonia from the other dysarthrias are described by Darley et al. (1969a, 1969b, 1975), and by Duffy (2005) in his review of supportive studies in the literature, as imprecision and irregular breakdowns of articulation, inappropriate variability of loudness and rate, strained harshness, transient breathiness, and audible inspiration (as in chorea, all due to the variable and transient pattern of unpredictable movements).

Those speech deviations, along with the speaker's apparent attempt to avoid the interruptions or to compensate for them, as in chorea, can result in slow rate, prolonged intervals and phonemes, inappropriate silences, and excessive and insufficient stress patterns.

Respiration and Phonation Symptoms

Golper, Nutt, Rau, and Coleman (1983) described the speech management program for 10 patients with focal cranial dystonia who showed a slow hyperkinetic dysarthria. Some patients showed some loudness problems, which may be indicative of disturbed breathing movements or a compensation for phonatory stenosis. LaBlance and Rutherford (1991) found that the decreased speech intelligibility in their generalized dystonia subjects was strongly related to decreased breathing patterns.

Aronson (1990) noted that in the hyperkinetic dysarthria of dystonia, the laryngeal-phonatory characteristics include the following: slow, continuous changes in strained-hoarse quality, breathiness, excess loudness variations, voice arrests, monopitch, monoloudness, reduced stress, and excess and equal stress on ordinarily unstressed syllables and words. Sudden uncontrolled adductor and abductor laryngeal spasms can result in strained hoarseness and breathiness, and occasionally paroxysmal inhalatory stridor. The physical appearance of the vocal folds is normal in structure and function, although there can be intermittent hyperadduction.

Mathers-Schmidt (2001), in her tutorial, noted that in paradoxical vocal fold motion (PVFM), the vocal folds adduct during inhalation and/or exhalation, thereby restricting the airway opening. Patients typically present with episodic or recurrent symptoms of dyspnea and/or stridor. Often patients complained of a tightness localized to the laryngeal area, and sometimes they reported a feeling of being choked. It occurs more in females, and the etiology of PVFM includes such factors as psychological condition, upper airway sensitivity, laryngeal irritants, and a form of laryngeal dystonia. Other etiologies include brainstem compression, cortical or upper motor neuron injury, and nuclear or lower motor neuron injury. Speech-language pathologist (SLP) treatment involves patient education, supportive counseling, instruction in tension identification and control, and instruction in "relaxed target breathing."

Koufman and Block (2008) provided an overview of paradoxical vocal fold movement by drawing from 30 years of clinical and research experience. In their experience, the most common causes of PVFM in order of frequency are (1) laryngopharyngeal reflux (LPR), (2) respiratory-type laryngeal dystonia, (3) asthma or hyperimmunity-associated PVFM, (4) brainstem abnormalities, (5) drug-induced dystonic reactions, and (6) psychogenic stridor. The authors noted that brainstem abnormalities, severe closed head injury, Chiari malformations I and II, meningomyelocele, and cerebrovascular accidents (strokes of the posterior circulation) may all produce PVFM. They also presented the differential diagnosis of PVFM and its distinguishing features. Finally, at the diagnosis, the authors recommended counseling and training (breathing recovery exercises) to be administered by the SLP. Treatment techniques include "Sniff in through your nose quickly, and then blow out slowly through your mouth," respiratory exercises that focus on exhalation, rhythmic abdominal movement patterns, and resonant voice and easy-onset voice exercises to reduce associated hyperfunctional voice behaviors.

Duffy (2005), in his summary of respiratory and phonatory findings in the hyperkinetic dysarthria of dystonia (based on the literature), confirmed the presence of the respiratory-phonatory symptom of audible inspiration, the respiratory-phonatory-prosody symptom of inappropriate variability of loudness and rate, and the phonatory symptoms of strained harshness and transient breathiness as distinguishing features.

Articulation and Prosody Symptoms

Duffy (2005), in his summary of articulatory and prosody findings in the hyperkinetic dysarthria of dystonia (based on the literature), confirmed the presence of the articulatory symptoms of imprecision and irregular breakdowns of articulation, the articulatory-prosody symptom of slow rate, and the prosody symptoms of prolonged intervals and phonemes, inappropriate silences, and excessive and insufficient stress patterns as distinguishing features.

Additional hyperkinetic dysarthrias (Aronson, 1990; Darley et al., 1975; Duffy, 2005) have been found in the following neurologic disorders: organic (essential) voice tremor, palatopharyngolaryngeal myoclonus, Tourette syndrome, athetosis, spasmodic torticollis, action myoclonus, and spasmodic dysphonia (spastic dysphonia). Cimino-Knight and Sapienza (2001) found that there is a need for describing phonatory instability and performance consistency as separate entities with regard to neurologic voice disorders (e.g., patients with adductor spasmodic dysphonia).

Bender, Cannito, Murry, and Woodson (2004) found that speakers with adductor spasmodic dysphonia (ADSD) were significantly more intelligible in the post-Botox condition than in the pre-Botox condition. The results also indicated that healthy speakers were significantly more intelligible than the speakers in both the pre- and post-Botox conditions. In general, these results indicated that intelligibility is affected in severe ADSD and the use of Botox injection in ADSD improves intelligibility scores. However, the results also indicated that the use of Botox injection does not result in speech intelligibility equivalent to that of normal, non-ADSD speakers.

Ataxic Dysarthria

The fifth type of dysarthria is described as ataxic dysarthria and is found in neurologic cerebellar disorders. The cerebellum regulates the force, speed, range, timing, and direction of movements arising from the other motor systems. The other motor systems generally start movements in excess of actual need, and the major role of the cerebellum is to dampen or inhibit such overactivity.

Quite often, ataxic dysarthria occurs because of bilateral or generalized damage to the cerebellum. The affected muscles tend to be hypotonic, voluntary movements are slow, and the force, range, timing, and direction of movements are inaccurate. For speech production, the important features of cerebellar disease are inaccuracy of movement, slowness of movement, and hypotonia.

Duffy (2005) noted that the etiologies of 107 cases of ataxic dysarthria seen at the Mayo Clinic were as follows: degenerative (34%), vascular (16%), demyelinating (15%), undetermined (14%), toxic/metabolic (7%), traumatic (6%), inflammatory (5%), tumor (3%), multiple (1%), and other (1%).

Speech Symptoms

Following is a sampling of some of the studies and reports related to the speech symptoms found in ataxic dysarthria. Additional references are noted in the "Diagnosis" and "Therapy" sections of this chapter.

Darley et al. (1969a, 1969b, 1975), in their study of 30 patients with cerebellar lesions, found that the most prominent speech deviations (from most to least severe) were imprecise consonants, excess and equal stress, irregular articulatory breakdown, distorted vowels, harsh voice quality, prolonged phonemes, prolonged intervals, monopitch, monoloudness, excess loudness variations, and voice tremor.

Kent et al. (2002) concluded that ataxic dysarthria reflects a global impairment of the respiratory, laryngeal, and articulatory subsystems of speech, although individual variations may be seen in the relative severity of these impairments in any given system. In addition, it appears likely that there is a subtle difference in ataxic dysarthria between males and females. A task/measure (sustained phonation, AMR, sentence recitations, conversation) analysis was found to be a suitable means for the detailed study of the speech disturbances in this speech disorder.

The speech deviations that best distinguish ataxic dysarthria from the other dysarthrias are described by Darley et al. (1969a, 1969b, 1975), and by Duffy (2005) in his review of supportive studies in the literature, as irregular articulatory breakdowns, irregular speech AMRs (both resulting from inaccurate direction of movement and dysrhythmia of repetitive movement of the articulators), excess and equal stress (resulting from slowness of individual and repetitive movements that places stress on all syllables in a word, including those that are normally produced in an unstressed manner), distorted vowels (resulting from inaccurate direction of movement and dysrhythmia of repetitive movement of the articulators), and prolonged phonemes (resulting from slowness of individual and repetitive movements of the articulators).

Respiration and Phonation Symptoms

Murdoch, Chenery, Stokes, and Hardcastle (1991) found that respiratory abilities were reduced in speakers with cerebellar disease. These participants had reduced vital capacities and had a breakdown in the coordination of the rib cage and abdomen while speaking. In particular, these irregularities affected their prosody.

Aronson (1990) noted that in ataxic dysarthria, the perceptual laryngeal-phonatory characteristics include frequently normal phonation, but others can have harsh voice quality, monopitch, monoloudness, excess and equal stress on ordinarily unstressed words or syllables, excess loudness, bursts of loudness, and coarse voice tremor. The physical appearance of the vocal folds is normal in structure and function.

Murry (1984) found that Friedreich ataxia involves more explosive speech than cerebellar ataxia. Phonatory characteristics are more bizarre, in that there is a rough or harsh quality along with a strained-strangled quality.

Articulation and Prosody Symptoms

Ackerman, Hertrich, and Scharf (1995) found that patients with cerebellar disease had an impaired ability to increase muscular forces in order to produce articulatory gestures of short duration. In a study by Hirose, Kiritani, Ushijima, and Sawashima (1978), electromyography (EMG) findings showed physiological evidence of inconsistency in the articulatory movement of a speaker with ataxic dysarthria. This pattern seems to be compatible with the characteristic of irregular articulatory breakdown in ataxic dysarthria.

However, Sheard, Adams, and Davis (1991) found that in ratings of ataxic dysarthric speech samples with varying intelligibility, judges agreed mostly on imprecise consonants, excess and equal stress, and harsh voice. They agreed, but less so, on distorted vowels and irregular articulatory breakdown.

Dworkin and Aronson (1986) noted the slowness of speech AMRs in participants with ataxic dysarthria. Gentil (1990) described slow speech rate and slow speech AMRs in 14 participants with Friedreich disease. Linebaugh and Wolfe (1984) found that speakers with ataxic dysarthria had significantly longer mean syllable duration than did neurotypical participants. Portnoy and Aronson (1982) observed that speakers with ataxic dysarthria had a significantly slower and more variable rate in repetition tasks than neurotypical participants.

Paslawski, Duffy, and Vernino (2005) noted that paraneoplastic cerebellar degeneration (PCD) is an autoimmune disease that can be associated with cancer of the breast, lung, and ovary. The clinical presentation of PCD commonly includes ataxia, visual disturbances, and dysarthria. The speech disturbances associated with PCD have not been well characterized, despite general acceptance that dysarthria is often part of the initial presentation. A retrospective study was conducted of the speech, language, and swallowing concerns of patients with PCD evaluated at the Mayo Clinic between 1990 and 2001. Prospective speech and language assessments were then conducted with five patients who had PCD. While ataxic dysarthria was the most common speech diagnosis, a spastic component was recognized frequently enough to suggest that the subacute (days to weeks) emergence and progression of an ataxic or mixed ataxic-spastic dysarthria in the setting of a more diffuse cerebellar ataxia should raise suspicions of a possible immune-related etiology, rather than a malignancy that is due to the direct effects of invasion of a tumor, infection, or vascular complications.

The authors of this text remember one such female patient whose main speech problems were excess high pitch and excess and equal stress that appeared almost suddenly, and well before her medical diagnosis of ovarian cancer.

Duffy (2005), in his summary of articulatory and prosody findings in ataxic dysarthria (based on the literature), confirmed the presence of the articulatory symptoms of irregular articulatory breakdowns and irregular speech AMRs, the articulatory-prosody symptoms of distorted vowels and prolonged phonemes, and the prosody symptom of excess and equal stress as distinguishing features.

Unilateral Upper Motor Neuron Dysarthria

A sixth type of dysarthria has been studied and reviewed by Duffy (2005) and is called unilateral upper motor neuron (UUMN) dysarthria. The most common cause of this dysarthria is stroke, followed by tumors, and then trauma that can damage upper motor neurons unilaterally.

The outstanding speech characteristics of UUMN dysarthria are imprecise consonants and irregular articulatory breakdown. Harshness, reduced loudness, and mild hypernasality are present in some cases.

Mixed Dysarthria

A seventh type of dysarthria is described as mixed dysarthria and is, for example, found in the neurologic disorder called *amyotrophic lateral sclerosis* (ALS). In ALS there is a progressive degeneration of both upper and lower motor neurons. Damage to these neurons produces symptoms from both systems, although the appearance of one or the other may predominate depending on the stage of the disease.

Symptoms of upper motor neuron damage (spastic paralysis, hypertonia, hyperreflexia, little or no atrophy, no fasciculations, etc.) are present unless the symptoms of lower motor neuron damage (flaccid paralysis, hypotonia, hyporeflexia, marked atrophy, fasciculations, etc.) predominate. The important features of ALS are weakness of the musculature, very slow production of single and repetitive movements, and reduced range of motion.

Duffy (2005) noted that the etiologies of 300 cases of mixed dysarthria seen at the Mayo Clinic were as follows: degenerative (63%), out of which ALS accounted for 41%; vascular (12%); demyelinating (6%); traumatic (5%); tumor (4%); undetermined (4%); multiple causes (4%); toxic/metabolic (1%); and inflammatory (1%).

Speech Symptoms

Following is a sampling of some of the studies and reports related to the speech symptoms found in ALS. Additional references are noted in the "Diagnosis" and "Therapy" sections of this chapter.

Darley et al. (1969a, 1969b, 1975), in their study of 30 patients with ALS, found that the most prominent speech deviations (from the most to the least severe) were imprecise consonants, hypernasality, harsh voice quality, slow rate, monopitch, short phrases, distorted vowels, low pitch, monoloudness, excessive and equal stress, prolonged intervals, reduced stress, prolonged phonemes, strained-strangled quality, breathiness, audible inspiration, inappropriate silences, and nasal emission.

The speech deviations that best distinguish the mixed dysarthria (flaccid and spastic) in ALS from the other dysarthrias are described by Darley et al. (1969a, 1969b, 1975), and by Duffy (2005) in his review of supportive studies in the literature, as labored and very slowly produced speech with short phrases and intervals between words and phrases and grossly defective articulation (both resulting from articulators that move sluggishly with a reduction of range, as well as weakness), short phrases and intervals between words and phrases (resulting from air wastage due to inefficient valving of the vocal folds, the palatopharyngeal area, and the oral area), marked hypernasality (resulting from incomplete palatopharyngeal closure), severe harshness and strained-strangled quality (resulting from hyperadduction of the vocal folds, which produces glottic restriction and resistance to exhalatory airflow), and monopitch and monoloudness (resulting from restricted range of movement of the speech muscles where normal peaks of accent cannot be attained).

Respiration, Phonation, and Resonation Symptoms

Putnam and Hixon (1984), in their study of patients with motor neuron disease, found that chest wall muscle weakness produced low lung volume, which resulted in reduced loudness and short phrases. Mulligan et al. (1994) found a greater decrease in forced vital capacity in patients who had dysarthria with ALS than in patients without dysarthria.

Aronson (1990) noted that in mixed dysarthria of ALS, the perceptual laryngeal-phonatory characteristics include hoarseness or harshness having a strained-strangled quality resulting from hyperadduction of the true and false vocal folds, and a "wet" or "gurgly" sounding hoarseness due to accumulation of saliva on the vocal folds because of a reduced frequency of swallowing. In addition, a rapid tremor or flutter is noted on vowel prolongation. If there is a strong flaccid component, a breathy voice is present due to hyperadduction of the vocal folds. Monopitch and monoloudness can be present, and loudness can be reduced. Audible inhalation can also be present.

The physical appearance of the vocal folds is normal. The vocal folds appear to adduct normally, or may hyperadduct along with the false vocal folds if the prime component is spasticity. Adduction of the vocal folds may be bilaterally symmetric, or one vocal fold may adduct less than the other. The vocal folds may adduct or abduct with less than normal excursions if there is a prime flaccid component.

Kent et al. (1991) identified hypernasality and harshness as major characteristics in the breakdown of intelligibility in a single patient with ALS. Renout, Leeper, Bandur, and Hudson (1995) found reduced and aperiodic vocal fold diadochokinesis in 12 participants who had ALS with bulbar signs, and 14 participants who had ALS with nonbulbar signs of the disease.

Duffy (2005), in his summary of phonatory and resonatory findings in the mixed (flaccid and spastic) dysarthria of ALS (based on the literature), confirmed the presence of the phonatory symptoms of severe harshness and strained-strangled quality, the phonatory-resonatory-articulatory symptom of labored and very slowly produced speech with short phrases and intervals between words and phrases, and the resonatory symptom of hypernasality as distinguishing features.

Articulation and Prosody Symptoms

DePaul and Brooks (1993) found that impairment of the tongue was the most critical feature when compared to impairment of the lips and jaw in ALS speakers. Dworkin, Aronson, and Mulder (1980) concluded that participants who had ALS had lower tongue force than neurotypical participants. Negative correlations existed between tongue force and severity of articulation. Langmore and Lehman (1994) also found that impairment of the tongue was more crucial than impairment of the jaw and lips in participants who had ALS.

Kent et al. (1990) studied the speech intelligibility in men with ALS. They found that the most disrupted phonetic features involved phonatory function (voicing contrast), velopharyngeal valving, place and manner of articulation for lingual consonants, and regulation of tongue height for vowels. Those five features correlated highly with intelligibility. In a follow-up study, Kent et al. (1992) concluded that women with ALS showed results similar to men with ALS, with the exception that men were more likely to have impairments of voicing with syllables in the initial position.

Kent et al. (1991) found that imprecise consonants were a major characteristic in the breakdown of intelligibility in a single patient with ALS. Mulligan et al. (1994) found slower diadochokinetic rates and decreased intelligibility in participants who had ALS with dysarthria than in those without dysarthria. Samlan and Weismer (1995) looked at articulatory precision and rhythmic consistency as part of a diadochokinetic evaluation, and their relationship to overall speech intelligibility in 15 men with ALS. They found that diadochokinetic judgment was weakly related to overall speech intelligibility in their participants.

Riddel, McCauley, Mulligan, and Tandan (1995) studied the phonetic breakdown of 29 patients (18 women and 11 men) with early ALS. They found that voicing errors, vowel distortions, longer vowel durations, and contrast errors involving fricatives versus affricates and alveolar fricatives versus palatal fricatives were the significant features of phonetic breakdown in early ALS. They noted that the men appeared more vulnerable to this breakdown than did the women. Turner, Tjaden, and Weismer (1995) found that vowel space area was an important component of global estimates of speech intelligibility in 9 participants with ALS.

Dworkin, Aronson, and Mulder (1980) found that participants who had ALS with dysarthria had slower syllable repetitions than neurotypical participants. Negative correlations existed between syllable rate and severity of articulation in ALS. Turner and Weismer (1993) concluded that participants who had ALS with dysarthria had more difficulty in changing speaking rate than did neurotypical participants.

Duffy (2005), in his summary of articulatory and prosody findings in the mixed dysarthria (flaccid and spastic) of ALS (based on the literature), confirmed the presence of the articulatory symptom of grossly defective articulation and the prosody symptoms of monopitch and monoloudness.

Additional mixed dysarthrias have been found in the following neurologic disorders: Multiple sclerosis (MS) (Darley et al. 1975; Darley, Brown, & Goldstein, 1972) most frequently showed a mixture of ataxic and spastic dysarthric components, although each component can be present alone. Because of the unpredictability of MS, in some patients any other single type of dysarthria or other mixture can be present. Hartelius, Buder, and Strand (1997) reported on the long-term phonatory instability of 20 individuals with MS, including those who had ataxic and spastic components.

Wilson disease (Berry, Darley, Aronson, & Goldstein, 1974; Darley et al., 1975; Day & Parnell, 1987) showed ataxic, spastic, and hypokinetic dysarthric components in different mixtures, although each component can be present alone in some patients.

Shy-Drager syndrome (Linebaugh, 1979) showed ataxic, hypokinetic, and spastic dysarthric components in different mixtures, although each component can be present alone in some patients.

Progressive supranuclear palsy (reviewed by Duffy, 2005) most frequently showed hypokinetic and spastic dysarthric components alone or as a mixture. However, ataxic dysarthric components, typically in combination with hypokinetic or spastic components, can also be present in some patients.

Friedreich ataxia (reviewed by Duffy, 2005) showed ataxic dysarthria as the most frequently occurring type, followed by spastic dysarthria, and then by scattered other types. The most common mixture would be that of ataxic and spastic components.

Olivopontocerebellar atrophy (reviewed by Duffy, 2005) showed ataxic, spastic, or flaccid dysarthric components, or various mixtures of all three. This atrophy also may be associated with Parkinsonian features, so there is a possibility that a hypokinetic dysarthric component may be present.

Liss, Krein-Jones, Wszolek, and Caviness (2006) described the speech characteristics of individuals with a neurodegenerative syndrome called pallido-ponto-nigral degeneration (PPND). The dysarthria is mixed, with hypokinetic, spastic, and flaccid features. Throughout the disease, vocal signs (stability and modulation deficits) exceed articulatory deficits. Key features include vocal instability (tremor and flutter), vocal modulation deficits (monopitch), and speech rate deficits (typically slowing). Speech abnormalities can appear early, even preceding the onset of other clinical indicators of disease. Cognitive and behavioral factors influence communication in the later stages of the disease, with decreased voluntary speech output, verbal and vocal perseverations, and eventual mutism.

Undetermined Dysarthria

An eighth type of dysarthria, called undetermined dysarthria (Duffy, 2005), indicates that a neurogenic motor speech disorder is present but that its perceptual symptoms are very subtle, complicated, or unusual. In that case, a diagnosis of "motor speech disorder, type undetermined" might be warranted.

Diagnosis

The model of health status and functioning called the *International Classification of Functioning* (ICF) (WHO, 2001) provides a framework that may increase awareness of the multidimensional nature of disabling conditions. The treatment outcomes measures should consider not only impairment and activity limitations of disease or injury, but also effects on societal participation. The ICF can be applied to an individual with dysarthria and reduced speech intelligibility (Dykstra et al., 2007). According to the American Speech-Language-Hearing Association (ASHA), the ICF model should be adopted as outlined in the *Scope of Practice in Speech-Language Pathology* (ASHA, 2001) and *Preferred Practice Patterns for the Profession of Speech-Language Pathology* (ASHA, 2004).

The *Communication Effectiveness Survey* (Donovan et al., 2007, 2008) may be an alternative to a lengthy comprehensive assessment. Individuals with dysarthria or their caregivers are asked eight questions about how effective their speech is, using a four-point scale ranging from not at all effective to very effective. For example, the individual would score 1 for not at all effective or 4 for very effective for the situation, "Having a conversation with a family member or friends at home." Psychometric evaluation of the survey is ongoing.

Diagnostic procedures for determining dysarthria can involve (1) establishing background information, (2) giving a neurologic evaluation, (3) perceptual evaluation of the speech and voice characteristics, (4) assessing the oral mechanism at rest and during nonspeech activities, and (5) evaluation through instrumentation.

Establishing Background Information and the Neurologic Evaluation

These procedures can be found at the beginning of the "Diagnosis" part of the section on aphasia.

Perceptual Evaluation of the Speech and Voice Characteristics

Lass, Ruscello, and Lakawicz (1988) and Lass, Ruscello, Harkins, and Blankenship (1993) found that listener perception of dysarthric speech adversely affected their notion of the speaker's personality and physical appearance. Garcia and Dagenais (1998) studied the sentence intelligibility of 4 speakers with dysarthria. They found that an audio plus video presentation, rather than an audio-only presentation, enhanced listener understanding for all speakers. They also found that the contributions of relevant signal-independent information (gestures and message predictiveness) were greater for the speakers with more severely impaired intelligibility. Tjaden and Wilding (2004) found that the loud condition was associated with improved intelligibility for the group with Parkinson disease, relative to their habitual and slow conditions. Speakers with multiple sclerosis were most intelligible in the habitual condition. For individuals with the lowest intelligibility scores, secondary to PD, scores for transcribed sentences from videotapes (auditory-visual, or AV) were significantly higher than from listening (auditory-only, or AO) to the speakers (Keintz et al., 2007). Correctly identified words were significantly higher for the AV presentation mode than for the AO mode when 224 listeners transcribed speech samples from 7 speakers with dysarthria (Hustad et al., 2007), but only slightly higher when 80 listeners provided word-by-word transcriptions for 4 speakers with dysarthria (Hustad, 2006a, 2006b)

Finally, Pannbacker (2004) has noted that SLPs are often involved in the diagnosis and treatment of velopharyngeal incompetence (VPI). The purpose of her article was to (1) review SLP standards and qualifications, (2) provide reasons for identifying qualified SLPs, and (3) identify strategies for reduction of risks involved in the delivery of speech-language services for people with VPI.

Following are several informal tests used in a perceptual evaluation of dysarthria. — therapy 1

A systematic perceptual evaluation of dysarthria requires a sample of several types of speech and voice production. The clinician should look for the symptoms described under each type of dysarthria. As suggested by Darley et al. (1975), a checklist of dysarthric symptoms might be used as a guideline and form sheet (see **Table 8.1**). Symptoms can be evaluated

TABLE 8.1

Checklist of Dysarthric Symptoms

A. **Respiration**
   1. Reduced loudness
   2. Excessive loudness
   3. Monoloudness
   4. Intermittent loudness
   5. Loudness decay
   6. Forced inhalation or exhalation
   7. Grunt at end of exhalation
   8. Loudness level overall
B. **Phonation**
   1. Breathiness
   2. Strained strangled
   3. Harshness
   4. Hoarseness
   5. Pitch breaks
   6. Tremors
   7. Monopitch
   8. Audible inhalation
   9. Voice stoppages
   10. Pitch level overall
C. **Resonance**
   1. Hypernasality
   2. Nasal emission
   3. Nasality overall
D. **Articulation**
   1. Distortion, omissions, substitutions, and additions of consonants
   2. Distortions, omissions, substitutions, and additions of vowels and diphthongs
   3. Articulation level overall
E. **Prosody**
   1. Monotone
   2. Excessive and equal stress
   3. Inappropriate silences
   4. Stress or vocal variety level overall
   5. Slow rate
   6. Short rushes of speech
   7. Rate level overall

according to their intelligibility (clarity) and bizarreness (understandable but varying very much from standard production). A 7-point scale can be used for evaluating each symptom in the checklist (Table 8.1): 1 = normal, 2 = mild, 3 = mild to moderate, 4 = moderate, 5 = moderate to severe, 6 = severe, 7 = very severe to unintelligible.

The patient can be asked to do the following:

1. Prolong /ah/, /ee/, and /oo/ separately, as long, as clearly, and as steadily as possible. Normal speakers can sustain the vowel /ah/ anywhere from 10 to 34.6 seconds (reviewed by Duffy, 2005).

    Numbers 2, 3, and 4 represent evaluation through AMR, which can check the speed and consistency of alternating movements of the lips, tongue, and jaw. Current technology, e.g., the Diadochokinetic Rate Analysis computer program, has clinical limitations, in that the program cannot execute more than one-third of the samples (Wang et al., 2009b). Still, the concept shows potential for clinical use if performance can be improved.

2. Repeat /puh/ as rapidly as possible.
3. Repeat /tuh/ as rapidly as possible.
4. Repeat /kuh/ as rapidly as possible. The AMR for typical speakers for /puh/, /tuh/, and /kuh/ ranges from 5 to 7 repetitions per second, with repetition of /kuh/ somewhat slower (reviewed by Duffy, 2005). Dworkin and Aronson (1986) found that speakers with dysarthria showed weaker tongue strength and slower AMR than did typical speakers. Nishio and Niimi (2006) found speaking rate, articulation rate, and AMR were all lower in speakers with dysarthria than in controls. Yunusova, Weismer, Westbury, and Lindstrom (2008) found that dysarthric speakers were slower in speaking than healthy controls, with the tongue experiencing a more significant impact of the neurological condition.

    Number 5 represents evaluation through sequential motion rate (SMR), which can check the rapid movement of one sound to another in sequence.

5. Repeat /puh-tuh-kuh/ as rapidly as possible. The SMR for neurotypical speakers for /puh-tuh-kuh/ ranges from 3.6 to 7.5 repetitions per second (as reviewed by Duffy, 2005). Scores on the SMR speech tend to be significantly lower for individuals with dysarthria associated with Friedreich ataxia, and is also correlated with disease progression (Friedman et al., 2010; Singh et al., 2010).
6. Repeat "snowman."
7. Repeat "gingerbread."
8. Repeat "impossibility."

Patients can be asked to respond out loud to action pictures, read out loud a phonetically balanced passage (e.g., grandfather passage), and respond out loud to standardized articulation tests or tests used specifically for dysarthria patients.

Tikofsky and Tikofsky (1964) and Yorkston and Beukelman (1980b) proposed that dysarthric patients read lists of words; based upon their intelligibility, the clinician can determine degrees of impairment. In a later study, Yorkston and Beukelman (1981b) found that speaking rate and intelligibility can distinguish the speech of individuals with mild dysarthria from those who are typical speakers.

Beukelman and Yorkston (1980) also found that speech-language pathologists overestimated intelligibility of dysarthric speech, possibly because of familiarity with the passage. In a later study, Yorkston and Beukelman (1983) found that familiarization with the speaker who had dysarthria did not increase intelligibility scores.

Kent, Weismer, Kent, and Rosenbek (1989) created a word intelligibility test for use with speakers who have dysarthria. Their test is designed to examine 19 acoustic-phonetic contrasts that are likely to (1) identify dysarthric impairment, and (2) contribute significantly to speech intelligibility.

The following are two formalized tests used in a perceptual evaluation of dysarthria.

Assessment of Intelligibility of Dysarthric Speech (Yorkston and Beukelman, 1981a) is a tool for quantifying single-word intelligibility, sentence intelligibility, and speaking rate of adult and adolescent speakers with dysarthria. Measures of speech intelligibility and speaking rate serve as an index of dysarthric severity, thus enabling the clinician to rank different speakers with dysarthria, compare performance of a single speaker with dysarthria to typical performance, and monitor changing performance over time.

The *Frenchay Dysarthria Assessment* (Enderby, 1983) is another test that can be used for evaluation of dysarthria. This test is divided into 11 sections: Reflex, Respiration, Lips, Jaw, Palate, Larynx, Tongue, Intelligibility, Rate, Sensation, and Influencing Factors (hearing, sight, teeth, language, mood). The patient is asked to perform designated tasks (e.g., "Say 'ah' for as long as possible" and "Count to 20 as quickly as possible") on 8 of the sections. Scoring is based on a patient's second attempt at each task; a 9-point rating scale is used. This examination was designed for use in categorically diagnosing dysarthria. Sample profiles are provided for five types of dysarthria: upper motor neuron lesion, mixed upper and lower motor neuron lesions, extrapyramidal disorders, cerebellar dysfunction, and lower motor neuron lesion.

Assessing the Oral Mechanism at Rest and During Nonspeech Activities

Duffy (2005) noted that examination of the oral mechanism at rest and during nonspeech activities can provide confirmatory evidence and information about the size, strength, symmetry, range, tone, sturdiness, speed, and accuracy of orofacial structures and movements. He described in detail how observation of the face (lips, mouth, cheeks, eyes), jaw, tongue, velopharynx, larynx, and respiration are made at rest, during sustained postures and movements, and in response to tests for neurotypical and primitive reflexes.

Assessment procedures of voluntary versus automatic nonspeech movements of the speech mechanism are described when nonverbal oral apraxia is a possibility. The following are two formalized tests for assessment of the oral mechanism at rest and during nonspeech activities.

The *Dworkin-Culatta Oral Mechanism Examination* (Dworkin & Culatta, 1980) includes 10 subtests that evaluate facial appearance, oral musculature, dentition and gingiva, hard palate, velopharyngeal mechanism, tongue, laryngeal mechanism, and oral and speech praxis. After administering the full examination, abnormal signs are noted on a checklist. The signs are then compared to the error profiles of 23 conditions. Each of the 23 conditions is described on the basis of site of neurologic involvement (e.g., extrapyramidal system, basal ganglia) or of anatomical abnormality (e.g., velum, tongue), and the tests and subcategories of tests that yielded the abnormal signs. The protocols also contain six sample reports of patients who manifested dysarthrias of the spastic, flaccid, hyperkinetic, and mixed spastic-ataxic types; oral apraxia and apraxia of speech; and physiologic disorders associated with structural and physiological abnormalities.

The *Oral Speech Mechanism Screening Examination, Revised Edition* (St. Louis & Ruscello, 1987) provides a quick method for performing oral speech mechanism examinations. Requiring 5 to 10 minutes to administer, this test examines the lips, tongue, jaw, teeth, hard palate, soft palate, pharynx, velopharyngeal functions, breathing, and diadochokinetic rates.

Three interpretations are possible for each of the structures or functions evaluated: normal, abnormal with referral to another specialty for additional assessment, and further testing to verify and more fully describe the disorder. Separate numerical subscores for structure and function, as well as a total score, permit comparison of individual clients with normal speakers. Included in the protocols is a detailed description of the importance of each structure to speech production, its appearance, and typical deviations.

Hill et al. (2006), in their pilot study, found that online assessment of motor speech disorders (in this study, 19 speakers with dysarthria), using an Internet-based telerehabilitation system, is both feasible and possible.

Evaluation Through Instrumentation

Simmons (1983) performed cineradiographic and spectrographic analysis to study the speech production of a participant who presented the classic neurological signs of cerebellar lesion and had speech characteristics similar to those that have been reported for ataxic dysarthria. Barlow, Cole, and Abbs (1983) described a head-mounted, lip-jaw movement transduction system for the study of motor speech disorders, and Barlow and Abbs (1983) further described the use of force transducers for the evaluation of labial, lingual, and mandibular motor impairments.

Hixon et al. (1983) discussed the use of a kinematic procedure in measuring speech production in a patient with flaccid paralysis of the rib cage, diaphragm, and abdomen. O'Dwyer, Neilson, Guitar, Quinn, and Andrews (1983) noted the use of EMG in evaluating the activity of orofacial and mandibular muscles of participants with dysarthria during nonspeech tasks.

Protocols were presented by Hixon and Hoit for use by the speech-language pathologist in conducting a physical examination of the diaphragm (1998), abdominal wall (1999), and rib cage (2000). A worksheet is provided to guide the speech-language pathologist in the examination of the status and function of the breathing apparatus.

Barlow and Burton (1990) and Wood, Hughes, Hayes, and Wolfe (1992) studied the use of lip force as a neuromotor assessment tool. Wit, Maassen, Gabreels, and Thoonen (1993) proposed the use of Maximum Performance Tests, which include maximum sound prolongation, fundamental frequency range, and maximum repetition rate as tools for detecting spastic dysarthria.

Liss et al. (2000) confirmed the ability of rhythm metrics to distinguish the speech of neurotypical controls from those with dysarthria, and to discriminate the dysarthria subtypes (hyperkinetic, hypokinetic, mixed flaccid-spastic, and ataxic). The authors claimed that rhythm metrics show promise for use as a rational and objective clinical tool. Narayana et al. (2009) explained the use of noninvasive functional imaging and "virtual" lesion techniques to study the neural mechanisms underlying motor speech disorders in Parkinson disease. They found evidence, in their case report of a patient with Parkinson disease, that impaired speech production accompanying subthalamic-nucleus–deep brain stimulation (STN-DBS) may result from unintended activation of the left dorsal premotor cortex. Clinical application of functional imaging and transcranial magnetic stimulation may lead to optimizing the delivery of STN-DBS to improve outcomes of speech production as well as general motor abilities. Liss, LeGendre, and Lotto (2010) concluded that the dysarthrias can be characterized by quantifiable temporal patterns in acoustic output. Because envelope modulation spectra (EMS), which quantifies the rhythmicity of speech within specified frequency bands, is automated and requires no editing or linguistic assumptions, it shows promise as a clinical and research tool.

Netsell (1994) noted that the best candidates for instrumentation testing and special procedures are patients with severe dysarthria who have unintelligible speech and may have the potential to regain intelligibility. Netsell stated that the best instruments are (1) those involving aerodynamics, where changes in airflow and pressure can be measured by rhinometers, and lung volume levels and air expired during speech by motorized spirometers; (2) video fluoroscopy, which is used in swallowing detection, to visualize the lips, tongue, jaw, and velopharynx during speech (if a microphone is added, speech can be seen and heard at the same time); and (3) videonasoendoscopic systems, which can be used to see the superior aspects of the velopharynx and the larynx.

Therapy

The Academy of Neurologic Communication Disorders and Sciences (ANCDS) writing committee on dysarthria searched 30 years of databases covering 5800 journals, using key words paired with the term *dysarthria*, and identified 51 intervention studies focusing on loudness (N = 21), speaking rate (N = 19), prosody (N = 10), and general instructions (N = 6), with some articles placed in more than one category.

In general, statistically significant improvement in loudness was found for participants with Parkinson disease who completed the 16-session protocol for Lee Silverman Voice Treatment (LSVT) (Yorkston et al., 2007, p. 19). Although statistical analysis related to acoustic variables, there were also improvements noted on physiologic and perceptual measures. Rate control treatments included delayed auditory feedback (DAF), pacing board, metronome, computer training, behavioral instructions, and biofeedback. Outcome measures were most often based on perceptual ratings of such variables as intelligibility. The research generally supports a relationship between reduced speaking rate and increased intelligibility.

Prosodic or suprasegmental features that were studied in the literature included stress patterning, intonation, and rate/rhythm. Prosodic disturbances are particularly noted in ataxic dysarthria, and refer to a complex interaction of rate loudness and pitch adjustments (Yorkston et al., 2007, p. 26). Acoustic parameters of fundamental frequency contours, intensity, and duration of speech production were the most frequent outcome measures analyzed in prosodic studies. Interpretation of outcomes was limited by the heterogeneity of the individuals in treatment, the small number of studies, and the fact that most investigations were case reports.

The final category of general instructions included many techniques telling patients to produce clear speech and providing feedback about the clarity of utterances. Perceptual ratings of clarity, intelligibility, and precision of articulation were the outcomes in the great majority of studies. Results do not provide strong evidence that there is an important benefit of instructing individuals with dysarthria to speak clearly.

The first goal of therapy is to inform the patient and the caretaker(s) about the nature and the consequences of the disorder.

The patient with dysarthria has a motor speech disorder that involves paralysis within the vocal tract. The speech components affected can involve respiration, phonation, resonation, articulation, and prosody in any combination. Typically, thinking abilities are normal or near normal, and language should be normal.

Prognosis

Netsell (1984) suggested six factors that influence treatment outcome with patients with dysarthria:

1. *Neurologic status and history.* Bilateral subcortical or brainstem lesions, and degenerative diseases such as ALS, offer the poorest prognosis. Love, Hagerman, and Taimi (1980) found that individuals who had cerebral palsy with more frequent dysphagic symptoms tended to present lower scores of overall speech proficiency and poor articulation scores. Neurologic history should be observed to see if developmental (e.g., cerebral palsy) or acquired dysarthria is present. Treatment procedures geared specifically to the cause would offer a better prognosis.

2. *Age.* Persons experiencing neurological insults during the development of the neocortical system might be expected to have, or to develop, better speech motor skills than those in whom the lesion occurred at a later age. The implication is that intact reticulo-limbic systems can support the more innate early motor skills. Younger children have a better chance to "grow out of" their lesions than adults. Elderly patients are negatively affected by age.

3. *"Automatic" adjustments.* In response to a lesion, automatic adjustments can be adaptive or maladaptive, intended or unintended, and reactive or "obligatory" (always the same). Incorporating automatic adjustments that are useful and minimizing those that are not offers a better prognosis.

4. *Treatment effects.* Treatment, especially combined (speech, medical, physical, behavioral) is better than no therapy or noncoordinated therapy.

5. *Personality and intelligence.* Those who were optimistic and purposeful before injury have a better prognosis than those who were not. Understanding premorbid levels of intelligence should aid in therapy.

6. *Support systems.* Treatment is enhanced if support is given by "significant others" and if the prospects for making contributions to society, however modest, are realistic.

The second goal of therapy is to provide the appropriate treatment approaches and techniques.

Efficacy of Therapy for Dysarthria

Yorkston (1996) reviewed a number of treatment efficacy studies of dysarthria. She found that several treatment techniques have been successfully applied to dysarthria caused by Parkinson disease, stroke and traumatic brain injury, cerebral palsy, and some other etiologies.

In Parkinson disease, the treatment studies ranged from retrospection to group to individual, with programs designed to improve voice loudness, intonation, articulation, and phonation. In the late 1960s and early 1970s, the broad-based speech improvement programs seemed to bring improvement during the treatment session, but these gains were not maintained outside the clinical setting. In the late 1970s and early 1980s, success was reported in the use of pacing boards and portable delayed auditory feedback devices.

During the 1980s, studies designed to improve respiration, voice, articulation, rate, intonation, intelligibility, and prosody showed success during the treatment session and some maintenance of progress. In the 1990s, several well-controlled group studies showed that treatment focusing on respiratory-phonatory function is more effective in changing the speech of patients with Parkinson disease than is treatment focusing on respiratory function alone. A systematic review of 51 articles on interventions for dysarthria indicated that the strongest evidence for efficacy was in modification of loudness in speakers with hypokinetic dysarthria secondary to Parkinson disease (Yorkston et al., 2007).

The Lee Silverman Voice Treatment protocol targets vocal loudness to increase vocal effort and improve coordination across the subsystems of respiration, phonation, resonation, and articulation. Training only vocal loudness often results in distributed effects of improved articulation, facial expression, and swallowing (Fox et al., 2006). The program requires intensive treatment, but similar treatment gains may occur when individuals are treated over the Internet (Howell et al., 2009).

For stroke and traumatic brain injury, Yorkston (1996) noted that group studies of persons with dysarthria following brain injury are not common because the pattern and severity of the dysarthria vary so extensively in this population. A number of case studies have shown that effective treatment for patients with dysarthria includes physiologic approaches (neuromuscular exercises), feedback of acoustic information, and rate control and breath patterning. Studies have shown that important changes in speech can occur many years post onset of traumatic brain injury (TBI) and suggest that long-term follow-up is necessary for brain-injured individuals with severe dysarthria.

Devices such as alphabet boards and palatal lifts also have been efficacious with individuals who have dysarthria. Outcomes of these studies are measured in several ways, including improvement in muscle strength or control, reduction in a selected deviant feature (e.g., consonant imprecision), and changes in overall features such as speech intelligibility, speaking rate, or naturalness. Hustad and Beukelman (2001) provided severely dysarthric and 72 nondisabled speakers with visual images containing alphabet, topic, combined (alphabet and topic together), and no cues. Findings showed that combined cues resulted in richer intelligibility scores than any other cue condition, and that alphabet cues were better than topic cues. Hustad and Beukelman (2002) noted findings consistent with intelligibility results of their previous study (2001), and their present study also found that, in severe dysarthria, combined cues resulted in higher comprehension scores than any other condition. Patel (2002) found that speakers with severe dysarthria were able to exert sufficient control to signal the question–statement contrast.

Hustad, Jones, and Dailey (2003) found that alphabet cues and combined cues (alphabet cues and topic cues) can have an important effect on intelligibility for speakers with severe dysarthria. Hustad and Gearhart (2004) found, in 7 speakers with dysarthria (spastic and mixed), that alphabet cues, rather than topic cues, and combined cues (alphabet and topic) were better than habitual speech in improving ratings of listener attitudes. The relationship between intelligibility scores and attitude ratings for each speaker was strong and positive, indicating that positive attitude seems to increase linearly with intelligibility scores. Hustad and Garcia (2005) found that when listeners were presented with simultaneous audio and visual information, both alphabet cues and hand gestures resulted in higher intelligibility scores and higher helpfulness ratings than the no-cues control condition for each of the three speakers with dysarthria. Alphabet cues used experimentally have resulted in improved identification of initial and final phonemes relative to a no-cues control condition (Hustad, 2006c). This improvement was maintained even when there was only partial cueing with alphabet supplementation (Hanson & Beukelman, 2006), and even when normal natural speech was electronically distorted to reduce intelligibility (Hanson et al., 2010).

Yorkston (1996) noted that reports on the efficacy of speech treatment for individuals with cerebral palsy are scarce. Some evidence suggests that speakers with cerebral palsy are able to modify their speech behaviors when faced with communication failure, or when using breath-group treatment strategy. Many published reports related to the effectiveness of treatment in cerebral palsy involve application of augmentative and alternative communication. It is beyond the scope of this text to report on the success of treatment using augmentative or alternative communication approaches in individuals with cerebral palsy and dysarthria. For this information, the reader is referred to the review of treatment efficacy in dysarthria by Yorkston (1996).

Concerning other etiologies, Yorkston (1996) noted that effective speech treatments for individuals with amyotrophic lateral sclerosis involved having the patient stay in the community, enhancing the quality of life, and providing modeling and instructions. Treatment effectiveness was also reported for the following types of individuals: in intensive or acute medical care units; with Wilson's disease; with multiple sclerosis; with Moebius syndrome, characterized by bilateral facial paralysis; with progressive nuclear palsy; with Shy-Drager syndrome; and with oral movement disorders.

General Principles

Darley et al. (1975) suggested the following general principles that underlie therapy for the motor speech disorders:

1. *Compensation.* The patient learns to make maximum use of the remaining potential and to "work around" the impairment that has altered his lifelong speech habits.
2. *Purposeful activity.* The patient learns to do on purpose what she had been doing automatically before. The patient must develop an awareness of where her articulators are and of what they are doing, of how word sequences fall into phrase groupings, of how breath supply can be coordinated with the onset of speech effort and adjusted to the appropriate phrase units, and of how her voice varies in loudness.
3. *Monitoring.* The patient learns to listen to himself talk (perhaps by listening to tape recordings of his speech performances from time to time), noting specific ways in which he falls short of his standard, whether in audibility, intelligibility, or emphasis.
4. *An early start.* The patient gets a head start in compensation, purposeful activity, and monitoring before her skills have deteriorated and it becomes next to impossible to sustain the effort to speak well.
5. *Motivation.* The patient is reassured that his effort is worthwhile. The clinician plans a sensible sequence of activities graduated in difficulty, with an optimistic manner that encourages the patient to do his best.

Indirect and Direct Treatment

Brookshire (2007) noted that treatment for dysarthria can be indirect, direct, or most likely a combination of the two. Indirect approaches would include sensory stimulation, muscle strengthening, modifying muscle tone, changing the posture and speaking position, and modifying respiration.

The purpose of sensory stimulation is to heighten motor control by increasing the patient's awareness of sensory feedback from the oral mechanism. Stimulation techniques may include brushing, stroking, vibration, or applying ice to the patient's lips, tongue, pharynx, or soft palate. The value of sensory stimulation is still debatable.

The purpose of muscle strengthening is to improve the patient's speech by increasing movements of weakened muscles. Muscle strengthening exercises work best for patients with severe dysarthria, where there is little intelligible speech. For the mild or moderately impaired patient, the value of muscle strengthening is debatable.

Maas et al. (2008) stated that the purpose of their tutorial was to introduce principles that enhance motor learning for nonspeech motor skills, and to examine the degree to which these principles apply in the treatment of motor speech disorders. After their review of relevant literature, they concluded that evidence from nonspeech motor learning suggests that these principles hold promise for treatment of motor speech disorders.

Defects in muscle tone can be manifested as hypertonicity (e.g., spastic dysarthria) or as hypotonicity (e.g., flaccid dysarthria). The modification of muscle tone in hypertonicity primarily includes techniques that relax the muscles (e.g., progressive relaxation, chewing exercises). The modification of muscle tone in hypotonicity can include techniques that increase the level of muscle tension (e.g., pushing and pulling exercises).

Changing the posture and speaking position of the patient can sometimes improve speech production. These changes are most beneficial for the weak or flaccid patient who has difficulty sitting up and keeping the head in an upright position. Cervical collars, body braces, slings, restraints, girdles, stomach bands, and stomach boards are among the items used to assist the patient in achieving this change.

Modifying respiration capacity is most beneficial for patients with a generalized weakness. Treatment can include postural and positioning adjustments, muscle strengthening of the respiratory muscles, increasing muscle tone with pushing exercises, and controlled exhalation techniques. Rosenbek and LaPointe (1985) presented in full detail the modification procedures for posture, muscle tone, and strength for general purposes, and for respiration, phonation, resonation, and articulation specifically.

Direct treatment procedures involve controlling respiration, phonation, resonation, articulation, and prosody in any combination during speech production. In the following pages are some of the indirect and direct treatment procedures for problems in articulation, hypernasality, strained-strangled voice, breathiness, prosody impairment (varying pitch, controlling rate), and loudness impairment, and for severe dysarthria. In some cases, indirect and direct treatment techniques are combined, and in other cases the entire approach is either direct or indirect. The concept of indirect and direct treatment procedures will be mentioned specifically only in the section dealing with therapy for articulation disorders. However, the concept should apply to all the other forms of therapy for dysarthria.

Schulz, Dingwall, and Ludlow (1999) found that cerebellar pathology did not interfere with practice effects for speech oral movements, suggesting that treatment involving either speech or oral movements would not be detrimentally affected in persons with cerebellar pathology. However, they found that practice on oral movement tasks may not be related to practice on speech tasks for patients with cerebellar atrophy. McCauley et al. (2009), in their review of the literature, found that there is insufficient evidence to support or refute the use of oral motor exercises, defined as nonspeech activities that involve sensory stimulation to or actions of the lips, jaw, tongue, soft palate, larynx, and respiratory muscles intended to influence the physiological underpinnings of the oropharyngeal mechanism to improve its functions. They may include activities described as active muscle exercise, muscle stretching, passive exercise, or sensory stimulation.

Articulation

For problems in articulation, mobility and stretching techniques may be used as indirect treatment. Duffy (2005) stated that stretching exercises of the lips, tongue, and jaw may have some effect on increasing range of motion and decreasing spasticity in speech. Because stretching of the articulators is necessarily voluntary and not passive, it may also contribute to increasing strength. Stretching may work best for those with spasticity and rigidity, and the possible strengthening effect of stretching might help some patients with weakness.

It must be noted that vigorous exercises of the articulators are contraindicated for conditions such as myasthenia gravis, where such exercises would produce a further weakening of the musculature (Darley et al., 1975; Rosenbek & LaPointe, 1985).

Duffy (2005) stated that nonspeech strengthening exercises should be used only after ascertaining that weakness is clearly related to the speech impairment. Although there is some controversy concerning the efficacy of strengthening exercises to improve articulation in patients with dysarthria (see Duffy, 2005), strengthening exercises have been recommended by Dworkin (1991) and Solomon and Stierwalt (1995).

The following exercises numbered 1–5, 7–11, and 13–17 are examples of mobility and stretching activities. Exercises numbered 6 (lips) and 12 (tongue) are examples of strengthening activities. Exercises numbered 1–17 are examples (Kilpatrick & Jones, 1977) of indirect treatment. Exercises 18–21 are examples of direct treatment using alternating motion rate activities.

A mirror should be used to do these exercises. The patient should do each exercise 5 times (fewer if necessary) and gradually, over a number of lessons, work up to 10 times. All exercises should be done 3 times (fewer if necessary) a day. The clinician should demonstrate each exercise.

1. Open and close mouth slowly; be sure lips are fully closed; hold, relax, and repeat.
2. Pucker lips, as for a kiss; hold, relax, and repeat.
3. Spread lips into a big smile; hold, relax, and repeat.
4. Pucker, hold, smile, hold; relax and repeat.
5. Open mouth, then try to pucker with mouth wide open, don't close jaw; hold, relax, and repeat.
6. Close lips tightly and press together; hold, relax, and repeat.
7. Close lips; suck tongue as if it were candy.
8. Open mouth and stick out tongue; be sure tongue comes straight out of your mouth and doesn't go off to the side; hold, relax, and repeat. Work toward sticking tongue out farther each day, but still pointing straight ahead.
9. Stick out tongue and move it slowly from corner to corner of your lips; hold it in each corner; relax and repeat. Be sure tongue actually touches each corner each time.
10. Stick out tongue and try to reach chin with the tongue tip; hold at farthest point; relax, repeat.
11. Stick out tongue and try to reach nose with the tongue tip; pretend to lick a popsicle or clean off some jelly from top lip (don't use bottom lip or fingers as helpers); give it a good stretch; hold, relax, and repeat.
12. Using tongue blade or spoon, stick out tongue; hold spoon against the tip of tongue and try to push the spoon even farther away with tongue while hand is holding the spoon steadily in place (hold the spoon like a popsicle or a sucker upright and not in mouth); relax and repeat.
13. Stick out tongue; pretend to lick a sucker, moving the tongue tip from near the chin to near the nose; go slowly and use as much movement as possible; relax and repeat.
14. Stick tongue out and pull it back, then repeat as quickly as you can; repeat.
15. Move tongue from corner to corner as quickly as you can; repeat.
16. Move tongue all around lips in a circle as quickly and as completely as you can, touching all of both upper lip and corner, lower lip and corner, in circle; repeat.
17. Open and close mouth as quickly as possible; be sure lips close each time; repeat.
18. Say "mah-mah-mah-mah" as quickly and accurately as you can without losing the "mah" sound; be sure there's an /m/ and an /ah/ each time.
19. Say "lah-lah-lah-lah" as quickly and accurately as possible; be sure there's an /l/ and an /ah/ each time; repeat.
20. Say "kah-kah-kah-kah" as quickly and accurately as you can; be sure there's a /k/ and an /ah/ each time; repeat.

21. Say "kahlah-kahlah-kahlah" as quickly and accurately as you can; be sure there's a /k/ and an /ah/ and an /l/ and an /ah/ each time; repeat.

To round out the above list, one can add exaggerated chewing exercises (indirect treatment) and production of sequential motion rate exercises (direct treatment) of /puh-puh-puh/ tuh-tuh-tuh/kuh-kuh-kuh/, and /puh-tuh-kuh/. Occasionally, the above exercises will have to be adapted in some way. For example, one patient with dysarthria did not want to smile when asked because she was in no mood to smile. She was gloomy and depressed about her condition and related matters, and could not bring herself to produce even the faintest of smiles. However, when asked to "Show me your teeth," she did, and one would think the sun had burst through the clouds.

Therapy that focuses on phoneme production (direct treatment) can include the following:

1. The phonetic placement method of describing the correct manner and place of articulation, and the correct voiced and voiceless components of target phoneme production, uses both visual and verbal instruction.

2. The motokinesthetic approach, which is the manual manipulation of the articulators to produce the correct sound, can also be employed. This approach should be used with some caution because a study by Creech, Wertz, and Rosenbek (1973) showed patients with dysarthria to be somewhat deficient in stereognostic abilities.

3. The phonetic derivation method (Rosenbek, 1985) achieves the correct production of sounds from intact nonspeech or speech gestures. For example, biting the lower lip produces /f, v/, puckering the lips produces /oo, oh, aw, w/, smiling produces /ee, eh/, yawning produces /ah, uh/, and wiping one's mouth produces /m, p, b/.

4. Using the above three approaches, the sound is worked on in isolation (most likely with the patient with severe dysarthria) and then with real words or with nonsense syllables (e.g., "ah, ay, ee, aw, oh, oo"), unconnected syllables (e.g., "s-ah"), and in connected form (e.g., "sah"). After this is achieved, the sound is employed in the initial, final, medial, and blend positions in words, phrases, sentences, and eventually controlled conversations.

5. Once the patient has achieved some success in producing consonant sounds, the use of minimal contrasts in single words (e.g., "tea—key"), phrases (e.g., "tan coat"), and sentences (e.g., "Ted can tell Kay about the two cars") can be used to bolster each individual consonant and to differentiate between consonants that are close. Keith and Thomas (1989) provided practice material for the vowels, diphthongs, and consonants for contrast purposes. Listed below are examples of contrasting pairs of words and phrases.

tea—key	tea cup
till—kill	Tim came
ten—Ken	tell Kay
tan—can	tan coat
tall—call	tall cow
top—cop	Tom cat
take—cake	take care
two—coo	two keys
tub—cub	tough call
toad—code	toll call

6. Another technique to achieve overall intelligibility requires the patient to read aloud lists of single words, sentences, or paragraphs; describe a picture; or engage in controlled conversation. The clinician can either face the patient or not, and tries to discern the intelligibility of what the patient is saying. If the patient is unclear, imitation

of the clinician can be effective in producing intelligibility. This technique can also be used with patients who have loudness, phonatory, nasality, rhythm, or rate problems.

7. Slowing the rate of speech is another procedure that might increase intelligibility in articulation (see Berry, 1984; Darley et al., 1975). Yorkston, Hummen, Beukelman, and Traynor (1990) found that slow rate helped sentence but not phoneme intelligibility in speakers with dysarthria. They also found that slowed rate affected the naturalness in neurotypical speakers, but not so much in speakers with dysarthria. In addition to slowing the rate of speech, Darley et al. (1975) advocated consonant exaggeration (e.g., "important, because") and a syllable-by-syllable approach (e.g., "af-ter sup-per, when-ev-er pos-sible") as a means of increasing intelligibility in articulation.

Medical, Pharmacological, and Prosthetic Management

Duffy (2005) reviewed the use of the following as aids in articulation therapy: surgical management (neural anastomosis, which with patients with dysarthria usually involves connecting the XII nerve to the damaged VII nerve to restore function; Botox injections for treatment of hemifacial spasm, spasmodic torticollis, and oral mandibular dystonia), pharmacological management, and prosthetic management (bite block made of acrylic or putty material that is custom fitted to be held between the lateral upper and lower teeth to inhibit uncontrolled jaw movements).

Schulz, Peterson, Sapienza, Greer, and Friedman (1999) found that unilateral pallidotomy surgery helped the speech and voice characteristics of six adults who had Parkinson disease with hypokinetic dysarthria. The patients with mild hypokinetic dysarthria benefited more than those with moderate dysarthria.

Hypernasality

The following are some suggestions for therapy.

1. Because hypernasality is caused by insufficient movement of the velum, one intervention approach involves stimulating the muscles of the soft palate:
   A. Sip through a straw with the other end sealed.
   B. Produce a very long (pull-in) kiss with a loud smack at the end.
   C. Perform pushing exercises (Boone et al., 2005; Froeschels, Kastein, & Weiss, 1955), which require the patient to push with both arms and hands down against a table top, upward under a table, hand against hand, or in a parallel downward motion against the air. This motion is accompanied by the /ah/ sound. With the sudden voluntary contraction of one group of muscles, other muscle groups tend to contract, reinforcing the function of the first group (muscles of the soft palate).
   D. Repeat /ah/ strongly and rapidly without pushing.
   E. Exercise for the back of the tongue (e.g., "kah, kay, kee" and "ahk, ayk, eek") can also be employed in stimulating the muscles of the soft palate; here, the production of linguavelar consonants provides the stimulation to the soft palate.
2. Another technique for reducing hypernasality involves directing the airstream through the oral cavity:
   A. Straws (putting a straw in water and blowing bubbles), bubble pipes, oral-nasal cardboard platforms, ping-pong balls, horns, whistles, musical instruments, pinwheels, candles, balloons, feathers, and paper have all been used to refocus the direction of the airstream.
   B. A sheet of paper with a hole or bull's-eye in the center can be held close to the patient's lips. The patient is instructed to hit the hole or bull's-eye with the /oo/ sound

produced through the oral cavity. The clinician slowly moves the paper away as the patient keeps phonating. The paper can be moved only if the patient produces the correct /oo/ sound through the oral cavity. This technique might be applicable as a breathing exercise in that it helps to prolong the breath stream.

Both the techniques of stimulating the muscles and of directing the airstream should be instituted with some caution, because some studies reviewed by Duffy (2005) have shown that these procedures may have little or no value in reducing hypernasality.

3. Tongue exercises (rotation, in and out) and lip exercises (pursing, puckering, retracting, biting down or up) are used to achieve flexibility. Also, because a raised mandible and retracted tongue tend to isolate the oral cavity, thereby increasing the hypernasality, tongue and lip exercises are used to prevent such movement. Appropriate exercises should open up the oral cavity as a resonator and combat the patient's attempts to retract the tongue or raise the mandible in an effort to reduce hypernasality.

Strained-Strangled Voice

The problem of strained-strangled voice is due to overadduction of the vocal folds. Therefore, a major thrust of therapy is attaining soft and easy onset of phonation. Suggestions for therapy include the following:

1. The yawn-sigh technique, in which the patient is taught to produce phonation in an easy, relaxed yawn. The rationale for this technique is that yawning opens up the entire vocal tract, thereby cutting down on hyperadduction of the vocal folds. Initially, the patient yawns and releases a sigh on exhalation.

2. Another technique is to teach the patient to initiate phonation with the phoneme /h/, since this phoneme is produced with the vocal folds abducted, and can eventually be employed to initiate the production of words and phrases.

3. Relaxation exercises centered around the head and neck area can also be used. In this instance, the patient imagines that his head is a heavy iron ball and lets it drop on his chest. Then he slowly rotates his head in a front-to-back motion and emits phonation while rotating his head. The relaxation of the head and neck area should help bring about easy onset of phonation.

   Rubow, Rosenbek, Collins, and Celesia (1984) reported that EMG biofeedback, as a method for producing relaxation, successfully reduced the strained-strangled quality in a patient with hemifacial spasm and dysarthria. Nemec and Cohen (1984) found that EMG biofeedback was an effective treatment technique in a case of hypertonic spastic dysarthria.

4. Chewing exercises, which are based on the concept of eating, can be used for attaining relaxation and proper muscular tonus in the vocal tract. In a graduated series of steps, the patient is taught exaggerated chewing movements without and then with phonation. Using these movements, the patient progresses from single-word phonation to conversational speech. Eventually, the exaggerated movements are reduced to where she can chew mentally. Chewing exercises are described in detail by their originator, Froeschels (1952), and by Boone et al. (2005).

Chiefly for spastic dysarthria, Aten (1984) suggested that all movements should be relaxed and slow, to avoid triggering the spastic contractions and to retreat to a relaxed baseline whenever spasticity occurs. To reduce hyperadduction of the vocal folds, the patient starts with a relaxed, breathy sigh of short duration, proceeds to short words beginning with /h/, then to open-mouth vowels, and then to a nasal consonant or continuant. Plosives and affricates should be avoided because of the excessive pressure and musculature movement involved. Murry (1984) suggested the use of nasal and liquid sounds to help "defuse" the explosive (strained-strangled) phonatory characteristics of Friedreich's ataxia. Duffy (2005) noted that laryngeal massage may help strained-strangled voices.

Duffy (2005) reviewed the management of the pseudobulbar effect (pathologic crying and laughing), which occurs more frequently in spastic dysarthria than in other types of dysarthria. Drug therapy and the modification of head turning that precedes crying were successful in some cases. The authors remember working with a dysarthric patient who exhibited pseudobulbar crying on almost every utterance. Therapy that included overall relaxation and prolonged pausing on a word-to-word basis seemed to help this patient.

Breathiness

The problem of breathiness results from insufficient glottal closure. Therefore, a main approach to therapy attempts to close the glottis during phonation. Some suggestions follow:

1. Coughing, clearing the throat, and counting in a hard manner.
2. The previously described pushing exercises (pulling apart interlocked fingers while saying "ee" or "oo").
3. Another technique based upon the pushing technique is the glottal attack using a phoneme. In this instance, the patient is taught to start hard contact phonation with a vowel or diphthong (/ah, ay, ee, aw, oh, oo/). This manner of initiating phonation is then applied to the production of words, phrases, and sentences.

   At first, with the pushing or glottal attack method, the patient may produce a string of vowels or diphthongs with half fully phonated and the others not; or a single word may be half breathy and half normal; or a group of words, sentences, and paragraphs may be half and half. The back and forth nature of clear or breathy voice can go on for a number of sessions. Eventually, if successful, all of the patient's output will be fully phonated.
4. In cases of unilateral vocal fold paralysis, Teflon and silicon injections (Hammarberg et al., 1984; Reich & Lerman, 1978) have been used to bolster or increase the size of the paralyzed fold. When the paralyzed fold is brought closer to the midline, better vocal fold vibration is frequently possible. The use of collagen injections (Duffy, 2005) may be recommended for the same purpose as Teflon. Collagen may be preferable because it is structurally similar to the natural collagen in the vocal folds and is subject to only limited absorption.

Prosody Impairment

Prosody, which involves intonation and rate, can be inferior in the speaker with dysarthria, as compared to neurotypical speakers (see LeDorze, Ouellet, & Ryalls, 1994). Ziegler, Hartmann, and Hoople (1993) found that syllabic timing was related to severity and intelligibility in speakers with dysarthria. Frequently, impairments in prosody can be alleviated by varying the patient's pitch and controlling the rate. Patel (2003) found that speakers with severe dysarthria may benefit from intervention aimed at improving prosodic control.

Varying Pitch

Exercises can help the patient discriminate auditorily while directing the pitch higher and lower. This therapy can begin with utterance of simple notes of the scale, then expand the vocalization to individual words, phrases, and then sentences. Although some of the following exercises have been suggested for dysarthria caused by Parkinson disease (American

Parkinson Disease Association, n.d.), they can be employed with most speakers with dysarthria regardless of the cause.

In the following example, key words in a sentence are stressed to clarify and change meaning. After the clinician does it first, the patient says the same sentence several times, changing word stress and noting how the meaning may change.

<u>I</u> don't want that gray coat. I <u>don't</u> want that gray coat. I don't <u>want</u> that gray coat. I don't want <u>that</u> gray coat. I don't want that <u>gray</u> coat. I don't want that gray <u>coat</u>.

In the next example, after the clinician does it first, the patient practices asking questions and giving answers. The patient raises and lowers his or her voice as indicated by the arrows.

Q. Are you going?↑ A. No, I'm not.↓
Q. Do you know her?↑ A. I think I do.↓
Q. Is it fixed?↑ A. I guess it is.↓
Q. Can you talk clearly?↑ A. I am trying hard.↓
Q. Have you seen my sweater?↑ A. It's in the closet.↓
Q. Can you help her?↑ A. Yes, I can.↓
Q. Do you think he needs it?↑ A. Yes, he might.↓
Q. Where is my book?↑ A. It's on the desk.↓

Controlling Rate

Most patients with dysarthria will have a slower than normal speaking rate because of the physiologic limitations within the vocal tract. Some speakers will be so slow that it reduces intelligibility or interferes greatly with the naturalness of speech. One patient with dysarthria complained about the impatience of people who hung up during a phone call. She was told to start her phone conversations by saying, "I speak slowly because of a condition. Please bear with me." This preface seemed to help in future phone conversations.

It may seem counterintuitive to treat a patient with a slower than normal speaking rate by further decreasing both articulation rate and overall speaking rate. However, decreasing rate is associated with clinically significant improvements in intelligibility for up to half of the participants with different types of dysarthria (Van Nuffelen et al., 2009, 2010). The most effective therapy techniques were use of an alphabet board, hand tapping, pacing board, and, for some, voluntary rate control.

To achieve intelligibility, slowing down the speaker's rate should bring about more control in the patient's attempts at consonant exaggeration. Yorkston, Beukelman, and Bell (1988) pointed out that naturalness of speaking should be preserved as much as possible; otherwise it will hinder intelligibility beyond any benefits achieved by slowing down the rate. The patient mentioned above is an example of how an extremely slow rate interfered with intelligibility.

Duffy (2005) described the techniques used in slowing down the rate for a speaker with dysarthria. They include the following:

1. Delayed auditory feedback—the patient wears earphones, enabling him to hear his own feedback at a slower rate.
2. Pacing board—while speaking, the patient uses a board with raised portions at measured intervals; each raised portion can indicate when a syllable or word should be spoken.
3. Metronomes—each beat can be used to indicate a syllable or word marker.
4. Pointing on an alphabet board to the first letter of each word spoken—this can increase the intelligibility of sounds, words, or sentences.

5. Flashing lights—each flash can signal a syllable or word marker.
6. Hand or finger tapping—each tap represents a syllable or word.
7. Rhythmic cueing—the clinician points to words in a rhythmic manner while the patient is reading a passage.
8. Visual feedback—this appears on a computer screen when the patient reads a passage.

Loudness Impairment

Loudness can be varied through the use of breathing exercises. Specifically, the patient can be taught to be aware of the breathing cycle and then to control the exhalation phase during phonation. For example, the patient may initially be told to say "one-two" on one exhalation. Once this easy task is accomplished, the patient progresses to "three" and so on, until he or she has gained the required control of both phonation and exhalation. From there, the patient can vary the loudness of his or her voice commensurate with the degree of breath control.

Intermittent loudness and inaudibility can be controlled by teaching the patient to slow down the rate of speech and speak syllable by syllable. Auditory training is essential to the development of self-monitoring skills for loudness levels. Because the respiratory process supplies the energy or force for speech, any impairment in this process should be properly evaluated and modified. However, stimulating increased levels of vocal loudness does not necessarily reduce nasalance (McHenry & Liss, 2006).

Most neurotypical speakers pause for breath at appropriate phrase and idea points in an utterance. With many speakers with dysarthria, the reduction in movement and control of respiratory muscles requires more frequent pauses between words. Several patients with dysarthria with whom the first author has worked had to take a breath before each word spoken. This may have been laborious, but for these patients it was the only way they could communicate in a relatively normal manner. Patients need to achieve a compromise between the usual pattern of word groupings and the number of words they can say clearly before pausing for breath. With the following set of exercises (American Parkinson Disease Association, n.d.), the clinician should always demonstrate what has to be done.

The clinician then instructs the patient to do the following:

1. To become aware of control over inhalation and exhalation, feel the movement of the stomach muscles as one breathes in and out (e.g., place hands on stomach; inhale slowly; exhale slowly; repeat several times; try to establish a regular pattern).
2. Coordinate the breath stream with saying vowel sounds. Inhale and then produce a continuous tone as one exhales. Hold each sound as long as the voice continues to be strong. Do not extend the time if the voice trails off (e.g., inhale and then say "ah" on exhalation; rest; repeat with other vowels and diphthongs).

   Timing the length of each sound will provide the average time each sound can be maintained and indicate if there is improvement. Sustaining a strong steady tone for seven to eight seconds is an average range.
3. Counting is a good way to practice breath control (e.g., hold palm of hand about 5 inches away from mouth to feel the airstream as one speaks; count from 1 to 10, inhaling and exhaling after each number; try to say each number with a firm, strong tone). The same exercise can be done with individual alphabet letters. Build up to as many numbers or alphabet letters as possible on one exhalation without fading. It is better to say 1 or 2 words clearly than to say 4 or 5 words that are unintelligible.
4. Practice breath control with short phrases. Inhale first and then say each word separately on exhalation (e.g., "read /a/ book, brush /your/ hair, walk /the/ dog, knife /and/

fork, gang /of/ men, change /the/ time, reach /the/ park, push /and/ pull, jump /for/ joy, lots /of/ fun").

5. Practice additional short phrases. Try to say the whole phrase on one exhalation (e.g., "can of soup," "go to sleep," "pot of gold," "just for fun," "cup of soup," "pinch of salt," "time to go," "next in line," "come for brunch," "join the crowd").

6. Practice phrasing with short sentences. Pause between phrases where marked (e.g., "we need/more soup, it's time/for brunch, Meg broke/the plate, please get/my hat, Jack lost/the new book, turn right/at the light, bring the bag/to the yard, Pat can come/ later on, Ted caught/a big fish, put my shirt/on the table").

7. Practice modulating voice from soft to loud. Say "ah" in a soft tone and gradually increase the loudness. Repeat several times. Inhale each time at start of exercise and stop when voice fades.

8. Practice short phrases using three levels of loudness for each phrase. Imagine talking to listeners in different settings, first to a listener sitting opposite, then to a listener across the room, then to a listener in another room. Read across, not down, with each of the following:

   To a Listener Opposite (softly):
   I won't . . . you can't . . . don't try . . . sit down . . . stop here
   TO A LISTENER ACROSS THE ROOM (A LITTLE LOUDER): I WON'T . . . YOU CAN'T . . . DON'T TRY . . . SIT DOWN . . . STOP HERE
   TO A LISTENER IN ANOTHER ROOM (MUCH LOUDER): I WON'T . . . YOU CAN'T . . . DON'T TRY . . . SIT DOWN . . . STOP HERE

don't rush	DON'T RUSH	**DON'T RUSH**
he's okay	HE'S OKAY	**HE'S OKAY**
keep still	KEEP STILL	**KEEP STILL**
so long	SO LONG	**SO LONG**

9. Practice short sentences, using the same procedure as in number 8 to practice 3 levels of loudness.

   To a Listener Opposite (softly):
   Look, Bill's awake.
   Is that Mary?
   I've got a nickel.
   TO A LISTENER ACROSS THE ROOM (A LITTLE LOUDER):
   GO TO SLEEP.
   BRING ME MY PEN.
   CLOSE THE BOOK.
   TO A LISTENER IN ANOTHER ROOM (MUCH LOUDER):
   THE MAILMAN JUST CAME.
   WHO WANTS PIE?
   YOU HAVE A PHONE CALL.

10. Say each of the following phrases twice in succession, as if repeating a command; on the second phrase, speak louder. Inhale before each phrase.
    keep quiet . . . don't go . . . go slow . . . be still . . . sit up . . . hurry up . . . look out first down . . . come back . . . move away
    KEEP QUIET . . . DON'T GO . . . . GO SLOW . . . BE STILL . . . SIT UP HURRY UP . . . LOOK OUT . . . FIRST DOWN . . . COME BACK . . . MOVE AWAY

For those patients with dysarthria who need it, Duffy (2005) reviewed the factors for increasing respiratory support (producing consistent subglottal air pressure, postural adjustments) and for prosthetic assistance (abdominal binders or corsets, expiratory boards or paddles). Watson and Hixon (2001) found that abdominal trussing may be useful in improving speech in individuals with a paralyzed or paretic abdomen whose breathing function for speech is diminished.

McNamara (1983) noted that a biofeedback instrument with visual feedback improved vocal loudness in a patient with dysarthria. Particularly for ataxic dysarthria, Murry (1984) suggested that loudness is rarely worked on alone. Proper phrasing and breathing, and multisyllabic words, are used to control loudness.

Ramig (1995) outlined the Lee Silverman Voice Treatment (LSVT) program for Parkinson disease. Much of that program centers around techniques for improving loudness, some of which have been described previously in this treatment section. Studying a single patient with Parkinson disease, Dromey, Ramig, and Johnson (1995) found that vocal intensity treatment not only helped to increase his vocal loudness, but also led to better articulation, which was not targeted in treatment.

Ramig, Countryman, Thompson, and Horii (1995) observed that intensive voice and respiration treatment, focusing on increased vocal fold adduction and respiration exercises, was more effective for improving vocal intensity in 45 patients with Parkinson disease than was respiration treatment alone.

Analyzing the same 45 patients with Parkinson disease, Ramig and Dromey (1996) found that the combination of increased vocal fold adduction and subglottal pressure is a key in generating posttreatment increases in vocal intensity in idiopathic Parkinson disease. Countryman, Hicks, Ramig, and Smith (1997) found that vocal fold adduction therapy increased vocal loudness, decreased supraglottic hyperadduction, and improved intonation and overall voice quality in an individual with Parkinson disease who had reduced vocal loudness and supraglottic hyperadduction.

Kleinow, Smith, and Ramig (2001) found that speaking loudly is associated with a spatial and temporal organization that closely resembles that used in habitual speech, which may contribute to the success of LSVT. Sapir, Spielman, Ramig, Story, and Fox (2007) found that the LSVT on vowel articulation, along with previous findings, add further support to the generalized therapeutic impact of intensive voice treatment on orofacial functions (speech, swallowing, facial expression) and respiratory and laryngeal functions in individuals with idiopathic Parkinson disease. Solomon, McKee, and Garcia-Barry (2001) found that LSVT, combined with respiration and physical therapy, was successful with a young man diagnosed with mixed hypokinetic-spastic dysarthria 20 months after sustaining a traumatic brain injury. Fox, Morrison, Ramig, and Sapir (2002) presented a comprehensive overview of the LSVT for individuals with idiopathic Parkinson disease and other neurological disorders. Sapir et al. (2003), in studying a single patient with ataxic dysarthria, found that LSVT resulted in short- and long-term improvement in phonatory and articulatory functions, speech intelligibility, and overall communication. Spielman et al. (2007) found that when 12 participants with idiopathic Parkinson disease were given an extended version of the Lee Silverman Voice Treatment (LSVT-X), they successfully increased vocal sound pressure levels, consistent with improvements following traditional LSVT: decreased perceived voice handicap and improved functional speech. The traditional LSVT had 4 one-hour sessions per week for 4 weeks, and the LSVT-X had 2 one-hour sessions per week for 8 weeks. However, the LSVT had a total of 40 homework assignments, and the LSVT-X had a total of 96 homework assignments.

Duffy (2005), Netsell (1994), and Rosenbek and LaPointe (1985) reviewed the instrumentation (biofeedback devices such as water manometers, air pressure transducers, etc.) and speech methods (postural adjustments, muscle strengthening, controlled exhalation, etc.) used in the diagnosis and treatment of respiratory problems.

Severe Dysarthria

For the speaker with severe dysarthria, Binger and Kent-Walsh (2010), Kangas and Lloyd (2006), Owens and House (1984), Shane and Bashir (1980), and Silverman (1989) offered criteria for determining candidacy for an augmentative or alternative system. They included a consideration of cognitive, oral reflex, language, motor, intelligibility, emotional, chronological age, previous therapy, imitative, and environmental factors. Roy, Leeper, Blomgren, and Cameron (2001) presented a case report that described the recovery of an individual with severe spastic dysarthria and illustrated the close relationship between intelligibility measures and acoustic and physiological parameters.

Kangas and Lloyd (2006), Shane and Sauer (1986), and Silverman (1989) reviewed the augmentative or alternative communication strategies that have been used with patients who have dysarthria. These include manual sign languages, gestural Morse code, nonelectronic communication (or conversation boards), electronic communication systems, computerized devices, eye-gaze systems, Blissymbolics (electronic and nonelectronic), and laptop computers with specialized software.

In cases of severe velopharyngeal incompetency, a palatal lift may be used to aid in producing closure of that area. This prosthesis is attached to the teeth and is made in the shape of a bulb obturator, with a hard plastic shelf attached to the posterior section of the palatal portion. This shelf projects posteriorly under the soft palate and maintains the palate in an elevated position (see Hardy, Netsell, Schweiger, & Morris, 1969).

With the use of a palatal lift, there has been success in reducing hypernasality and nasal emission and in increasing the overall intelligibility of speech in children with dysarthria (Kent & Netsell, 1978), in children with developmental delay (Shaughnessy, Netsell, & Farrage, 1983), and in adults with dysarthria (Brand, Matsko, & Avart, 1988; Netsell, 1995). Duffy (2005) noted the use of pharyngeal flap surgery as a means for managing velopharyngeal incompetence in speakers with dysarthria, although the much preferred method is a palatal lift prosthesis.

Solomon et al. (2000) found that pallidal stimulation and medication helped three men with severe Parkinson disease in motor function (better mobility, reduced tremor and dyskinesia), but responses for speech varied from improvement to worsening. Farrell, Theodoros, Ward, Hall, and Silburn (2005) found that neurologic intervention (pallidotomy, thalamotomy, and deep brain stimulation) did not significantly change the perceptual speech dimensions or oromotor function despite significant postoperative improvements in ratings of general motor function and disease severity in participants with Parkinson disease.

Additional types, reviews of evaluation procedures, and speech methods used in the treatment of dysarthria can be found in Boone et al. (2005), Duffy (2005), and Freed (2000). Reviews of nonspeech communication can be found in Kangas and Lloyd (2006), Shane and Sauer (1986), and Silverman (1989).

The third goal of therapy is to encourage the patient and the caretaker(s) to continue the rehabilitative process outside of the clinical setting.

Carryover, or the ability to use the correction consistently in normal conversation, is achieved by making the patient aware of his or her error while speaking, and motivating him or her to practice. Some techniques used in achieving carryover are giving the patient a clear understanding of the problem; objectifying progress through tape recordings, graphs, and charts; giving assignments with practice; and enlisting the family or caretaker's help.

For example, the patient can practice reading aloud lists of words, phrases, sentences, and paragraphs. One patient with dysarthria, who had articulation and projection problems, was a former nonprofessional singer who had performed in churches, at family get-togethers, and just for fun. As a result of her interest in singing, she had a vast repertoire of popular music. After each therapy session, her assignment was to choose two songs and to concentrate on the articulation and projection. We called this practice assignment with singing "Stump the Clinician," which she accomplished about 50% of the time.

Another patient with dysarthria, a retired high school teacher, had misarticulations and a weak, monotonous voice. She loved poetry, and her assignment was to pick out her favorite passages of poetry and recite them aloud. The instructions were to imagine auditioning for a radio program and to concentrate on the proper articulation, projection, and vocal variety.

A third patient was a mostly Spanish-speaking woman with dysarthria, who had articulation and loudness problems. The SLP (one of the present authors) knew some Spanish and gave her materials to practice, written in Spanish. They included repeating the following after the SLP: counting 1–10; reciting days of the week and months of the year; and singing well-known Spanish songs learned premorbidly. The patient's clergyman came early one day, heard the SLP say to the patient, "Besame, besame mucho," and was taken aback. He thought the SLP was coming on to the patient. After an explanation, it all ended happily.

The point was that all three patients practiced, which was the purpose. The suggestions listed here for achieving carryover may be applied, with adaptations, to the other speech problems described in this section and in the chapter on apraxia of speech.

Improving Comprehensibility

Yorkston, Strand, and Kennedy (1996) suggested some techniques for improving comprehensibility (listener understanding of speech in a communicative setting) between the speaker with dysarthria and the listener.

What the listener can do to aid comprehensibility is:

- Know the general topic of the conversation (e.g., encourage the dysarthric speaker to let the listener know beforehand, through any means, what the theme will be)
- Watch for turn-taking signs (e.g., look at verbal, gestural, and body language signs that the patient with dysarthria shows when wanting to speak)
- Give the speaker undivided attention
- Pick the right time and place for communication (e.g., not when the patient is tired or upset)
- Look at the speaker with dysarthria
- Avoid talking when not in the same room
- Determine and use strategies for resolving communication breakdowns by the speaker with dysarthria (e.g., repeating misunderstood words, rephrasing, verbal spelling, writing)

What the speaker with dysarthria can do to aid comprehensibility is:

- Provide the listener with the context of the topic (e.g., through writing or spelling of the topic heading)
- Avoid shifting topics abruptly
- Choose proper turn-taking signals (e.g., eye gaze, a breathing pattern, a body movement, a gesture, verbal interjection)
- Get the listener's attention (e.g., saying listener's name)

- Use predictable wording and sentences (e.g., avoid unusual idioms, slang, and longer, grammatically complicated sentences)
- Accompany speech with simple gestures (e.g., use index finger to make a circle, use hand to indicate a traffic cop's stop signal)
- Avoid extended talking when not in same room as listener (e.g., use a buzzer or bell to get listener's attention)
- Have a handy backup system in case of difficulty (e.g., alphabet boards, pencil and paper)
- Use the previously mentioned repair strategies for resolving communication breakdowns

In light of the above suggestions, Garcia and Cannito (1996) found that when signal fidelity is poor, as with the speaker who has severe, flaccid dysarthria, differing combinations of signal-independent information (gestures, predictiveness of message content, relatedness of sentences to specific situational contexts, and prior familiarity with the speaker) may be employed to enhance listener understanding of the spoken message. Garcia, Cannito, and Dagenais (2000) reviewed the nature of hand gestures (gesticulations) in typical communicative interactions to examine their potential role as a compensatory communicative strategy in dysarthria rehabilitation. DePaul and Kent (2000) found that a highly familiar listener was superior to an unfamiliar listener in judging the severity and intelligibility of a speaker with progressive dysarthria.

Hustad and Cahill (2003) found that audiovisual information did not enhance intelligibility relative to audio-alone information for four of the five speakers with dysarthria. Those four speakers had a mild dysarthria. The one speaker whose intelligibility was enhanced by audiovisual information had severe dysarthria. All five speakers showed that with repeated speaker-specific familiarization, there was a significant improvement in intelligibility. Bunton, Kent, Duffy, Rosenbek, and Kent (2007) found that levels of listener agreement indicate that auditory-perceptual ratings show promise during clinical assessment for identifying salient features of dysarthria for speakers with various etiologies. Hustad (2008) found that listener comprehension of dysarthric speech is not based solely on intelligibility. For example, a speaker may sound very impaired and listeners may have difficulty in transcribing sentences produced by that speaker, but in situations in which contextual cues and world knowledge are available, the information-bearing capability (i.e., listener's ability to comprehend the message) of that same speech signal may be adequate for the exchange of meaning.

Advanced Study

Members of the ANCDS group studying dysarthria (Spencer, Yorkston, & Duffy, 2003, p. 40) described a flowchart that they hoped would help in clinical decision making. Management options were placed in the context of the support that might be available for these options. The evidence basis for support of a particular management technique came from published literature on intervention for dysarthria as well as from expert opinion. Assessment and management sections evaluated strategies related to respiratory and phonatory dysfunction, including decreased respiratory support, decreased respiratory-phonatory coordination and control, and reduced phonatory function.

Management of reduced function focused on improving respiratory support through nonspeech tasks, such as exercises to increase subglottal air pressure to support phonation. These exercises are unnecessary and inappropriate if the patient can perform speech exercises to reach goals of treatments (Spencer et al., 2003). Postural adjustments, especially for individuals in wheelchairs, can impact respiratory support for speech, but efficacy of treatment is not known at present. Such prosthetic assistance as abdominal binding or trussing may either support weak abdominal muscles and facilitate more efficient speech breathing or restrict inspiration and cause pneumonia. Medical supervision and approval are required before instituting strategies of prosthetic assistance. Targeting actual speech production to improve respiratory support focuses on modifying inhalation and exhalation patterns through instruction or biofeedback.

Improvement in coordination and control may similarly be addressed through nonspeech and speech tasks. One nonspeech task used for management of dysarthria in cerebral palsy is timing breathing to the beat of a metronome. Therapy with evidence-based support include breathing against resistance (such as a blow bottle), pushing and pulling exercises, and biofeedback of chest wall movement. There are no studies providing evidenced-based support for postural adjustments, and only one (abdominal trussing) for prosthetic assistance. There is also evidence-based support for biofeedback of targeted air pressure levels (Spencer et al., 2003, p. 51).

Evidence-based (EB) support for improving coordination and control of respiration and phonation is found only in the nonspeech and speech tasks that incorporate biofeedback therapy. EB support for improving phonatory function is found in the techniques of effort closure as well as Lee Silverman Voice Treatment, and the speech task of reducing tension through strategies such as easy onset of phonation. In some instances, the best intervention may be augmentative-alternative communication (AAC), which we describe in detail in the section on apraxia of speech.

CASE DESCRIPTION

One of the authors was waiting with HS behind a glass partition of a four-wall handball court at a local YMCA. HS described how his symptoms of Parkinson disease were reduced in the physical exertion of playing ball. While he had some relief of the classical triad of symptoms—tremor, rigidity, and bradykinesia—as a result of medication, HS and the author both noted rest tremors.

We followed HS over the years as his condition, unfortunately, worsened. He developed a waxy (shiny, yellowish) facial complexion, showed little change of expression, and evidenced almost no eye blinking. When HS tried to lift his feet off the floor or lift his hands up from his lap or from a table, he said it felt as if there were glue on the soles of his feet or the palms of his hands, and that they were stuck to the surfaces. His walking started with slow, small steps, and then accelerated. He eventually had to use a walker with bicycle-type hand brakes to help his shuffling feet stop, once he got moving; otherwise, he might not stop until he made contact with a wall.

HS was not deemed to be a candidate for deep brain stimulation, and the effectiveness of medication decreased. We visited him in his home, where he lived alone except for four hours of daily home attendant service. His articulation was characterized by a verbal form of the festination (palilalia) that we had observed in his gait, as well as reduced excursion of the articulators, which resulted in imprecise consonant formation and disfluency similar to stuttering. Breathing was shallow, with a poor shift from the vegetative pattern (slow inhalation through the nose, slightly longer exhalation, with a latency between respiratory cycles) to speech breathing (short, deep inhalation through the mouth, controlled exhalation with a checking action to modify airflow); it appeared that he attempted to speak while maintaining the vegetative breathing pattern. Vocal volume was reduced, and there was a lack of variety in pitch and volume. He did not respond well to a variation of Lee Silverman Voice Treatment (LSVT), claiming that the effort to "think loud" exhausted him. LSVT is the most thoroughly researched and statistically significantly effective treatment for hypokinetic dysarthria secondary to Parkinson disease. So why didn't it work better? The patient did not qualify for home-care SLP services, and received therapy only when one of the authors visited him. Success in LSVT is based on a 16-week treatment protocol, which was not followed. Finally, HS had few occasions to speak, and insisted that the listener, who felt fine, should be the one to make more of an effort.

Discussion Questions: Theory

1. Why might it be more appropriate to refer to "the dysarthrias" rather than dysarthria?

2. What is meant by an upper motor neuron impairment?

3. What is meant by a lower motor neuron impairment?

4. What are the types of mixed dysarthria?

5. What is the difference between intelligibility and comprehensibility?

Discussion Questions: Therapy

1. How does the SLP treat imprecise consonant formation?

2. How does the SLP treat hypernasality?

3. How does the SLP treat strain-strangled voice?

4. How does the SLP treat monopitch and monoloudness?

5. How does the SLP treat reduced excursion of the articulators?

Assignment: Write a multiple-choice question with five options. Explain why the key option is correct, and why the distractors or decoys are incorrect. Avoid using forms such as, "All of the following are (in)correct *except*" in the stem, and "All (or none) of the above" in the options.

Example: Which of the following characterizes dysarthria more than apraxia of speech?
  a. Substitution errors
  b. Inconsistent errrors
  c. Neurological evidence of slowness, weakness, incoordination, and alteration of tone
  d. Phonemic reapproaches and other self-correction efforts
  e. A planning or programming disorder

The correct answer is *c*: Dysarthria is caused by weakness or paralysis of the speech mechanism, due to brain damage. *a* is incorrect because dysarthric errors tend to be distortions or omissions; *b* is incorrect because dysarthric errors tend to be consistent; *d* and *e* are incorrect because individuals with dysarthria do not use phonemic reapproaches or other reprogramming strategies.

References

Ackerman, H., Hertrich, L., & Scharf, G. (1995). Kinemic analysis of lower lip movements in ataxic dysarthria. *Journal of Speech and Hearing Research, 38,* 1252–1259.

American Speech-Language-Hearing Association. (2001). Scope of practice in speech-language pathology. Retrieved from http://www.asha.org/docs/html/SP2007-00283.html.

American Speech-Language-Hearing Association. (2004). Preferred practice patterns for the profession of speech-language pathology. Retrieved from http://www.asha.org/docs/html/PP2004-00191.html.

Aronson, A. (1990). *Clinical voice disorders.* New York, NY: Thieme.

Aten, J. (1984). Treatment of spastic dysarthria. In W. Perkins (Ed.), *Dysarthria and apraxia* (pp. 69–77). New York, NY: Thieme-Stratton.

Baker, K., Ramig, L., Johnson, A., & Freed, C. (1997). Preliminary voice and speech analysis following fetal dopamine transplants in 5 individuals with Parkinson disease. *Journal of Speech-Language-Hearing Research, 40,* 615–626.

Barlow, S., & Abbs, J. (1983). Force transducers for the evaluation of labial, lingual, and mandibular motor impairments. *Journal of Speech and Hearing Research, 26,* 616–621.

Barlow, S., & Burton, M. (1990). Ramp-and-hold force control in the upper and lower lips: Developing new neuromotor assessment applications in traumatically brain injured adults. *Journal of Speech and Hearing Research, 33,* 660–675.

Barlow, S., Cole, K., & Abbs, J. (1983). A new head-mounted lip-jaw movement transduction system for the study of motor speech disorders. *Journal of Speech and Hearing Research, 26,* 283–288.

Bellaire, K., Yorkston, K., & Beukelman, D. (1986). Modification of breath patterning to increase naturalness of a mildly dysarthric speaker. *Journal of Communication Disorders, 19,* 271–280.

Bender, B., Cannito, M., Murry, T., & Woodson, G. (2004). Speech intelligibility in severe adductor spasmodic dysphonia. *Journal of Speech, Language, and Hearing Research, 47,* 21–32.

Berry, W. (1984). Treatment of hypokinetic dysarthria. In W. Perkins (Ed.), *Dysarthria and apraxia* (pp. 91–99). New York, NY: Thieme-Stratton.

Berry, W., Darley, F., Aronson, A., & Goldstein, N. (1974). Dysarthria in Wilson's disease. *Journal of Speech and Hearing Research, 17,* 169–183.

Beukelman, D. R., & Yorkston, K. M. (1980). Influence of passage familiarity on intelligibility estimates of dysarthric speech. *Journal of Communication Disorders, 13,* 33–41.

Binger, C., & Kent-Walsh, J. (2010). *What every speech-language pathologist/audiologist should know about augmentative and alternative communication.* Boston, MA: Pearson.

Boone, D., McFarlane, S., & Von Berg, S. (2005). *The voice and voice therapy.* Boston, MA: Allyn & Bacon.

Brand, H., Matsko, T., & Avart, H. (1988). Speech prosthesis retention problems in dysarthria. *Archives of Physical Medicine and Rehabilitation, 69,* 213–214.

Brookshire, R. (2007). *An introduction to neurogenic communication disorders* (7th ed.). St. Louis, MO: Mosby Yearbook.

Bunton, K., Kent, R., Duffy, J., Rosenbek, J., & Kent, J. (2007). Listener agreement for auditory-perceptual ratings of dysarthria. *Journal of Speech, Language, and Hearing Research, 50,* 1481–1495.

Bunton, K., & Weismer, G. (2001). The relationship between perception and acoustics for a high-low vowel contrast produced by speakers with dysarthria. *Journal of Speech, Language, and Hearing Research, 44,* 1215–1228.

Caligiuri, M. (1989). The influence of speaking rate on articulatory hypokinesia in Parkinsonian dysarthria. *Brain and Language, 36,* 493–502.

Canter, G., & Van Lancker, D. (1985). Disturbances of the temporal organization of speech following bilateral thalamic surgery in a patient with Parkinson's disease. *Journal of Communication Disorders, 18,* 329–349.

Caviness, J., Liss, J., Adler, C., & Evidente, V. (2006). Analysis of high-frequency electroencephalographic-electromyographic coherence elicited by speech and oral nonspeech tasks in Parkinson's disease. *Journal of Speech, Language, and Hearing Research, 49,* 424–438.

Chen, H., & Stevens, K. (2001). An acoustic study of the fricative /s/ in the speech of individuals with dysarthria. *Journal of Speech, Language, and Hearing Research, 44,* 1300–1314.

Cimino-Knight, A., & Sapienza, C. (2001). Consistency of voice produced by patients with adductor spasmodic dysphonia: A preliminary investigation. *Journal of Speech, Language, and Hearing Research, 44*, 793–802.

Countryman, S., Hicks, J., Ramig, L., & Smith, M. (1997). Supraglottal hyperadduction in an individual with Parkinson disease: A clinical treatment note. *American Journal of Speech-Language Pathology, 6*, 74–84.

Creech, R., Wertz, R., & Rosenbek, J. (1973). Oral sensation and perception in dysarthric adults. *Perceptual and Motor Skills, 37*, 167–172.

D'Alatri, L. Paludetti, G., Contarino, M. F., Galla, S., Marchese, M. R., & Bentivoglio, A. R. (2008). Effects of bilateral subthalamic nucleus stimulation and medication on Parkinsonian speech impairment. *Journal of Voice, 22*, 365–372.

Darby, J., Simmons, N., & Berger, P. (1984). Speech and voice parameters of depression: A pilot study. *Journal of Communication Disorders, 17*, 75–85.

Darkins, A., Fromkin, V., & Benson, D. (1988). A characterization of the prosodic loss in Parkinson's disease. *Brain and Language, 34*, 315–327.

Darley, F., Aronson, A., & Brown, J. (1969a). Clusters of deviant speech dimensions in the dysarthrias. *Journal of Speech and Hearing Research, 12*, 462–496.

Darley, F., Aronson, A., & Brown, J. (1969b). Differential diagnostic patterns of dysarthria. *Journal of Speech and Hearing Research, 12*, 246–269.

Darley, F., Aronson, A., & Brown, J. (1975). *Motor speech disorders*. Philadelphia, PA: Saunders.

Darley, F., Brown, J., & Goldstein, N. (1972). Dysarthria in multiple sclerosis. *Journal of Speech and Hearing Research, 15*, 229–245.

Day, L., & Parnell, M. (1987). Ten-year study of a Wilson's disease dysarthric. *Journal of Communication Disorders, 20*, 207–218.

DePaul, R., & Brooks, R. (1993). Multiple orofacial indices in amyotrophic lateral sclerosis. *Journal of Speech and Hearing Research, 36*, 1158–1167.

DePaul, R., & Kent, R. (2000). A longitudinal case study of ALS: Effects of listener familiarity and proficiency on intelligibility judgments. *American Journal of Speech-Language Pathology, 9*, 230–240.

Donovan, N. J., Kendall, D. L., Young, M. E., & Rosenbek, J. C. (2008). The communicative effectiveness survey: Preliminary evidence of construct validity. *American Journal of Speech-Language Pathology, 17*, 335–347.

Donovan, N. J., Velozo, C. A., & Rosenbek, J. C. (2007). The communicative effectiveness survey: Investigating item-level psychometric properties. *Journal of Medical Speech-Language Pathology, 15*, 433–447.

Dromey, C., Ramig, L., & Johnson, A. (1995). Phonatory and articulatory changes associated with increased vocal intensity in Parkinson disease: A case study. *Journal of Speech and Hearing Research, 38*, 751–764.

Duffy, J. R, (2005). *Motor speech disorders: Substrates, differential diagnosis, and management* (2nd ed.). St. Louis, MO: Elsevier Mosby.

Dworkin, J. (1991). *Motor speech disorders: A treatment guide*. St. Louis, MO: Mosby.

Dworkin, J., and Aronson, A. (1986). Tongue strength and alternate motion rates in normal and dysarthric subjects. *Journal of Communication Disorders, 19*, 115–132.

Dworkin, J., Aronson, A., & Mulder, D. (1980). Tongue force in normals and in dysarthric patients with amyotrophic lateral sclerosis. *Journal of Speech and Hearing Research, 23*, 828–837.

Dworkin J., & Culatta, R. (1980). *Dworkin-Culatta oral mechanism examination*. Vero Beach, FL: The Speech Bin.

Dykstra, A. D., Hakel, M. E., & Adams, S. G. (2007). Application of the ICF in reduced speech intelligibility in dysarthria. *Seminars in Speech and Language, 28*, 301–311.

Enderby, P. (1983). *Frenchay dysarthria assessment*. San Diego, CA: College Hill Press.

Farrell, A., Theodoros, D., Ward, E., Hall, B., & Silburn, P. (2005). Effects of neurosurgical management of Parkinson's disease on speech characteristics and oromotor function. *Journal of Speech, Language, and Hearing Research, 48*, 5–20.

Forrest, K., & Weismer, G. (1995). Dynamic aspects of lower lip movement in Parkinsonian and neurologically normal geriatric speakers' production of stress. *Journal of Speech and Hearing Research, 38*, 260–272.

Fox, C. (2002). Current perspectives on the Lee Silverman Voice Treatment (LSVT) for individuals with idiopathic Parkinson disease. *American Journal of Speech-Language Pathology, 11*, 111–123.

Fox, C., & Ramig, L. (1997). Vocal sound pressure level and self-perception of speech and voice in men and women with idiopathic Parkinson disease. *American Journal of Speech-Language Pathology, 6*, 85–94.

Fox, C. M., Ramig, L. O., Ciucci, M. R., Sapir, S., McFarland, D. H., & Farley, B. G. (2006). The science and practice of LSVT/LOUD: Neural plasticity-principled approach to treating individuals with Parkinson disease and other neurological disorders. *Seminars in Speech and Language, 27*, 283–299.

Freed, D. (2000). *Motor speech disorders: Diagnosis and treatment.* Clifton Park, NY: Delmar Cengage Learning.

Friedman, L. S., Farmer, J. M., Perlman, S., Wilmot, G., Gomez, C. M., Bushara, K. O., . . . Lynch, D. R. (2010). Measuring the rate of progression in Friedreich ataxia: Implications for clinical trial design. *Movement Disorders, 25*, 426–432.

Froeschels, E. (1952). Chiming method as therapy. *Archives of Otolaryngology, 56*, 427–434.

Froeschels, E., Kastein, S., & Weiss, D. (1955). A method of therapy for paralytic conditions of the mechanisms of phonation, respiration, and glutination. *Journal of Speech and Hearing Disorders, 20*, 365–370.

Gallena, S., Smith, P., Zeffiro, T., & Ludlow, C. (2001). Effects of levodopa on laryngeal muscle activity for voice onset and offset in Parkinson disease. *Journal of Speech, Language, and Hearing Research, 44*, 1284–1294.

Garcia, J., & Cannito, M. (1996). Influence of verbal and non-verbal contexts on the sentence intelligibility of a speaker with dysarthria. *Journal of Speech and Hearing Research, 39*, 750–760.

Garcia, J., Cannito, M., & Dagenais, P. (2000). Hand gestures: Perspectives and preliminary implications for adults with acquired dysarthria. *American Journal of Speech-Language Pathology, 9*, 107–115.

Garcia, J., & Dagenais, P. (1998). Dysarthric sentence intelligibility: Contribution of iconic gestures and message predictiveness. *Journal of Speech-Language-Hearing Research, 41*, 1282–1293.

Gentil, M. (1990). Dysarthria in Friedreich disease. *Brain and Language, 3*(8), 438–448.

Golper, L., Nutt, J., Rau, M., & Coleman, R. (1983). Focal cranial dystonia. *Journal of Speech and Hearing Disorders, 48*, 128–134.

Halpern, H., Hochberg, I., & Rees, N. (1967). Speech and hearing characteristics in familial dysautonomia. *Journal of Speech and Hearing Research, 10*, 361–366.

Hammarberg, B., Fritzell, B., & Schiratzki, H. (1984). Teflon injection in 16 patients with paralytic dysphonia: Perceptual and acoustic evaluation. *Journal of Speech and Hearing Disorders, 49*, 78–82.

Hammen, V., Yorkston, K., & Minifie, F. (1994). Effects of temporal alterations on speech intelligibility on Parkinsonian dysarthria. *Journal of Speech and Hearing Research, 37*, 244–253.

Hanson, E. K., & Beukelman, D. R. (2006). Effect of omitted cues on alphabet supplemented speech intelligibility. *Journal of Medical Speech-Language Pathology, 14*, 185–196.

Hanson, E. K., D. R. Beukelman, Heidemann, J. K., & Shutts-Johnson, E. (2010). The impact of alphabet supplementation and word prediction on sentence intelligiblity of electronically distorted speech. *Speech Communication, 52*, 99–105.

Hardy, J., Netsell, R., Schweiger, J., & Morris, H. (1969). Management of velopharyngeal dysfunction in cerebral palsy. *Journal of Speech and Hearing Disorders, 34*, 123–136.

Hartelius, L., Buder, E., & Strand, E. (1997). Long-term phonatory instability in individuals with multiple sclerosis. *Journal of Speech, Language, and Hearing Research, 40*, 1056–1072.

Hill, A., Theodoros, D., Russell, T., Cahill, L., Ward, E., & Clark, K. (2006). An interest-based telerehabilitation system for the assessment of motor speech disorders: A pilot study. *American Journal of Speech-Language Pathology, 15*, 45–56.

Hirose, H. (1986). Pathophysiology of motor speech disorders (dysarthria). *Folia Phoniatrica, 34*, 106–112.

Hirose, H., Kiritani, S., & Sawashima, M. (1982). Patterns of dysarthric movement in patients with amyotrophic lateral sclerosis and pseudo-bulbar palsy. *Folia Phoniatrica, 34*, 106–112.

Hirose, H., Kiritani, S., Ushijima, T., & Sawashima, M. (1978). Analysis of abnormal articulatory dynamics in two dysarthric patients. *Journal of Speech and Hearing Disorders, 43*, 96–105.

Hixon, T., & Hoit, J. (1998). Physical examination of the diaphragm by the speech-language pathologist. *American Journal of Speech-Language Pathology, 7*, 37–45.

Hixon, T., & Hoit, J. (1999). Physical examination of the abdominal wall by the speech-language pathologist. *American Journal of Speech-Language Pathology, 8*, 335–346.

Hixon, T., & Hoit, J. (2000). Physical examination of the rib cage wall by the speech-language pathologist. *American Journal of Speech-Language Pathology, 9*, 176–196.

Hixon, T., Putnam, A., & Sharp, J. (1983). Speech production with flaccid paralysis of the rib cage, diaphragm, and abdomen. *Journal of Speech and Hearing Disorders, 48*, 315–327.

Hoit, J., Banzett, R., Brown, R., & Loring, S. (1990). Speech breathing in individuals with cervical spinal cord injury. *Journal of Speech and Hearing Research, 33*, 798–807.

Hoodin, R., & Gilbert, H. (1989). Nasal airflow in Parkinsonian speakers. *Journal of Communication Disorders, 22*, 169–180.

Howell, S., Tripoliti, E., & Pring, T. (2009). Delivering the Lee Silverman Voice Treatment (LSVT) by Web camera: A feasibility study. *International Journal of Language & Communication Disorders, 44*, 287–300.

Huber, J., & Darling, M. (2011). Effect of Parkinson's disease on the production of structured and unstructured speaking tasks: Respiratory physiologic and linguistic considerations. *Journal of Speech, Language, and Hearing Research, 54*, 33–46.

Hustad, K. C. (2006a). A closer look at transcription intelligibility for speakers with dysarthria: Evaluation of scoring paradigms and linguistic errors made by listeners. *American Journal of Speech-Language Pathology, 15*, 268–277.

Hustad, K. C. (2006b). Estimating the intelligibility of speakers with dysarthria. *Folia Phoniatrica et Logopaedica, 58*, 217–228.

Hustad, K. C. (2006c). Influence of alphabet cues on listeners' ability to identify sound segments in sentences produced by speakers with moderate and severe dysarthria. *Journal of Medical Speech-Language Pathology, 14*, 249–252.

Hustad, K. (2007). Contribution of two sources of listener knowledge to intelligibility of speakers with cerebral palsy. *Journal of Speech, Language, and Hearing Research, 50*, 1228–1240.

Hustad, K. (2008). The relationship between listener comprehension and intelligibility scores for speakers with dysarthria. *Journal of Speech, Language, and Hearing Research, 51*, 562–573.

Hustad, K., & Beukelman, D. (2001). Effects of linguistic cues and stimulus cohesion on intelligibility of severely dysarthric speech. *Journal of Speech, Language, and Hearing Research, 44*, 497–510.

Hustad, K., & Beukelman, D. (2002). Listener comprehension of severely dysarthric speech: Effects of linguistic cues and stimulus cohesion. *Journal of Speech, Language, and Hearing Research, 45*, 545–558.

Hustad, K., & Cahill, M. (2003). Effects of presentation mode and repeated familiarization on intelligibility of dysarthric speech. *American Journal of Speech-Language Pathology, 12*, 198–208.

Hustad, K. C., Dardis, C. M., & McCourt, K. A. (2007). Effects of visual information on intelligibility of open and closed class words in predictable sentences produced by speakers with dysarthria. *Clinical Linguistics and Phonetics, 21*, 353–367.

Hustad, K., & Garcia, J. (2005). Aided and unaided speech supplementation strategies: Effect of alphabet cues and iconic hand gestures on dysarthric speech. *Journal of Speech, Language, and Hearing Research, 48*, 996–1012.

Hustad, K., & Gearhart, K. (2004). Listener attitudes toward individuals with cerebral palsy who use speech supplementation strategies. *America Journal of Speech-Language Pathology, 13*, 168–181.

Hustad, K., Jones, T., & Dailey, S. (2003). Implementing speech supplementation strategies: Effects on intelligibility and speech rate of individuals with chronic severe dysarthria. *Journal of Speech, Language, and Hearing Research, 46*, 462–474.

Kangas, K., & Lloyd, L. (2006). Augmentative and alternative communication. In N. Anderson & G. Shames, (Eds.), *Human communication disorders: An introduction* (pp. 436–470). Needham Heights, MA: Allyn & Bacon.

Keintz, C. K., Bunton, K., & Hoyt, J. D. (2007). Influence of visual information on the intelligibility of dysarthric speech. *American Journal of Speech-Language Pathology, 16*, 222–234.

Keith, R., & Thomas, J. (1989). *Speech practice manual for dysarthria, apraxia, and other disorders of articulation*. Philadelphia, PA: Decker.

Kent, R., Duffy, J., Slama, A., Kent, J., & Clift, A. (2001). Clinicoanatomic studies in dysarthria: Review, critique, and directions for research. *Journal of Speech, Language, and Hearing Research, 44,* 535–551.

Kent, R., Kent, J., Duffy, J., Thomas, T., Weismer, G., & Stuntebeck, J. (2002). Ataxic dysarthria. *Journal of Speech, Language, and Hearing Research, 43,* 1275–1289.

Kent, J., Kent, R., Rosenbek, J., Weismer, G., Martin, R., Sufit, R., & Brooks, B. (1992). Quantitative description of the dysarthria in women with amyotrophic lateral sclerosis. *Journal of Speech and Hearing Research, 35,* 723–733.

Kent, R., Kent, J., Weismer, G., Sufit, R., Rosenbek, J., Martin, R., & Brooks, B. (1990). Impairment of speech intelligibility in men with amyotrophic lateral sclerosis. *Journal of Speech and Hearing Disorders, 55,* 721–728.

Kent, R., & Netsell, R. (1978). Articulatory abnormalities in athetoid cerebral palsy. *Journal of Speech and Hearing Disorders, 43,* 353–373.

Kent, R., Sufit, R., Rosenbek, J., Kent, J., Weismer, G., Martin, R., & Brooks, B. (1991). Speech deterioration in amyotrophic lateral sclerosis: Case study. *Journal of Speech and Hearing Research, 34,* 1269–1275.

Kent, R., Vorperian, H., & Duffy, J. (1999). Reliability of the multidimensional voice program for the analysis of voice samples of subjects with dysarthria. *American Journal of Speech-Language Pathology, 8,* 129–136.

Kent, R., Weismer, G., Kent, J., & Rosenbek, J. (1989). Toward phonetic intelligibility testing in dysarthria. *Journal of Speech and Hearing Disorders, 54,* 482–499.

Kilpatrick, K., & Jones, C. (1977). *Therapy guide for language and speech disorders.* Akron, OH: Visiting Nurse Service.

Kim, Y., Kent, R., & Weismer, G. (2011). An acoustic study of the relationships among neurologic disease, dysarthria type, and severity of dysarthria. *Journal of Speech, Language, and Hearing Research, 54,* 417–429.

Kim, Y., Weismer, G., Kent, R. D., & Duffy, J. R. (2009). Statistical models of F2 slope in relation to severity of dysarthria. *Folia Phoniatrica et Logopaedica, 61,* 329–335.

Kiran, S., & Larson, C. (2001). Effect of duration of pitch-shifted feedback on vocal responses in patients with Parkinson's disease. *Journal of Speech, Language, and Hearing Research, 44,* 975–987.

Kleinow, J., Smith, A., & Ramig, L. (2001). Speech motor stability in IPD: Effects of rate and loudness manipulations. *Journal of Speech, Language, and Hearing Research, 44,* 1041–1051.

Koufman, J., & Block, C. (2008). Differential diagnosis of paradoxical vocal fold movement. *American Journal of Speech-Language Pathology, 17,* 327–334.

LaBlance, G., & Rutherford, D. (1991). Respiratory dynamics and speech intelligibility in speakers with generalized dystonia. *Journal of Communication Disorders, 24,* 141–156.

Langmore, S., & Lehman, M. (1994). Physiologic deficits in the orofacial system underlying dysarthria in amyotrophic lateral sclerosis. *Journal of Speech and Hearing Research, 37,* 28–37.

LaPointe, L., & Katz, R. (1998). Neurogenic disorders of speech. In G. Shames, E. Wiig, & W. Secord (Eds.), *Human communication disorders: An introduction* (pp. 434–471). Needham Heights, MA: Allyn & Bacon.

Lass, N., Ruscello, D., Harkins, K., & Blankenship, B. (1993). A comparative study of adolescents' perceptions of normal-speaking and dysarthric children. *Journal of Communication Disorders, 26,* 3–12.

Lass, N., Ruscello, D., & Lakawicz, J. (1988). Listeners' perceptions of non-speech characteristics of normal and dysarthric children. *Journal of Communication Disorders, 21,* 385–391.

LeDorze, G., Ouellet, L., & Ryalls, J. (1994). Intonation and speech rate in dysarthric speech. *Journal of Communication Disorders, 27,* 1–18.

Linebaugh, C. (1979). The dysarthrias of Shy-Drager syndrome. *Journal of Speech and Hearing Disorders, 44,* 55–60.

Linebaugh, C., & Wolfe, V. (1984). Relationships between articulation rate, intelligibility, and naturalness in spastic and ataxic speakers. In M. McNeil, J. Rosenbek, & A. Aronson (Eds.), *The dysarthrias: Physiology, acoustics, perception, management* (pp. 195–205). San Diego, CA: College Hill Press.

Liss, J., Krein-Jones, K., Wszolek, Z., & Caviness, J. (2006). Speech characteristics of patients with pallido-pontal-nigral degeneration and their application to presymptomatic detection in at-risk relatives. *American Journal of Speech-Language Pathology, 15,* 226–235.

Liss, J., LeGendre, S., & Lotto, A. (2010). Discriminating dysarthria type from envelope modulation spectra. *Journal of Speech, Language, and Hearing Research, 53*, 1246–1255.

Liss, J., White, L., Mattys, S., Lansford, K., Lotto, A., Spitzer, S., & Caviness, J. (2009). Quantifying speech rhythm abnormalities in the dysarthrias. *Journal of Speech, Language, and Hearing Research, 52*, 1334–1352.

Logemann, J., & Fisher, H. (1981). Vocal tract control in Parkinson's disease: Phonetic feature analysis of misarticulations. *Journal of Speech and Hearing Disorders, 46*, 348–352.

Logemann, J., Fisher, H., Boshes, B., & Blonsky, E. (1978). Frequency and cooccurrence of vocal tract dysfunctions in the speech of a large sample of Parkinson patients. *Journal of Speech and Hearing Disorders, 43*, 47–57.

Love, R., Hagerman, E., & Taimi, E. (1980). Speech performance, dysphagia and oral reflexes in cerebral palsy. *Journal of Speech and Hearing Disorders, 45*, 59–75.

Ludlow, C., Hoit, J., Kent, R., Ramig, L., Shrivastav, R., Strand, E., . . . Sapienza, C. (2008). Translating principles of neural plasticity into research on speech motor control recovery and rehabilitation. *Journal of Speech, Language, and Hearing Research, 51*, S240–S258.

Ma, J., Whitehill, T., & So, S. (2010). Intonation contrast in Cantonese speakers with hypokinetic dysarthria associated with Parkinson's disease. *Journal of Speech, Language, and Hearing Research, 53*, 836–849.

Maas, E., Robin, D., Austermann-Hula, S., Freedman, S., Wolf, G., Ballard, K., & Schmidt, R. (2008). Principles of motor learning in treatment of motor speech disorders. *American Journal of Speech-Language Pathology, 17*, 277–298.

MacPherson, M., Huber, J., & Snow, D. (2011). The intonation-syntax interface in the speech of individuals with Parkinson's disease. *Journal of Speech, Language, and Hearing Research, 54*, 19–32.

Marshall, R., & Karow, C. (2002). Retrospective examination of failed rate-control intervention. *American Journal of Speech-Language Pathology, 11*, 3–16.

Mathers-Schmidt, R. (2001). Paradoxical vocal fold motion: A tutorial on a complex disorder and the speech-language pathologist's role. *American Journal of Speech-Language Pathology, 10*, 111–125.

McCauley, R., Strand, E., Lof, G., Schooling, T., & Frymark, T. (2009). Evidence-based systematic review: Effects on nonspeech oral motor exercises on speech. *American Journal of Speech-Language Pathology, 18*, 343–360.

McHenry, M. (2003). The effect of spacing strategies on the variability of speech movement sequences in dysarthria. *Journal of Speech, Language, and Hearing Research, 46*, 702–710.

McHenry, M. A., & Liss, J. M. (2006). The impact of stimulated vocal loudness on nasalance in dysarthria. *Journal of Medical Speech-Language Pathology, 14*, 197–205.

McNamara, R. (1983). A conceptual holistic approach to dysarthria treatment. In W. Berry (Ed.), *Clinical dysarthria* (pp. 191–201). San Diego, CA: College Hill Press.

Mulligan, M., Carpenter, J., Riddel, J., Delaney, M., Badger, G., Krusinski, P., & Tandan, R. (1994). Intelligibility and the acoustic characteristics of speech in amyotrophic lateral sclerosis (ALS). *Journal of Speech and Hearing Research, 37*, 496–503.

Murdoch, B., Chenery, H., Stokes, P., & Hardcastle, W. (1991). Respiratory kinematics in speakers with cerebellar disease. *Journal of Speech and Hearing Research, 34*, 768–780.

Murray, L. (2000). Spoken language production in Huntington's and Parkinson's diseases. *Journal of Speech, Language, and Hearing Research, 43*, 1350–1366.

Murray, L., & Stout, J. (1999). Discourse comprehension in Huntington's and Parkinson's diseases. *American Journal of Speech-Language Pathology, 8*, 137–148.

Murry, T. (1978). Speaking fundamental frequency characteristics associated with voice pathologies. *Journal of Speech and Hearing Disorders, 43*, 374–379.

Murry, T. (1984). Treatment for ataxic dysarthria. In W. Perkins (Ed.), *Dysarthria and apraxia* (pp. 75–89). New York, NY: Thieme-Stratton.

Narayana, S., Jacks, A., Robin, D., Poizner, H., Zhang, W., Liotti, M., . . . Fox, P. (2009). A noninvasive imaging approach in understanding speech changes following deep brain stimulation in Parkinson's disease. *American Journal of Speech-Language Pathology, 18*, 146–161.

Natsopoulos, D., Katsarov, Z., Bostantzopoulou, S., Grovious, G., Mentenopoulos, G., & Logothetis, J. (1991). Strategies in comprehension of relative clauses by Parkinsonian patients. *Cortex, 27*, 255–268.

Neel, A. (2008). Effects of loud and amplified speech on sentence and word intelligibility in Parkinson disease. *Journal of Speech, Language, and Hearing Research, 52,* 1021–1033.

Neel, A. T., Palmer, P. M., Sprouls, G., & Morrison, L. (2006). Tongue strength and speech intelligibility in oculopharyngeal muscular dystrophy. *Journal of Medical Speech-Language Pathology, 14,* 273–277.

Nemec, R., & Cohen, K. (1984). EMG biofeedback in the modification of hypertonia in spastic dysarthria: Case report. *Archives of Physical Medicine and Rehabilitation, 65,* 103–104.

Netsell, R. (1984). A neurobiologic view of the dysarthrias. In M. McNeil, J. Rosenbek, & A. Aronson (Eds.), *The dysarthrias: Physiology, acoustics, perception, management* (pp. 1–36). San Diego, CA: College Hill Press.

Netsell, R. (1994). Instrumentation and special proceedings for individuals with dysarthria. *American Journal of Speech-Language Pathology, 3,* 9–11.

Netsell, R. (1995). Speech rehabilitation for individuals with unintelligible speech and dysarthria: The respiratory and velopharyngeal systems. *Neurophysiology and Neurogenic Speech and Language Disorders, 5*(4). (Special Interest Division 2 Newsletter, 6–9). Rockville, MD: American Speech-Language-Hearing Association.

Nishio, M., & Niimi, S. (2006). Comparison of speaking rate, articulation rate and alternating motion rate in dysarthric speakers. *Folia Phoniatrica et Logopaedica, 58,* 114–131.

O'Dwyer, N., Neilson, P., Guitar, B., Quinn, P., & Andrews, G. (1983). Control of upper airway structures during nonspeech tasks in normal and cerebral palsied subjects: EMG findings. *Journal of Speech and Hearing Research, 26,* 162–170.

Owens, R., & House, L. (1984). Decision-making processes in augmentative communication. *Journal of Speech and Hearing Disorders, 49,* 18–25.

Palmer, R., Enderby, P., & Hawley, M. (2007). Addressing the needs of speakers with long-standing dysarthria: computerized and traditional therapy compared. *International Journal of Language and Communication Disorders 42*(Suppl 1), 61–79.

Pannbacker, M. (2004). Velopharyngeal incompetence: The need for speech standards. *American Journal of Speech-Language Pathology, 13,* 195–201.

Paslawski, T., Duffy, J., & Vernino, S. (2005). Speech and language findings associated with paraneoplastic cerebellar degeneration. *American Journal of Speech-Language Pathology, 14,* 200–207.

Patel, R. (2002). Prosodic control in severe dysarthria: Preserved ability to mark the question–statement contrast. *Journal of Speech, Language, and Hearing Research, 45,* 858–870.

Patel, R. (2003). Acoustic characteristics of the question–statement contrast in severe dysarthria due to cerebral palsy. *Journal of Speech, Language, and Hearing Research, 46,* 1401–1415.

Patel, R., & Campellone, P. (2009). Acoustic and perceptual cues to contrastive stress in dysarthria. *Journal of Speech, Language, and Hearing Research, 52,* 206–222.

Portnoy, R. (1979). Hyperkinetic dysarthria as an early indicator of impending tardive dyskinesia. *Journal of Speech and Hearing Disorders, 44,* 214–219.

Portnoy, R., & Aronson, A. (1982). Diadochokinetic syllable rate and regularity in normal and in spastic and ataxic dysarthric subjects. *Journal of Speech and Hearing Disorders, 47,* 324–328.

Putnam, A., & Hixon, T. (1984). Respiratory kinematics in speakers with motor neuron disease. In M. McNeil, J. Rosenbek, & A. Aronson (Eds.), *The dysarthrias: Physiology, acoustics perception, management* (pp. 36–67). San Diego, CA: College Hill Press.

Ramig, L. (1995). Speech treatment for individuals with Parkinson disease. *Neurophysiology and Neurogenic Speech and Language Disorders, 5*(4). (Special Interest Division 2 Newsletter). Rockville, MD: American Speech-Language-Hearing Association.

Ramig, L., Countryman, S., Thompson, L., & Horii, Y. (1995). Comparison of two forms of intensive speech treatment for Parkinson disease. *Journal of Speech and Hearing Research, 38,* 1232–1251.

Ramig, L., & Dromey, C. (1996). Aerodynamic mechanisms underlying treatment related changes in vocal intensity in patients with Parkinson disease. *Journal of Speech and Hearing Research, 39,* 798–807.

Reich, A., and Lerman, J. (1978). Teflon laryngoplasty: An acoustical and perceptual study. *Journal of Speech and Hearing Disorders, 43,* 496–505.

Renout, K., Leeper, H., Bandur, D., & Hudson, A. (1995). Vocal fold diadochokinetic function of individuals with amyotrophic lateral sclerosis. *American Journal of Speech-Language Pathology,* 73–80.

Riddel, J., McCauley, R., Mulligan, M., & Tandan, R. (1995). Intelligibility and phonetic contrast errors in highly intelligible speakers with amyotrophic lateral sclerosis. *Journal of Speech and Hearing Research, 38,* 304–314.

Rosen, K. M., Goozee, J. V., & Murdoch, B. E. (2008). Examining the effects of multiple sclerosis on speech production: Does phonetic structure matter? *Journal of Communication Disorders, 41,* 49–69.

Rosen, K., Kent, R., Delaney, A., & Duffy, J. (2006). Parametric quantitative acoustic analysis of conversation produced by speakers with dysarthria and healthy speakers. *Journal of Speech, Language, and Hearing Research, 49,* 395–411.

Rosenbek, J. (1985). Treating apraxia of speech. In D. Johns (Ed.), *Clinical management of neurogenic communicative disorders* (pp. 267–312). Boston, MA: Little, Brown.

Rosenbek, J., & LaPointe, L. (1985). The dysarthrias: Description, diagnosis, and treatment. In D. Johns (Ed.), *Clinical management of neurogenic communicative disorders* (pp. 97–152). Boston, MA: Little, Brown.

Roy, N., Leeper, H., Blomgren, M., & Cameron, R. (2001). A description of phonetic, acoustic, and physiological changes associated with improved intelligibility in a speaker with spastic dysarthria. *American Journal of Speech-Language Pathology, 10,* 274–290.

Rubow, R., Rosenbek, J., Collins, M., & Celesia, G. (1984). Reduction of hemifacial spasm and dysarthria following EMG biofeedback. *Journal of Speech and Hearing Disorders, 49,* 26–33.

Samlan R., & Weismer, G. (1995). The relationship of selected perceptual measures of diadochokinesis to speech intelligibility in dysarthric speakers with amyotrophic lateral sclerosis. *American Journal of Speech-Language Pathology, 4,* 9–13.

Sapir, S., Ramig, L. O., Spielman, J. L., & Fox, C. (2010). Formant centralization ratio: A proposal for a new acoustic measure of dysarthric speech. *Journal of Speech, Language, and Hearing Research, 53,* 114–125.

Sapir, S., Spielman, J., Ramig, L., Hinds, S., Countryman, S., Fox, C., & Story, B. (2003). Effects of intensive voice treatment (the Lee Silverman Voice Treatment [LSVT]) on ataxic dysarthria: A case study. *American Journal of Speech-Language Pathology, 12,* 387–399.

Sapir, S., Spielman, J., Ramig, L., Story, B., & Fox, C. (2007). Effects of intensive voice treatment (the Lee Silverman Voice Treatment [LSVT]) on vowel articulation in dysarthric individuals with idiopathic Parkinson disease: Acoustic and perceptual findings. *Journal of Speech, Language, and Hearing Research, 50,* 899–912.

Schulz, G., Dingwall, W., & Ludlow, C. (1999). Speech and oral motor learning in individuals with cerebellar atrophy. *Journal of Speech, Language, and Hearing Research, 42,* 1157–1175.

Schulz, G., Peterson, T., Sapienza, C., Greer, M., & Friedman, W. (1999). Voice and speech characteristics of persons with Parkinson's disease pre- and post-pallidotomy surgery: Preliminary findings. *Journal of Speech, Language, and Hearing Research, 42,* 1176–1194.

Shane, H., & Bashir, A. (1980). Election criterion for the adoption of an augmentative communication system, preliminary considerations. *Journal of Speech and Hearing Research, 45,* 408–414.

Shane, H., & Sauer, M. (1986). *Augmentative and alternative communication.* Austin, TX: Pro-Ed.

Shaughnessy, A., Netsell, R., & Farrage, J. (1983). Treatment of a four-year-old with a palatal lift prosthesis. In W. Berry (Ed.), *Clinical dysarthria* (pp. 217–230). San Diego, CA: College Hill Press.

Sheard, C., Adams, R., & Davis, P. (1991). Reliability and agreement of ratings of ataxic dysarthric speech samples with varying intelligibility. *Journal of Speech and Hearing Research, 34,* 285–293.

Silverman, F. (1989). *Communication for the speechless.* Englewood Cliffs, NJ: Prentice-Hall.

Simmons, N. (1983). Acoustic analysis of ataxic dysarthria: An approach to monitoring treatment. In W. Berry (Ed.), *Clinical dysarthria* (pp. 283–294). San Diego, CA: College Hill Press.

Simpson, M., Till, J., & Goff, A. (1988). Long-term treatment of severe dysarthria. *Journal of Speech and Hearing Disorders, 53,* 433–440.

Singh, A., Epstein, E., Myers, L. M., Farmer, J. M., & Lynch, D. R. (2010). Clinical measures of dysarthria in Friedreich ataxia. *Movement Disorders, 25,* 108–111.

Solomon, N., & Hixon, T. (1993). Speech breathing in Parkinson's disease. *Journal of Speech and Hearing Research, 36,* 294–310.

Solomon, N., McKee, A., & Garcia-Barry, S. (2001). Intensive voice treatment and respiration treatment for hypokinetic-spastic dysarthria after traumatic brain injury. *American Journal of Speech-Language Pathology, 10,* 51–64.

Solomon, N., McKee, A., Larson, K., Nawrocki, M., Tuite, R., Eriksen, S., . . . Maxwell, R. (2000). Effects of pallidal stimulation on speech in three men with severe Parkinson's disease. *American Journal of Speech-Language Pathology, 9,* 241–256.

Solomon, N., Robin, D., & Luschei, E. (2000). Strength, endurance, and stability of the tongue and hand in Parkinson disease. *Journal of Speech, Language, and Hearing Research, 43,* 256–267.

Solomon, N., & Stierwalt, J. (1995). Strength and endurance training for dysarthria. *Neurophysiology and Neurogenic Speech and Language Disorders, 5*(4). (Special Interest Division 2 Newsletter, 13–16). Rockville, MD: American Speech-Language-Hearing Association.

Spencer, K. A., Yorkston, K. M., & Duffy, J. R. (2003). Behavioral management of respiratory/phonatory dysfunction from dysarthria: A flowchart for guidance in clinical decision making. *Journal of Medical Speech-Language Pathology, 11,* 39–61.

Spielman, J., Ramig, L., Maher, L., Halper, A., & Gavin, W. (2007). Effects of an extended version of the Lee Silverman Voice Treatment on voice and speech in Parkinson's disease. *American Journal of Speech-Language Pathology, 16,* 95–107.

St. Louis, K., & Ruscello, D. (1987). *Oral speech mechanism screening examination* (rev. ed.). Austin, TX: Pro-Ed.

Tikofsky, R., & Tikofsky, R. (1964). Intelligibility measures of dysarthric speech. *Journal of Speech and Hearing Research, 7,* 325–333.

Tjaden, K. (2000). A preliminary study of factors influencing perception of articulatory rate in Parkinson disease. *Journal of Speech, Language, and Hearing Research, 43,* 997–1010.

Tjaden, K. (2003). Anticipatory coarticulation in multiple sclerosis and Parkinsin's disease. *Journal of Speech, Language, and Hearing Research, 46,* 554–566.

Tjaden, K., Rivera, D., Wilding, G. E., & Turner, G. (2005). Characteristics of the lax vowel space in dysarthria. *Journal of Speech, Language, and Hearing Research, 48,* 554–566.

Tjaden, K., & Wilding, G. (2004). Effect of rate production and increased loudness on acoustic measures of anticipatory measures of coarticulation in multiple sclerosis and Parkinson's disease. *Journal of Speech, Language, and Hearing Research, 48,* 261–277.

Turner, G., Tjaden, K., & Weismer, G. (1995). The influence of speaking rate on vowel and speech intelligibility for individuals with amyotrophic lateral sclerosis. *Journal of Speech and Hearing Research, 38,* 1001–1013.

Turner, G., & Weismer, G. (1993). Characteristics of speaking rate in the dysarthria associated with amyotrophic lateral sclerosis. *Journal of Speech and Hearing Research, 36,* 1134–1144.

Van Lancker Sidtis, D., Rogers, T., Codier, V., Tagliati, M., & Sidtis, J. (2010). Voice and fluency changes as a function of speech task and deep brain stimulation. *Journal of Speech, Language, and Hearing Research, 53,* 1167–1177.

Van Nuffelen, G., De Bodt, M., Vanderwegen, J., Van de Heyning, P., & Wuytsm F. (2010). Effect of rate control on speech production and intelligibility in dysarthria. *Folia Phoniatrica et Logopaedica, 62,* 110–119.

Van Nuffelen, G., De Bodt, M., Wuyts, F., & Van de Heyning, P. (2009). The effect of rate control on speech rate and intelligibility of dysarthric speech. *Folia Phoniatrica et Logopaedica, 61,* 69–75.

Walker, H., Phillips, D., Boswell, D., Guthrie, B., Guthrie, S., Nicholas, A., . . . Watts, R. (2009). Relief of acquired stuttering associated with Parkinson's disease by unilateral left subthalamic brain stimulation. *Journal of Speech, Language, and Hearing Research, 52,* 1652–1657.

Walsh, B., & Smith, A. (2011). Linguistic complexity, speech production, and comprehension in Parkinson's disease: Behavioral and physiological indices. *Journal of Speech, Language, and Hearing Research, 54,* 787–802.

Wang, Y-T., Kent, R. D., Duffy, J. R., & Thomas, J. E. (2009a). Analysis of diadochokinesis in ataxic dysarthria using the motor speech profile program. *Folia Phoniatrica et Logopaedica, 61,* 1–11.

Wang, Y-T., Kent, R. D., Kent, J. F., Duffy, J. R., & Thomas, J. E. (2009b). Acoustic analysis of voice in dysarthria following stroke. *Clinical Linguistics and Phonetics, 23,* 335–347.

Watson, P., & Hixon, T. (2001). Effects of abdominal trussing on breathing and speech in men with cervical spinal cord injury. *Journal of Speech, Language, and Hearing Research, 44,* 751–762.

Watterson, T., MacFarlane, S., & Menicucci, A. (1990). Vibratory characteristics of Teflon-injected and noninjected paralyzed vocal folds. *Journal of Speech and Hearing Disorders, 55*, 61–66.

Weismer, G. (2006). Philosophy of research in motor speech disorders. *Clinical Linguistics and Phonetics, 20*, 315–349.

Wit, J., Maassen, B., Gabreels, F., & Thoonen, G. (1993). Maximum performance tests in children with developmental spastic dysarthria. *Journal of Speech and Hearing Research, 36*, 452–459.

Wood, L., Hughes, J., Hayes, K., & Wolfe, D. (1992). Reliability of labial closure force measurements in normal subjects and patients with CNS disorders. *Journal of Speech and Hearing Research, 25*, 252–258.

World Health Organization. (2001). *International classification of functioning, disability and health.* Geneva, Switzerland: Author.

Yorkston, K. (1996). Treatment efficacy: Dysarthria. *Journal of Speech and Hearing Research, 39*, S46–S57.

Yorkston, K. M. (2007). The degenerative dysarthrias: A window into critical clinical and research issues. *Folia Phoniatrica et Logopaedica, 59*, 107–117.

Yorkston, K., & Beukelman, D. (1980a). An analysis of connected speech samples of aphasic and normal speakers. *Journal of Speech and Hearing Disorders, 45*, 27–36.

Yorkston, K., & Beukelman, D. (1980b). A clinician-judged technique for quantifying dysarthric speech based on single-word intelligibility. *Journal of Communication Disorders, 13*, 15–31.

Yorkston, K., & Beukelman, D. (1981a). *Assessment of intelligibility of dysarthric speech.* Tigard, OR: CC Publications.

Yorkston, K., & Beukelman, D. (1981b). Communication efficiency of dysarthric speakers as measured by sentence intelligibility and speaking rate. *Journal of Speech and Hearing Disorders, 46*, 296–301.

Yorkston, K., & Beukelman, D. (1983). The influence of judge familiarization with the speaker on dysarthric speech intelligibility. In W. Berry (Ed.), *Clinical dysarthria* (pp. 153–163). San Diego, CA: College Hill Press.

Yorkston, K., Beukelman, D., & Bell, K. (1988). *Clinical management of dysarthric speakers.* San Diego, CA: College Hill Press.

Yorkston, K., Beukelman, D., & Honsinger, M. (1989). Perceived articulatory adequacy and velopharyngeal function in dysarthric speakers. *Archives of Physical Medicine and Rehabilitation, 70*, 313–317.

Yorkston, K. M., Hakel, M., Beukelman, D. R., & Fager, S. (2007). Evidence for effectiveness of treatment of loudness, rate, or prosody in dysarthria: A systematic review. *Journal of Medical Speech-Language Pathology, 15*, 11–36.

Yorkston, K., Hammen, V., Beukelman, D., & Traynor, C. (1990). The effect of rate control on the intelligibility and naturalness of dysarthric speech. *Journal of Speech and Hearing Disorders, 55*, 550–560.

Yorkston, K., Klasner, E., & Swanson, K. (2001). Communication in context: A qualitative study of the experiences of individuals with multiple sclerosis. *American Journal of Speech-Language Pathology, 10*, 126–137.

Yorkston, K., Strand, E., & Kennedy, M. (1996). Comprehensibility of dysarthric speech: Implications for assessment and treatment planning. *American Journal of Speech-Language Pathology, 5*, 55–66.

Yunusova, Y., Weismer, G., Westbury, J., & Lindstrom, M. (2008). Articulatory movements during vowels in speakers with dysarthria and healthy controls. *Journal of Speech, Language, and Hearing Research, 51*, 591–611.

Ziegler, W., & Zierdt, A. (2008). Telediagnostic assessment of intelligibility in dysarthria: A pilot investigation of MVP-online. *Journal of Communication Disorders, 41*, 553–577.

Ziegler, W., Hartmann, E., & Hoople, P. (1993). Syllabic timing in dysarthria. *Journal of Speech and Hearing Research, 36*, 683–693.

Ziegler, W., & von Cramon, D. (1986). Spastic dysarthria after acquired brain injury: An acoustic study. *British Journal of Disorders of Communication, 21*, 173–187.

Apraxia of Speech

Definition

Apraxia of speech (AOS) is an articulation and prosody disorder that results from impairment, due to brain damage, of the capacity to order the positioning of the speech musculature and the sequencing of muscle movements for volitional production of phonemes and sequences of phonemes. It is not accompanied by significant weakness, slowness, or incoordination of these same muscles in reflex and automatic acts (Darley, 1964; Johns & Darley, 1970). If we eliminate the phrase "due to brain damage," and substitute the word *stuttering* for *apraxia of speech*, we have a pretty serviceable definition of stuttering (Goldfarb, 2006, p. 128).

Site of lesion following stroke is often observed to be in the left superior precentral gyrus of the insula (SPGI). However, there may be additional involvement of neighboring brain areas in more severe forms of AOS as well as in language deficits, such as aphasia (Ogar et al., 2006). According to Hillis et al. (2004), structural damage or low blood flow in the left posterior inferior frontal gyrus may result in poor drainage into the anterior insula. Reperfusion of the anterior insula will not relieve symptoms of apraxia of speech, which the authors describe as a motor programming speech disorder associated with left frontal lobe damage.

Theories of Phonetic Encoding

Speech output may be seen to be a result of putting together syllables or phrases segment by segment. AOS occurs when there is a disruption of these segmental routines. Ziegler, Thelen, Staiger, and Liepold (2008) found that error rate in AOS was influenced by the complexity of syllable constituents and the number of metrical feet in a word. Alternatively, Varley, Whiteside, Windsor, and Fisher (2004) proposed that the disorder stems from a failure to activate stored phonetic plans for words and utterances. An individual with AOS encodes speech by combining residual word plans with compensatory mechanisms, such as changing the code from auditory word representations to phonetic output. The authors considered direct and indirect encoding strategies, or a dual-route theory of speech control. The direct route would entail using stored phonetic plans, while the indirect route would use various assembly mechanisms.

There are also two ways of looking at the notion of stored phonetic plans. In one, the size of the stored phonetic plan corresponds directly to the number of syllables. In the other, frequency of usage is the determining factor of speech encoding, regardless of the size of the high frequency unit. According to the frequency of usage argument, movement sequences become chained together if they co-occur with some frequency. Whether the sequence is short, as in "Hi," or a bit longer, as in "How are you?" or even longer, as in "Have a nice day," the chains are produced with a stored phonetic plan of equal difficulty for the individual with AOS.

Conceptual-Programming Level of Motor Organization for Speech

The attempt to retrieve a word may activate associated areas that are responsible for motor planning. The articulatory-kinematic approaches usually followed in treating apraxia of speech require phoneme manipulation that may activate motor planning. If apraxia of speech results from a reduction of efficiency in making the transition from phonological plans to motor plans, then practice should involve both a plan for phoneme manipulation and self-monitoring of that plan. Recall that self-monitoring is a prerequisite for self-correction. Even repeated implicit practice of retrieving and internally monitoring sounds, such as thinking about rhymes and alliterations, may improve efficiency of transition from phonological plan to initial phase of motor planning to monitoring of that plan, as Davis, Farias, and Baynes (2009) showed in a single-subject multiple baseline study.

Apraxia of speech has been described by Darley, Aronson, and Brown (1975) as a planning or programming disorder that fits into a five-stage, conceptual-programming level of motor organization for speech.

The *first stage* is conceptualization, involving a desire to do something and establishing a plan of action to carry out that desire (e.g., thinking about calling a friend on the phone). In this stage, cortical activity is probably bilateral and widespread, and if interfered with can result, for example, in a cognitive thought disorder called *dementia*.

The *second stage* is spatial-temporal (linguistic planning), involving language (e.g., planning what one will say on the phone). In this stage, cortical activity for linguistic processes is located in the left hemisphere for the great majority of people, and if interfered with can result in aphasia.

The *third stage* is motor planning (programming), which is the bridge between the language formulation and the motor execution stage of the neuromuscular system (e.g., talking on the phone). This stage is responsible for connecting the inner language processes into the endless number of speech utterances. It has been surmised that about 100 different muscles, each containing about 100 motor units, are involved in speaking for 1 second.

If an individual averages about 14 phonemes per second, then there are 140,000 neuromuscular events for 1 second of speech. Because of the complexity and the almost instantaneous speed and timing of those movements needed for speech, it is postulated that these movements have been stored in the brain (preprogrammed), ready to be activated immediately.

The storage of these movements starts in early childhood, and their individual strength is determined by the frequency of usage over a lifetime of speaking. For example, the authors have heard a majority of patients say, "He could never make up his *filthy* mind" instead of the correct version, "He could never make up his *flighty* mind," when reading aloud the phonetically balanced passage called "Arthur the Young Rat." Apparently, "filthy mind" has been used more often (strong storage) than "flighty mind" (weaker storage).

In this stage, brain activity for motor planning is located for the great majority of people in the left hemisphere, involving Broca's area and its connections to the language portions of the temporal and parietal lobes, primary motor cortex (frontal lobe), supplementary motor area (frontal lobe), somatosensory cortex (parietal lobe), supramarginal gyrus (parietal lobe), and insula. If this stage is interfered with, the result can be apraxia of speech.

The *fourth stage* is performance, which is the motor execution portion of the neuromuscular system involved in speaking (e.g., talking on the phone). The brain activity is bilateral and involves activation pathways, the control circuits, the final common pathway, feedback from sensory pathways, and continuous commands from the motor speech programmer. If this stage is interfered with, it can result in dysarthria.

The *fifth stage* is feedback, which provides sensory information about ongoing and completed motor speech movements. The modification of presently occurring and future motor speech movements is based upon this sensory information (e.g., getting a shot of Novocaine and compensating for the numbness in your lip and/or tongue in order to speak). The brain activity may occur at the spinal and brainstem level, in the cerebellum, thalamus, basal ganglia, and cortex. If this stage is interfered with, the result can be dysarthria.

Symptoms

Apraxia of speech can affect timing, rate, or range of movement of the articulators, and selection of articulatory contact points along the vocal tract. Salient features include disturbed articulation (inconsistent trial-and-error misarticulations) and prosody (hesitations, slowness, groping, difficulty initiating speech, dysprosody) with pockets of correct speech. Most often, patients are aware of their errors and can become frustrated when they cannot correct themselves. This disorder can resemble the oral expressive language behavior of the patient with aphasia. For example, the phonemic groping of the patient with apraxia can resemble the word-finding difficulty of the patient with aphasia. Apraxia of speech can stand alone as a condition, coexist with aphasia, coexist with dysarthria, or coexist with aphasia and dysarthria.

Table 9.1 is an example of a patient with apraxia of speech repeating words, phrases, and sentences first spoken by the clinician (one of the authors).

TABLE 9.1

Patient with Apraxia of Speech Repeating Words, Phrases, and Sentences

Clinician	Patient
Snowman	Snugman-<u>smug</u>-snowman
Gingerbread	gingerbed
Impossibility	in-impossibility
Please sit down	Please sit down
Seventeen seventy-six	s<u>e</u>nerteen senerty-six-severteen seventy-six
Columbia Presbyterian Hospital	Columbia Pesbyterian Hostiple-Columbian Pres terian Host
Methodist Episcopal Church	Metho<u>diss</u> Epu<u>sle</u> Church-Methodist Episical Church
Will you answer the telephone?	Willee lloo lansit luh teleson-Will<u>ee</u> lloo lansit luh teletone?
No ifs, ands, or buts	No iss and or buts – No <u>its</u> and of buts
He lives in the third house from the corner.	He'd lived in the <u>t</u>ird ouse <u>f</u>om duh torner.

The following studies describe the symptoms of apraxia of speech. Many of the studies cited come from the review by Darley (1982), supplemented by the other literature listed.

1. Articulatory errors increase as the complexity of motor adjustment required of the articulators increases.
   A. Vowels evoke fewer errors than singleton consonants (Wertz, LaPointe, & Rosenbek, 1984). Odell, McNeil, Rosenbek, and Hunter (1991) found that no differences existed in number of errors between vowels and consonants among speakers with apraxia of speech. Jacks, Mathes, and Marquardt (2010) found that vowel production at the word level is unimpaired in speakers with AOS, supporting the previous studies that have shown vowel production is relatively intact in AOS.
   B. Of the singleton consonants, affricative and fricative phonemes evoke the most errors (Wertz et al., 1984).
   C. Most difficult of all are consonant clusters (Burns & Canter, 1977; Deal & Darley, 1972; Dunlop & Marquardt, 1977; Johns & Darley, 1970; LaPointe & Johns, 1975; Shankweiler & Harris, 1966; Trost & Canter, 1974; Wertz et al., 1984).
   D. Palatal and dental phonemes are significantly more susceptible to error than other phonemes classified according to place of articulation (LaPointe & Johns, 1975).
   E. In manner of articulation, fricatives and affricatives are least retained (Klich, Ireland, & Weidner, 1979).
   F. Repetition of a single consonant such as /puh/, /tuh/, or /kuh/ is ordinarily accomplished more easily than repetition of the sequence /puh-tuh-kuh/ (Rosenbek, Wertz, & Darley, 1973). In the latter task the patient is typically unable to maintain the correct sequence, even when he or she is repeatedly given a model to imitate.
   G. Klich et al. (1979), Marquardt, Reinhart, and Peterson (1979), and Wolk (1986) noted that patients with apraxia made a systematic effort to reduce the articulatory complexity in the production of consonants. Keller (1984) also found that patients with apraxia tended to reduce the proportion of phoneme sequences (e.g., consonant clusters and diphthongs) and to increase the proportion of single consonants and single vowels in their speech.
   H. Wertz et al. (1984) noted that a given sound can be correct in one position in a word but incorrect in another. They also noted that the production of easier consonants in place of more difficult ones is highly variable.
2. Position of phoneme within the word has an effect on articulatory errors.
   A. Consonants. Initial consonants tend to be misarticulated more often than consonants in other positions (Hecaen, 1972; Shankweiler & Harris, 1966; Trost & Canter, 1974). Burns and Canter (1977) found that five patients with conduction aphasia and five with Wernicke's aphasia (mostly with posterior lesions) made what the authors called "phonemic paraphasic errors" more frequently in the final than in the initial position of words.

   However, Johns and Darley (1970) reported that no single position in the word emerged as characteristically more difficult. LaPointe and Johns (1975) found error percentages for initial, medial, and final positions to be nearly equal, and Dunlop and Marquardt (1977) found phonemic position unrelated to occurrence of error. Klich et al. (1979) found that more substitutions were made in the initial word position. Wertz et al. (1984) concluded that sound position in a word may or may not have an influence on whether it will be produced accurately. Odell, McNeil, Rosenbek, and Hunter (1990) found that in consonant production by adults with apraxia of speech, most errors occurred in the medial position of words.

B. Vowels. In a follow-up study, Odell et al. (1991) found that in vowel production by adults with apraxia of speech, most errors occurred in the initial position of words.

3. On repeated readings of the same material, adults with apraxia of speech demonstrate a consistency effect, tending to make errors at the same loci from trial to trial; they also demonstrate some adaptation effect, tending to make fewer errors in successive readings (Deal, 1974). The amount of reduction of errors is not great, varying from subject to subject.

4. Phonemes occurring with relatively high gauge tend to be more accurately articulated than phonemes occurring less frequently (Trost & Canter, 1974; Wertz et al., 1984). These effects occur not only in single words, but also in spontaneous speech. For example, Staiger and Ziegler (2008) compared phoneme errors in the spontaneous speech (minimum of 1000 syllables spoken) of 3 adults with apraxia of speech and 15 neurotypical controls, and found that syllable frequency and syllable structure play a decisive role with respect to articulatory accuracy. In all 3 patients the proportion of errors was significantly higher on low- than on high-frequency syllables. However, syllable structure effects were found only for the low-frequency syllables in the spontaneous speech production of patients with AOS. Independently, Laganaro (2008) found a significant effect of syllable frequency in a participant with AOS and in a participant with conduction aphasia.

5. Numerous phonemic errors occur, including substitutions, omissions, additions, repetitions, and distortions, with a predominance of substitutions (Johns & Darley, 1970; LaPointe & Johns, 1975; LaPointe & Wertz, 1974; Trost, 1970; Wertz et al., 1984). Analysis of substitution errors made by adults with apraxia of speech, according to the system of distinctive features, indicates that the errors are variably related to the target sounds. In their review of the literature, Wertz et al. (1984) conclude that generally, "apraxic patients are in the ballpark, most of the time. One or two phonetic feature errors predominate" (pp. 53–57).

Wertz et al. (1984) further concluded that adults with apraxia of speech generally "make more substitutions of voiceless consonants for voiced ones rather than the opposite" (p. 57). However, Skenes and Trullinger (1988) found that speakers with apraxia made more errors on voiced than on voiceless consonants in tasks involving repetition of consonant-vowel-consonant. Odell et al. (1990) observed that distortion errors predominated in consonant production, and Odell et al. (1991) found that distortion errors predominated in the vowel production of speakers with apraxia.

6. When errors made by adults with apraxia of speech are analyzed with regard to sequential aspects, three types of errors are observed: anticipatory (prepositioning), reiterative (postpositioning), and metathesis (the order of two phonemes being reversed) (LaPointe & Johns, 1975). Wertz et al. (1984) noted that some patients display all three kinds of errors, with the anticipatory being the most frequent. However, all types of errors did not abound.

7. Adults with apraxia of speech display a marked discrepancy between their relatively good performance on automatic and reactive speech productions and their relatively poor volitional-purposive speech performance. "Words and phrases highly organized by practice and usage tend to sound normal" (Schuell, Jenkins, & Jimenez-Pabon, 1964, p. 265). Such islands of fluent, well-articulated speech appear in conversation, punctuated by episodes of effortful, off-target groping (LaPointe & Wertz, 1974; Wertz et al., 1984).

8. Imitative responses tend to be characterized by more articulatory errors than spontaneous speech production. This holds true for single monosyllabic words as well as for

material of greater length and complexity. Some patients display remarkably long latencies between the presentation of a stimulus word and their repetition of it (Johns & Darley, 1970; Schuell et al., 1964; Trost, 1970). On the other hand, Wertz et al. (1984) found imitation to be better than spontaneous speech.

9. Articulation errors increase as length of words increases (Deal & Darley, 1972; DiSimoni & Darley, 1977; Wertz et al., 1984). As the patient produces a series of words with increasing numbers of syllables (e.g., door, doorknob, doorkeeper, dormitory), more errors are noted in all longer words. Such errors typically occur in the syllable common to all of the words, not just in the added syllables (Johns & Darley, 1970).

   Odell et al. (1990) found no difference in the number of errors between consonant production of monosyllabic and polysyllabic words; Odell et al. (1991) found more errors in vowel production of monosyllabic than of polysyllabic words in apraxic speakers.

10. In oral reading of contextual material, articulatory errors do not occur at random; they are more frequent on words that carry linguistic or psychologic "weight" and that are more essential for communication (Deal & Darley, 1972; Hardison, Marquardt, and Peterson, 1977). The combination of word length and grammatical class is an especially important determinant of the loci of errors. The difficulty level of initial phonemes also has a particularly negative effect on articulatory accuracy, when combined with grammatical class.

   Grammatical class alone has not been found to be significantly related to occurrence of error (Deal & Darley, 1972; Dunlop & Marquardt, 1977; Wertz et al., 1984). Strand and McNeil (1996) observed that five adults with apraxia of speech consistently produced longer vowel and between-word segment durations in sentence contexts than in word contexts. In general, when the complexity of a required response is increased, more errors occur. Any single characteristic may be insufficient to elicit error, but if characteristics are combined, their joint effect may be powerful enough to induce inaccuracies.

11. Correctness of articulation is influenced by mode of stimulus presentation (Johns & Darley, 1970; Trost & Canter, 1974). Patients tend to articulate more accurately when speech stimuli are presented by a visible examiner (auditory-visual mode) than when they are presented by tape recorder (auditory mode) or printed on a card (visual mode). Wertz et al. (1984) noted that the influence of stimulus mode is highly variable and depends on the individual patient.

12. Johns and Darley (1970) found that attainment of the correct articulation target is facilitated more by repeated trials of a word than by increase in the number of stimulus presentations. Patients are more likely to be on target if they are given a model once and have three opportunities to imitate it, than if they are permitted a single trial or are given three presentations of a model but only one trial to imitate it. LaPointe and Horner (1976) and Warren (1977) concluded that adults with apraxia of speech were extremely variable in their ability to improve on repeated trials. Wertz et al. (1984) observed that the process of repeated trials to aid facilitation is highly variable and depends a good deal on the clinical process.

13. Accuracy of articulation in patients is not significantly influenced by a number of auditory, visual, and psychologic variables. For example, when patients perform a task under two conditions, one while observing themselves in the mirror and the other without such visual monitoring, the difference in the number of errors they produce is not statistically significant (Deal & Darley, 1972). Similarly, introduction of masking

noise that prevents patients from hearing their own speech does not significantly alter the number of articulation errors they make (Deal & Darley, 1972; Wertz et al., 1984).

Neither is articulatory accuracy influenced by the instructional set created in the speaker (Deal & Darley, 1972; Wertz et al., 1984). Patients do equally well (or poorly) in reading passages whether told that the passage is extremely easy, that it is loaded with hard words and phonemes and is extremely difficult, or that the degree of difficulty is unknown. Finally, incidence of errors is not significantly influenced by imposing upon the patient's speech an external auditory rhythm (metronome) (Shane & Darley, 1978; Wertz et al., 1984).

14. Aronson (1990) noted that in apraxia of speech, the laryngeal-phonatory characteristics include the following: phonation varies from normal sounding to mutism; mutism and other attempts at phonation (e.g., whispered speech) are due to the inability to voluntarily produce phonation or respiration on command, or to imitate, although patients can reflexively produce phonation (e.g., coughing) and respiration (e.g., for intake of oxygen and outgo of carbon dioxide). The physical appearance of the vocal folds is normal in structure and function.

Oral Apraxia

Apraxia of speech (AOS) and oral apraxia are related to each other in the sense that the speech musculature comes into play in both conditions. In apraxia of speech, the disturbance is in the speech musculature during speaking, whereas in oral apraxia the disturbance is in the speech musculature during nonspeaking activities.

Oral (also nonverbal or buccofacial) apraxia has been described as a difficulty in performing voluntary movements with the muscles of the lips, tongue, mandible, and larynx in nonspeech tasks (coughing, chewing, sucking, or swallowing), although automatic movements of the same muscles are preserved (Darley et al., 1975). Oral apraxia exists despite intact motor abilities, sensory function, and comprehension of the required task. Oral apraxia often accompanies AOS, but each of these disorders can also exist alone.

Benson and Ardila (1996) ascribed the sites of lesion that can produce oral apraxia (a form of ideomotor apraxia) as tissue damage (cortex or white matter pathways) involving (1) the supramarginal gyrus of the dominant parietal lobe, particularly the arcuate fasciculus; (2) the dominant hemisphere motor association cortex, or the white matter tissues underlying this region; and (3) the anterior corpus callosum and/or the pathways that traverse this interhemispheric connector. Oral apraxia is evaluated by having the patient perform oral postures (after demonstration) such as mouth open, tongue out, show teeth, and pucker lips, and oral movements (after demonstration) such as tongue in and out, pucker and smile, blow air, whistle, and cough (DiSimoni, 1989).

Apraxia of Speech Versus Dysarthria

In an effort to clarify the distinction between dysarthria and apraxia of speech, Darley (1982), Darley et al. (1975), Duffy (2005), Wertz (1985), and Wertz et al. (1984) noted the following:

1. Dysarthria generally involves all speech levels (respiration, phonation, resonance, articulation, and prosody), whereas apraxia of speech is primarily a disorder of articulation and prosody (may be caused by compensatory behaviors).
2. Usually dysarthria is characterized by distortion errors, whereas apraxia of speech is characterized by substitution errors.

3. Dysarthric errors are probably more consistent than apraxia of speech errors; however, mild dysarthria is probably less consistent than severe apraxia of speech.

4. Dysarthric speakers are relatively uninfluenced by the degree of automatic speech (counting, reciting days of the week or months of the year, etc.), speaking situation (spontaneous speech, reading aloud, imitation), or linguistic variables (word length, frequency of occurrence, meaningfulness). Speakers with apraxia of speech can do better with automatic speech as opposed to propositional speech; depending on the speaking situation, can show correct or incorrect responses; and can be influenced by linguistic variables.

5. In apraxia of speech, neurologic examination reveals no significant evidence of slowness, weakness, incoordination, or alteration of tone of the speech musculature as in dysarthria. Dysarthria does not occur with aphasia as often as does apraxia of speech.

6. In dysarthria, the presence of oral apraxia rarely occurs, whereas oral apraxia occurs more frequently with apraxia of speech.

7. Darley (1982) and Darley et al. (1975) further noted that at the onset of apraxia of speech, the patient may experience difficulty initiating phonation at will; once this difficulty passes, as it usually does in a few days, phonation and resonance are normal.

8. In dysarthria, the articulatory errors are characteristically errors of simplification (distortions and omissions). In apraxia of speech, there is a preponderance of errors that must be considered complications of speech (substitutions of other phonemes, additions of phonemes, substitutions of a consonant cluster for a single consonant, repetitions of phonemes, and prolongations of phonemes).

   Dysarthric patients usually do not grope for correct articulatory positions, nor are they successful at immediate self-correction. In contrast, patients with apraxia of speech typically show trial-and-error groping and attempts at self-correction that are sometimes immediately successful. Speakers with dysarthria probably show less variable disfluencies than speakers with apraxia of speech.

9. Rosenbek, Kent, and LaPointe (1984) noted that more distortion errors have crept into the symptomatology of apraxia of speech. In spite of this, their clinical rule is that dysarthria is the most likely diagnosis if a patient has a high proportion of relatively consistent distortions. Apraxia of speech is the likely diagnosis if distortions are mixed with what sound like substitutions, especially if such errors are relatively inconsistent.

10. Ludlow, Connor, and Bassich (1987) found that patients with dysarthria, who have Parkinson and Huntington diseases, were not impaired in speech planning or initiation, but had poor control over speech events. Conversely, apraxia of speech is viewed as a planning or programming disorder that can involve initiation disturbances.

11. Odell et al. (1991) found that in vowel production,
    A. Speakers with apraxia of speech and ataxic dysarthria both made more errors in initiating than in sequencing (usually apraxic patients make more such errors).
    B. There was no difference in number of errors between vowels and consonants (usually both groups make more errors on consonants).
    C. Groups with both apraxia and dysarthria made more distortion than substitution errors (usually patients with dysarthria make more such errors).
    D. Groups with both apraxia and dysarthria made more errors in initial position than in other positions (usually apraxic patients make more such errors).
    E. Both groups showed no difference in the number of errors between monosyllabic and polysyllabic words (usually patients with apraxia make more errors on polysyllabic words).
    F. Both groups made more errors on stressed syllables (usually patients with apraxia make more errors on stressed syllables).

Apraxia of Speech Versus Phonemic or Literal Paraphasia

Table 9.2 lists features that differentiate apraxia of speech from phonemic or literal paraphasia. A major proportion of the material comes from the reviews by Duffy (2005) and Wertz, LaPointe, and Rosenbek (1984), supplemented by the other literature listed.

Additional Studies That Compare AOS, Dysarthria, Aphasia, and Typical Speech

Halpern, Darley, and Brown (1973) found that when comparing the symptoms of participants with aphasia, AOS, confused language (traumatic brain injury [TBI]), and general intellectual impairment (dementia), the symptom that most differentiated AOS from the other disorders was fluency (pausing, halting, and groping for articulatory placement).

Square-Storer, Darley, and Sommers (1988) found that in nonspeech and speech processing skills, patients with pure apraxia performed as well as neurotypical participants, compared to patients with aphasia. This finding lends support to the position that apraxia of speech is a

---

TABLE 9.2

Differences Between Apraxia of Speech and Phonemic or Literal Paraphasia

Apraxia of Speech	Phonemic or Literal Paraphasia
A. Brain lesion usually in the frontal lobe of the left hemisphere.	A. Brain lesion usually in the temporal or parietal lobe of the left hemisphere.
B. CVA the predominant etiology.	B. CVA the predominant etiology.
C. A right hemiplegia is common.	C. Usually no hemiplegia is present.
D. Accompanying oral apraxia more common.	D. Accompanying oral apraxia less common.
E. If patient also has aphasia, it usually profiles as a Broca's aphasia. If patient does not have aphasia, then performance in the other language modalities should be normal.	E. The language deficits typically profile as a conduction or Wernicke's aphasia. Performance in the other language modalities should be impaired.
F. Accompanying unilateral upper motor neuron dysarthria is more common.	F. Accompanying unilateral upper motor neuron dysarthria is less common.
G. Speech characteristics:	G. Speech characteristics:
1. A lower proportion of sequencing errors.	1. A higher proportion of sequencing errors.
2. A higher proportion of positioning (initiation) errors.	2. A lower proportion of positioning (initiation) errors.
3. More predictable substitutions of sounds (slightly off-target) and more lawful in relation to manner and place of articulation, and voiced and voiceless features.	3. Less predictable substitutions of sounds (more off-target) and less lawful in relation to manner and place of articulation, and voiced and voiceless features.
4. More errors on sounds in the initial position.	4. More errors on sounds in the medial and final positions.
5. More nonfluent output, slow rate, and groping.	5. More fluent output, normal rate, and nongroping.
6. More distortion of suprasegmentals (stress).	6. Less distortion of suprasegmentals (stress).
* Because of 5 & 6 prosody is more abnormal.	* Because of 5 & 6 prosody is less abnormal.
7. Ability to repeat is equal or superior to spontaneous speech.	7. Ability to repeat is much worse than spontaneous speech.
8. More recognition and more attempts to self-correct articulatory errors.	8. Less recognition and fewer attempts to self-correct articulatory errors.
9. Speech production therapy (articulation and prosody) most effective.	9. Language stimulation therapy (comprehension and expression) most effective.

disorder distinct from aphasia. Li and Williams (1990) tested patients with conduction, Broca's, and Wernicke's aphasia in their ability to repeat phrases and sentences. Participants with conduction aphasia showed a greater number of phonemic attempts, word revisions, and word and phrase repetitions. Participants with Broca's aphasia showed more phonemic errors and omissions. Patients with Wernicke's aphasia showed more unrelated words and jargon.

McNeil, Liss, Tseng, and Kent (1990) measured the effects of speech rate on the absolute and relative timing of the sentence production of AOS and speakers with conduction aphasia. Their results showed that there was a phonetic-motoric component contributing to the speech patterns of both apraxia and conduction aphasia groups. McNeil, Weismer, Adams, and Mulligan (1990) found that speakers with dysarthria and apraxia showed greater instability on lip, jaw, and finger isometric force and static position control than did neurotypical speakers and those with conduction aphasia. Speakers with conduction aphasia fell somewhere between speakers with dysarthria and apraxia, and neurotypical speakers.

Odell et al. (1991) concluded that patients with conduction aphasia made more vowel substitutions than did patients with apraxia of speech and ataxic dysarthria; patients with conduction aphasia made more vowel errors on polysyllabic words than did those with apraxia of speech and ataxic dysarthria; patients with conduction aphasia made more vowel errors in the final position than did those with apraxia of speech and ataxic dysarthria; and patients with apraxia of speech and ataxic dysarthria made more vowel errors on stressed syllables than did those with conduction aphasia. Another study (Robin et al., 2008) compared adults with AOS and those with conduction aphasia on nonspeech visuomotor oral tracking of a moving target. Assessment of nonspeech movements of the speech production mechanism allows the analysis of motor control deficits without requiring linguistic processing. Tracking tasks are dynamic rather than static in nature, and tracking sinusoidal signals results in movement gestures with a peak velocity in the middle of the movement, similar to the pattern observed for speech movements. The findings suggest that motor control capabilities are impaired in AOS, but not in conduction aphasia, and that the impairment is based on motor programming deficits, not impaired motor execution.

Seddoh et al. (1996) found that in speech timing measures, patients with apraxia of speech had longer and more variable mean durations than did neurotypical subjects. Although patients with conduction aphasia had longer consonant-vowel and vowel durations, their productions were not more variable than those of neurotypical participants. The authors suggested that these findings support the view that apraxia of speech is a motor speech disorder, and that conduction aphasia is a phonological rather than a motoric condition.

Hough and Klich (1998) examined the timing relationships of EMG (electromyography) activity of lip muscles underlying vowel production in two neurotypical individuals and two individuals with marked to severe AOS. They found that the relative amounts of time devoted to onset and offset of EMG activity for lip rounding are disorganized in AOS. Word length appeared to affect the timing of the onset and offset of muscle activity for both the neurotpyical and the AOS speakers. The authors suggested that in AOS, termination of EMG activity may be at least as disturbed as the initiation of EMG activity.

Etiology

The etiology for apraxia of speech is brain damage—most likely a unilateral lesion in the language-dominant hemisphere, involving singly or in combination Broca's area (frontal lobe), the premotor cortex (frontal lobe), the supplementary motor area (frontal lobe), the somatosensory area (parietal lobe), the supramarginal gyrus (parietal lobe), or the insula (paralimbic area).

The frontal lobe is involved most often, followed by the parietal lobe. Sometimes the temporal lobe or subcortical areas are implicated.

Duffy, Peach, and Strand (2007) found that AOS can occur in motor neuron disease (MND), typically also with dysarthria, but not invariably with aphasia or other cognitive deficits. Thus a diagnosis of MND does not preclude the presence of AOS. More importantly, MND should be a diagnostic consideration when AOS is a prominent sign of degenerative disease.

Duffy (2005) noted that the etiologies of 107 cases of apraxia of speech (primary speech pathology diagnosis) seen at the Mayo Clinic were as follows: vascular (58%), composed of single left hemisphere stroke (48%) and multiple strokes including left hemisphere (10%); degenerative (16%); traumatic (15%), composed of neurosurgical (13%) and closed head injury (2%); tumor, left hemisphere (6%); other (5%); and multiple causes (1%).

Diagnosis

Diagnostic procedures for determining apraxia of speech can involve (1) establishing background information, (2) giving a neurologic evaluation, (3) employing informal tests, and (4) employing formal tests. A committee of the Academy of Neurologic Communication Disorders and Sciences (ANCDS) was charged with developing evidence-based treatment guidelines for acquired AOS. They reported (Wambaugh, 2006) the following concerns about diagnosis and description of individuals in the AOS treatment literature:

1. Description of participants in investigations was cited as a particularly problematic area.
2. Published reports did not include enough information about AOS diagnosis, the speech behaviors of participants, severity levels of impairment, and other speech-language disorders that co-occurred with AOS.
3. The profession does not yet agree on diagnostic standards for AOS.
4. More than half of the published reports of AOS were case studies, which lack scientific controls for internal and external validity.

Accordingly, the committee recommended that researchers detail the behaviors that characterize and support their diagnosis of AOS, and include the level of severity of the disorder. When aphasia co-occurs with AOS, investigators need to provide information about the language disorder and its impact on verbal production.

Establishing Background Information and the Neurologic Evaluation

These procedures can be found at the beginning of the "Diagnosis" part of the section on aphasia.

Informal Tests

In testing for apraxia of speech, the same alternating motion rate (AMR) and sequential motion rate (SMR) procedures can be used as described in the "Diagnosis" part of the section on dysarthria. The patient is asked to repeat sounds, syllables, words, and sentences after the examiner. For example, while looking for the previously described symptoms of apraxia of speech, the examiner asks the patient to do the following:

1. Prolong /ah/.
2. Prolong /ee/.
3. Prolong /oo/.
4. Repeat /puh/ rapidly.
5. Repeat /tuh/ rapidly.
6. Repeat /kuh/ rapidly.

7. Repeat /puh-tuh-kuh/ rapidly.
8. Repeat "snowman."
9. Repeat "gingerbread."
10. Repeat "impossibility."
11. Repeat "Please sit down."
12. Repeat "seventeen seventy-six."
13. Repeat "Columbia Presbyterian Hospital."
14. Repeat "Methodist Episcopal Church."
15. Repeat "Will you answer the telephone?"
16. Repeat "no ifs, ands, or buts."
17. Repeat "He lives in the third house from the corner."

Informal scoring can follow the guidelines proposed by Darley et al. (1975). The inability to begin any phonation at the laryngeal level may indicate apraxia of phonation, which is an early and transient problem. Severe AOS is indicated if the patient can produce only some sounds at the laryngeal level, or one or two words (often with correct articulation).

Sometimes the single word is used appropriately. For example, one patient who communicated in Spanish and English prior to his stroke was able to produce only the word "si" (yes), which he used appropriately. When a response of "si" was not called for, he could produce only incomprehensible language sounds as a response. At other times, the single word is used for all responses. One patient was able to produce only the word "time" or "time-time," which she used for every single oral response, regardless of what was called for. Another patient said "Bye, bye-bye, bye" continually, but every once in a while, he would produce "Evelyn" (his wife's name) in a crystal clear manner.

Moderate AOS is indicated if the patient produces inconsistent trial-and-error substitutions, omissions, distortions, or additions of phonemes; stuttering-like hesitations and blocking on phonemes; or groping for sounds and words, difficulty in starting speaking, disprosody, and pockets of correct articulation.

Mild AOS is indicated if the patient produces phonemes in a nearly normal manner in contextual speech, but shows apraxic phonemic errors when asked to produce more difficult multisyllabic words or those that include demanding consonant clusters.

Informal testing can also be accomplished by engaging the patient in normal conversation, or asking the patient to respond out loud to action pictures or to read aloud a phonetically balanced passage (e.g., grandfather passage). Particularly for these informal testing situations, the use of a tape recorder would be helpful. The clinician's knowledge of phonetic transcription is an asset too, especially when it is used to describe the highly unusual and inconsistent output of the AOS patient.

Formal Tests

The *Apraxia Battery for Adults* (Dabul, 1979) checks for apraxia of speech by having the patient produce a timed diadochokinetic task, repeat words of increasing length, name pictures within a specific time period, read out loud, produce automatic speech by counting, and engage in spontaneous speech. A quantified scoring method is incorporated in the test. Recent use of this instrument for 11 individuals with apraxia of speech indicated no significant differences in subtest scores for those assessed by telerehabilitation compared to face-to-face test environments (Hill et al., 2009).

Wertz et al. (1984) described their *Motor Speech Evaluation*, whose origin is spread throughout the literature. It is a screening tool that usually takes less than 20 minutes to administer. Scoring the test can be descriptive (e.g., A for apraxic productions, P for paraphasias, D for dysarthria, U for nondiagnostic errors, O for other errors, and N for neurotypical responses). Scoring can also be multidimensional (e.g., utilizing *PICA*, the *Porch Index of Communicative Ability* 16-point scale [Porch, 1981]) or use of narrow or broad phonetic transcription.

The tasks are traditional:

1. Conversation
2. Vowel prolongation
3. Repetition of monosyllables /puh/, /tuh/, /kuh/
4. Repetition of a sequence of monosyllables like /puh-tuh-kuh/
5. Repetition of multisyllabic words
6. Multiple trials with the same word
7. Repetition of words that increase in length (e.g., thick, thicken, thickening)
8. Repetition of monosyllabic words that contain the same initial and final sound (e.g., mom, judge)
9. Repetition of sentences
10. Counting forward and backward
11. Picture description
12. Repetition of sentences used volitionally to determine consistency of production
13. Oral reading

Wertz et al. (1984) further discussed sound-by-position tests, the influence of stimulus modes, and procedures for scoring and determining severity. Wertz (1984) noted some of the difficulties in assessing apraxia of speech. He advocated using a comprehensive set of tasks sensitive enough to tap the ambiguous patient.

The *Comprehensive Apraxia Test* (CAT) (DiSimoni, 1989) checks the following:

1. 20 oral volitional movements (e.g., after demonstration, the patient has to pucker lips, move tongue side to side)
2. Production of 33 phonemes (e.g., patient repeats /i/, /ai/, /p/)
3. Four sets of alternate motion rate (e.g., /pʌpʌpʌ/, /tʌtʌtʌ/)
4. Production of 10 syllables in nonsense words (e.g., patient repeats /m-i-m/) and 10 syllables in short, real words (e.g., patient repeats /m-a-m/)
5. 13 utterances of increasing length (e.g., patient repeats "cowboy," "exercise," "instructor")
6. 80 nonsense items in contextual inference (e.g., patient repeats /tug/, /tip/)

This test uses a multidimensional scoring system based on errors of phonemes in manner and place of articulation, and in voiced and voiceless contexts.

Duffy (2005) described a set of tasks that combine portions of the *Motor Speech Evaluation* (Wertz et al., 1984) and unpublished Mayo Clinic tasks for assessing apraxia of speech. It includes a scoring code that may be used to signify apraxia of speech response, for example, D for distortion, G for groping, S for substitution, SC for attempt at articulatory self-correction, DR for delayed response, AOE for awareness of errors, SE for sequencing errors, SR for slow rate, and SXS for syllable-by-syllable production of multisyllabic words or phrases.

Another scoring method for assessing apraxia of speech is the numeric code adapted from the *PICA* (Porch, 1981), where 15 = correct in all respects, 14 = distorted, 13 = delayed, 10 = self-corrected articulatory error, 9 = correct after a stimulus repetition, 7 = error clearly related to target, 6 = error unrelated to target, 5 = rejection or stated inability to respond, 4 = unintelligible but differentiated from other responses, 3 = unintelligible and relatively undifferentiated from other responses.

Duffy (2005) further suggested the use of broad or narrow transcription after the patient repeats vowels, diphthongs, consonants, words, words of increasing length (cat, catnip, catapult, catastrophe), the same word three times, and sentences. The patient is also asked to do the following: repeat /pʌpʌpʌ/, /tʌtʌtʌ/, /kʌkʌkʌ/, and /pʌtʌkʌ/ as fast and as steadily as possible; count from 1 to 10; and say the days of the week. As the patient sings "Happy Birthday," "Jingle Bells," or another familiar tune, the examiner makes note of how well the tune is carried and how adequate the articulation is. The examination also describes the patient's abilities in conversation, narrative speech, and reading aloud.

Katz and McNeil (2010) noted that electromagnetic articulography (EMA) is a method originally designed for the laboratory measurement of speech articulatory motion. They described the use of EMA as applied to the remediation of AOS. In this experimental technique, individuals with AOS are provided with real-time, visual information concerning the movement of the tongue during speech. From information sent via EMA sensors mounted on the tongue, patients are guided into hitting "targets" displayed on a computer monitor, designed to guide correct articulatory placement. The results of several studies suggest that augmented feedback-based treatment is efficacious and that this treatment follows principles of motor learning described in the limb motor literature.

Therapy

The first goal of therapy is to inform the patient and the caretaker(s) about the nature and the consequences of the disorder.

The patient with apraxia of speech has a motor speech problem that involves problems with articulation, prosody, and fluency, in any combination. Thinking abilities are normal or near normal, and language should be intact. If aphasia is present, as it often is, then language will be impaired.

Prognosis

Inclusion and exclusion criteria, regarding such variables as race and ethnicity, socioeconomic status and education, cognitive and hearing functioning, medications, and neuroimaging information have rarely been reported (Wambaugh, 2006). If reported consistently, this information could help assessment of prognosis for recovery.

Rosenbek (1984) and Wertz et al. (1984) noted that particular patients with apraxia of speech present symptoms that warrant a favorable prognosis. These patients have the following characteristics: are less than one month postonset, suffered a small lesion confined to Broca's area, have minimal coexisting aphasia, do not display significant oral or nonverbal apraxia, are in good health, and have the stamina for intensive treatment. In addition, the following combination of factors enhances the prognosis for improved speech: education, counseling, and drilling; the patient's ability to learn and to generalize; and the patient's willingness to practice. The authors noted that patients with untreated apraxia do not reach the same competence as do those who are treated. Thus, the prognosis for functional recovery is poor without treatment, fair with treatment for the severe patient, and good with treatment for the moderate to mild patient.

The second goal of therapy is to provide the appropriate treatment approaches and techniques.

Efficacy of Therapy for Apraxia of Speech

Duffy (2005) noted that efficacy-of-treatment studies for apraxia of speech consist primarily of case reports and single-subject design studies. These studies indicate that a number of approaches and techniques can be effective in treating apraxia of speech, particularly if aphasia is absent or not outstanding. However, there has been almost no research that compares treatments or examines effects of combining treatments (Wambaugh, 2006). The literature also lacks information about therapeutic "dosage," that is, optimal length of treatment sessions, number of sessions per week, and total duration of therapy needed to provide maximum positive outcomes.

The ANCDS writing committee on apraxia of speech (Wambaugh et al., 2006, p. 36) identified five general categories of treatments:

1. Articulatory kinematic
2. Rate/rhythm
3. Intersystemic facilitation/reorganization
4. Augmentative-alternative communication (AAC)
5. Other

Verbal production was a requisite goal for the 30 studies of articulatory kinematics to improve speech production. Most treatments used modeling/repetition, also called "integral stimulation," to elicit desired speech behaviors. In integral stimulation, the patient is instructed to "watch me, listen to me, and say it with me" (Wambaugh et al., 2006, p. 36). In many studies articulatory placement cues are also used to correct sounds produced in error. Other forms of stimulation include prompts for restructuring oral and muscular phonetic targets (PROMPT), which obliges the clinician to obtain specialized training, and written cues.

There were seven studies of rate or rhythm control for treatment of AOS. In all investigations, there was an external source of control, including metronomic pacing, computerized control using visual displays, and a pacing board. The present authors have found that it is easy, and much less expensive than buying commercially available types, to create a pacing board by wrapping rubber bands around the inch markers of a six-inch ruler.

There were eight investigations of effects of intersystemic facilitation/reorganization treatments. The most frequently studied type of treatment was gestural reorganization, often employing American Indian Hand Talk (Amer-Ind), with most treatments requiring vocalizations paired with the gestures. We discuss the code developed by Native Americans (Skelly, 1979) elsewhere in this section. There is some overlap between rate/rhythm and intersystemic facilitation/reorganization treatments, such as in singing and in vibrotactile stimulation.

The eight treatment studies that employed augmentative-alternative communication (AAC) focused on improving communication without using speech. As we note in the "Advanced Study" portion of this section, it is possible and often desirable to use AAC to stimulate vocal communication.

An additional five studies that could not fit into the other categories of treatment included a focus on communication partners, work on segmental and suprasegmental aspects of speech productions paired with head movements, and treatment that appeared to combine several approaches.

The ANCDS writing group (Wambaugh et al., 2006, p. 42) concluded that articulatory kinematic approaches were probably effective; rate/rhythm control approaches and intersystemic approaches were possibly effective, and AAC approaches could not be rated regarding likelihood of benefit, because of insufficient data.

Principles of motor learning that involve drill, self-learning and instruction, feedback, specificity of training, consistent and variable practice, and speed-accuracy tradeoff tasks are important in treatment. Motor-learning research shows that delaying or reducing the frequency of feedback promotes retention and transfer of skills, a finding recently supported experimentally (Austermann et al., 2008). Jacks (2008) compared production of three vowel sounds by five adults with apraxia of speech and aphasia and five neurotypical adults in a bite-block condition compared to unconstrained production of the same vowels. Differences between the two groups were apparent only in the unconstrained condition, where vowel accuracy was poorer for those with AOS. The author concluded that feedback control for vowel production was intact in the individuals with AOS and aphasia.

Maas (2010) reviewed a number of conditions of practice and feedback (sometimes referred to as principles of motor learning) in relation to treatment for AOS. He noted that one of the challenges in clinical management for AOS is that resources (including time) are limited, which means that one cannot treat all possible speech sounds or sequences indefinitely. Thus it becomes important to structure the available treatment time so as to maximize acquisition, maintenance, and generalization (maintenance and generalization being the primary indices of learning).

Evidence of treatment effects is limited because of lack of replication, either within or across the AOS literature (Wambaugh et al., 2006). Group studies have occurred so rarely that it is not possible to draw lessons from them. Especially because of the preponderance of single-subject studies, there should be at least three demonstrated replications before treatment efficacy is claimed. Outcome measures should address more than speech intelligibility, including speech in spontaneous or elicited discourse and the impact of therapy on the participant's activity limitations and restrictions.

Several specific programs of treatment (described later in this section) have been identified as effective. They include the following: the eight-step continuum for treating apraxia of speech, prompts for restructuring oral muscular phonetic targets, melodic intonation therapy, multiple input phoneme therapy, voluntary control of involuntary utterances, and a number of specific techniques not tied to any one program but associated with many of them (e.g., phonetic derivation, phonetic placement, minimal contrasts). As Duffy (2005) and Wambaugh and Doyle (1994), cited by Wambaugh, Kalinyak-Flisger, West, and Doyle (1998), pointed out in their reviews, more efficacy-of-treatment studies are needed that compare therapy programs and techniques.

General Principles

The general principles discussed in the "Therapy" portion of the section on dysarthria that underlie therapy for the motor speech disorders (Darley et al., 1975) are applicable here. Wertz et al. (1984) pointed out that therapy for apraxia of speech should concentrate on the disordered articulation and therefore differs from the language stimulation and auditory and visual processing therapies appropriate to the aphasias or the dysarthrias, where multiple problems due to paralysis exist (e.g., mobility exercises for a weak musculature would be appropriate for many patients with dysarthria, but is not called for in apraxia of speech).

Five speakers with apraxia of speech and nonfluent aphasia exhibited longer movement durations and, in some instances, larger tongue movements for consonant singletons and consonant clusters in single-syllable and two-syllable utterances (Bartle-Meyer, Carly, Goozee, & Murdoch, 2009). The study used electromagnetic articulography to measure lingual kinematics, such as tongue-tip and tongue-back movements. Two of the five participants were able to produce words comparable in length to those produced by control speakers. Bartle, Goozee, and Murdoch (2007) used electromagnetic articulography to record tongue movement for three consonants in monosyllabic words. The single participant with AOS used silent articulatory attempts and starters that contributed to her prolonged response latencies.

These behaviors, not observed in gender-matched controls, provide additional support for considering AOS as a motor speech disorder.

In general, a variety of phonetic conditions affect articulatory accuracy of the patient with AOS in fairly predictable ways. These phonetic conditions are as follows: consonants produce more errors than vowels; consonant clusters produce more errors than singletons; within singletons, affricates and fricatives produce the most errors; substitution errors are perceived more than distortions, omissions, additions, and repetitions, and these substitutions are complications rather than simplifications of the target phoneme.

Duffy (2005) noted that with substitutions, most errors are in place of articulation, followed by manner of articulation, then by the voiced–voiceless division, and finally by the oral–nasal division, which had the fewest errors. Within place of articulation, most errors occur on palatal and dental phonemes; bilabials and lingua-alveolar phonemes are least in error (Duffy, 2005). Within manner of articulation, affricates and fricatives produce the most errors. In addition, initial consonant or vowel in a word produce the most errors, performance is better on automatic speech than on nonautomatic speech, more errors occur on words that have linguistic or psychological weight, and real words are easier than nonsense words.

Additional factors are distance between successive phonemes, where likelihood of error increases as distance between successive points of articulation within an utterance increases; word length, where errors increase as words increase in length; and word frequency, where errors occur more readily on rare than on common words. Trost and Canter (1974) found that phonemes with relatively high frequency tend to be more accurately articulated than those that occur less frequently. Therapeutic principles derived from the phonetic conditions described above should be considered when beginning therapy.

Articulatory accuracy in apraxia of speech is influenced by mode of stimulus (Johns & Darley, 1970; Trost & Canter, 1974). Johns and Darley (1970) found that auditory-visual stimulation is better than auditory or visual stimulation alone—*visual* in this instance referring to watching the clinician speak. However, LaPointe and Horner (1976) observed no differences in correct production among single and combined modes of stimulation. Deal and Darley (1972) found that patients with apraxia do not achieve greater phonemic accuracy if they are allowed to monitor their own speech in a mirror. An evaluation of sound production treatments (Wambaugh, 2010) considered combinations of modeling, repetition, minimal pair contrast, integral stimulation, articulatory placement cueing, and verbal feedback, using a response-contingent hierarchy. Although there is strong response generalization to untrained exemplars of trained sounds, generalization across sounds is not expected unless sound errors and sound targets are closely related.

Auditory training does not necessarily precede production when instituting therapy. The patient with apraxia who has mild aphasia can show auditory perception difficulties, as Aten, Johns, and Darley (1971) demonstrated, or can have little or no auditory perception problems, as Square (1981) showed. Nor does therapy necessarily employ a motokinesthetic approach (manual manipulation of the articulators for correct production) when deficits in oral sensation and perception have been demonstrated (Rosenbek, Wertz, & Darley, 1973). Deutsch (1981) found that oral form identification deficits are not causally related to motor speech programming problems.

Therapy does emphasize the auditory and visual modalities, especially the visual, because these clinically appear to be the most potent in guiding the articulators. Although it has not been experimentally confirmed yet, it appears that establishing or strengthening "visual memory" is most important to therapeutic success with patients with apraxia. The phonetic placement method of describing the correct manner and place of articulation and the correct voiced and voiceless components of phoneme production is useful.

In his review, Duffy (2005) mentioned that in AOS, abnormalities occur in rate (e.g., slower than normal), prosody (e.g., equal stress on all syllables within a word), and fluency (e.g., groping for and/or repeating sounds and syllables).

Specific Phonemic Therapy Techniques

Aichert and Ziegler (2008) found that training of phonologically simple syllables, which were derived from more complex target syllables, showed a generalization effect on these target syllables. Response generalization of sound production treatment for acquired apraxia of speech was also strong for untrained exemplars of trained sounds (Wambaugh, 2010).

Wambaugh (2010, p. 72) proposed the following sound production treatment (SPT). The hierarchy is response-contingent, with steps used only as needed, and does not reverse directions.

SPT Treatment Hierarchy

1. The clinician says the target item and requests a repetition (e.g., "Say *sun*").
   a. If correct, the clinician requests 5 additional repetitions and then goes to Step 5.
   b. If incorrect, the clinician gives feedback, using a minimal pair item (e.g., "That's not quite right. Let's try a different word. Say *ton*."). This strategy is not used with sentence-level stimuli.
      i. If correct, the clinician gives feedback and says, "Let's go back to the other word," and goes to Step 2 with the target word.
      ii. If incorrect, the clinician gives feedback, attempts production with integral stimulation up to 3 times, and goes to Step 2 with the target word.
2. The clinician shows the printed letter representing the target sound, says the target word, and requests a repetition (e.g., "Let's focus on this sound on the card. Say *sun*.").
   a. If correct, the clinician requests 5 additional repetitions and goes to the next item.
   b. If incorrect, the clinician goes to Step 3.
3. The clinician uses integral stimulation up to 3 times to elicit the target word (e.g., "Watch me, listen to me, and say it with me").
   a. If correct, the clinician requests 5 additional repetitions and goes to the next item.
   b. If incorrect, the clinician goes to Step 4.
4. The clinician gives articulatory placement cues, and requests production of the target word again, after cueing using integral stimulation. Cues are dependent upon the errors produced by the client.
   a. If correct, the clinician requests 5 additional repetitions.
   b. If incorrect, the clinician goes to Step 5.
5. Go to the next item.

An Eight-Step Continuum for Treatment

Using the general principles mentioned above, Rosenbek, Lemme, Ahern, Harris, and Wertz (1973) advocate an eight-step integral stimulation method ("Watch me and listen to me") as an approach to therapy with patients with apraxia. The eight steps are presented below using "bat" (as in baseball bat) as an example of a target word.

1. After integral stimulation by the clinician, the patient and the clinician say "bat" at the same time.
2. There is integral stimulation by the clinician, then after a delay the clinician mimes or repeats "bat" soundlessly (visual cue only), and the patient tries to say it out loud.

3. There is integral stimulation by the clinician, and after a delay the patient tries to say "bat" without any visual cue.

4. There is integral stimulation by the clinician, and after a delay the patient tries to say "bat" several times consecutively without any intervening auditory or visual cues.

5. The patient reads out loud the written or printed word *bat*.

6. The patient sees the written or printed word *bat*, reads it silently, and then says it out loud after the word is removed.

7. The imitative model is abandoned, and the clinician provides conditions so that the target utterance can be used volitionally as the correct response to a question (e.g., clinician says, "What do we hit a baseball with?" and patient attempts the word "bat").

8. The patient provides the appropriate response in a role-playing situation (e.g., a mock ball game; clinician says, "You're at the plate with a _____" or "You're up next and swinging a _____").

Rosenbek et al. (1973) noted that the above steps can be employed on the syllable, word, phrase, or sentence level, and that patients need not go through all of the steps, especially those that are quite difficult. In addition, if integral stimulation does not work, other methods should be used (e.g., phonetic placement and phonetic derivation, which are described later). In a later study, Deal and Florance (1978) presented several successful cases that used a modified version of the eight-step continuum program.

Dabul and Bollier

Dabul and Bollier (1976) observed that the most characteristic problem for patients with apraxia is the sequencing of speech sounds. To improve this condition they advocated the following sequential steps:

1. Mastery of individual consonant phonemes.

2. Rapid repetition of each mastered consonant plus the vowel /a/.

3. Buildup of sounds into syllables using CV, CV combinations, such as /fa/, ta/, and CVC combinations such as /pap/.

4. After acquisition of a solid, basic "vocabulary" of articulatory positions, the patient attempts a difficult word by saying each phoneme in isolation and then blending the separate productions into syllables and words.

Dabul and Bollier (1976) advocated the use of nonmeaningful syllable combinations in order to focus the patient's attention on the necessary phoneme sequencing and away from the decision of whether movements were voluntary or automatic. They found that mastery of volitional control over nonmeaningful syllable combinations leads to improved articulation of meaningful words. However, Kahn, Stannard, and Skinner (1998), Rosenbek (1984), and Wertz et al. (1984) favored the use of meaningful stimuli because of clinical success.

Melodic Intonation Therapy

Sparks and Holland (1976) reported success in using melodic intonation therapy (MIT) with patients with nonfluent aphasia who exhibited relatively good auditory comprehension, frequent phonemic errors, and poor repetition skill. The intoned pattern is based on one of several speech prosody patterns that are reasonable choices for a given sentence, depending on the inference intended. The three elements are the melodic line, the rhythm, and points of stress. Through a gradual progression of carefully intoned sentences and phonemes, the patient is guided to normal prosody to aid speech return. A full discussion of this form of therapy can be found in Sparks (2008).

Rhythm Techniques

Rosenbek, Hansen, Baughman, and Lemme (1974) and Yoss and Darley (1974) found that various rhythmic techniques can facilitate the increase of articulatory accuracy. However, Shane and Darley (1978) found that auditory rhythmic stimulation (metronome) did not significantly improve articulatory accuracy. Keith and Aronson (1975) described the use of singing as a form of apraxia of speech therapy.

In Metrical Pacing Therapy (Ziegler et al., 2010), the target utterance becomes a rhythmical skeleton, represented as a sequence of short tones. There are repeated presentations through headphones, so the participant can internalize the target utterance. Then the patient synchronizes production of the word or phrase with the auditory signal. There is immediate feedback provided on a computer screen. Treatment is individualized for delivery rate of the rhythmical templates, length of the target utterance, and complexity of training materials. Treatment effects of Metrical Pacing Therapy were as follows:

1. Whole syllables generalized to two-syllable words containing the learned syllables.
2. Less complex syllables generalized to a more complex target.
3. Speaking rate and fluency improved, compared to a control therapy, but there were no differences between the two therapies for improvement in articulation accuracy.

Phonetic Derivation and Phonetic Placement

Rosenbek (1985) advocated using the phonetic derivation method, whereby target sounds are derived from intact nonspeech or speech gestures. For example, biting the lower lip produces /f/ and /v/; puckering the lips produces /u/, /ou/, /ɔ/, and /w/; smiling produces /i/ and /ɛ/; yawning produces /a/ and /ʌ/, and wiping one's mouth produces /m/, /p/, and /b/. The phonetic placement method of describing the correct manner and place of articulation, and the correct voiced and voiceless components of target phoneme production, uses both visual and verbal instruction.

Prompts for Restructuring Oral Musculature Phonetic Targets

Another approach is PROMPT (Square-Storer & Hayden, 1989), which stands for "prompts for restructuring oral musculature phonetic targets." This approach stresses the patient's kinesthetic awareness of speech movements or their prevention. The clinician provides tactile cues to various portions of the patient's vocal tract (e.g., touching patient's nose for a nasal sound or the lips for a bilabial sound, with the length of the touch determining the length of time the sound should be held). Once this heightened kinesthetic awareness is established, combinations of visual, auditory, and tactile input are used for the production of sounds, words, and short phrases. Because of the possibility of impaired oral stereognosis in apraxia of speech, a motokinesthetic approach (if it is used) should be combined with visual feedback, say with the clinician and client sitting next to each other and looking at a mirror.

Multiple Input Phoneme Therapy

Stevens (1989) described an approach called *multiple input phoneme therapy* (MIPT). Geared for patients with severe apraxia, this approach takes the involuntary verbal stereotypes and tries to bring them under voluntary control. First the clinician repeats the stereotypic utterance, then the patient repeats along with the clinician, and then both of them tap simultaneously along with the utterance. The initial phoneme of the utterance is stressed, and gradually the clinician fades the voice away and only mouths the words while the patient continues saying them. Other words beginning with that same phoneme are introduced, eventually leading to all phonemes, phrases, and short sentences. If all prior steps are successful, the repetitions are faded and patient responses are evoked, for example, by naming of pictures or reading cues.

Voluntary Control of Involuntary Utterances

Helm and Barresi (1980) developed the voluntary control of involuntary utterances (VCIU) for use with patients who have apraxia and aphasia. In this approach, the clinician writes down any real word the patient says in any speaking context. The clinician writes these words individually on cards for the patient to read aloud. If another real word is substituted for the target word, then the target word is scrapped and the substituted word is kept for future use as a target word.

Short, frequently used, easy initial phoneme, and emotion-laden words are suggested for building up a vocabulary. After the patient can read this vocabulary aloud, the next step would be having the patient name pictures or engage in controlled conversation that employs those words. All the while, any new words are added to the vocabulary.

Minimal Contrasts

Minimal contrasts in single words (e.g., "tea–key"), phrases, (e.g., "tan–coat"), and sentences (e.g., "Ted can tell Kay about the two cars") can be used to bolster each individual consonant and to differentiate between consonants that are close. Cognates are pairs of consonants that are alike in manner and place of articulation but differ in the voiced–voiceless category. Words beginning with cognate pairs (e.g., "pat–bat, to–do, fan–van, sue–zoo, Kay–gay") can also be used in contrast drills. Keith and Thomas (1989) provided practice materials for the vowels, diphthongs, and consonants for contrast purposes.

Wambaugh et al. (1998) studied the effects of a treatment for sound errors in three speakers with chronic apraxia of speech and aphasia. Treatment combined the use of minimal contrast pairs with traditional sound production training techniques such as integral stimulation and articulatory placement cueing, and was applied sequentially to sounds that were consistently in error before training. Results indicated increased correct sound productions for all speakers in trained and untrained words.

Contrastive stress refers to an aspect of prosody that can differentiate, for example, *ice cream* from *I scream*. According to Ballard et al. (2010), the pattern of equal stress across syllables in words and phrases observed in AOS arises from poor control of spatial and temporal aspects of movements of the articulators. The authors developed a treatment approach, which they called *rapid syllable transition treatment*, or ReST, which uses nonword multisyllable strings to help in the transition between syllables with varying stress patterns.

Traditional Therapy for the Patient with Severe Apraxia of Speech

To initiate phonation, the clinician (with the use of a mirror) should produce the sound /a/ and have the patient watch and listen and then imitate. If the patient is unable to imitate the sound, the clinician should place the patient's hand on the clinician's larynx while attempting to phonate. Sometimes it may be necessary for the clinician to manually open the patient's mouth and shape the lips. This procedure should be repeated numerous times. The auditory stimulation by the clinician and from the patient's own auditory feedback system, plus the tactile stimulation of holding the larynx, should facilitate controlled production. Some severely involved patients may have to work on oromotor control to achieve any sort of sound.

Dworkin (1991) and Dworkin, Abkarian, and Johns (1988) described a number of nonspeech oromotor exercises for the lips, tongue, jaw, and respiratory system. Aronson (1990) recommended that establishing response hierarchies by starting with a reflective sound such as a cough, clearing the throat, a moan, a grunt, a laugh, a sigh, or humming a tune, can facilitate the production of a volitional /a/ sound. Volitional sound production can also be augmented by having the patient shape his or her lips with his or her own fingers. Duffy (2005) suggested pairing a highly used symbolic gesture with its associated sound or word (e.g., placing the index finger to the lips to say /ʃ/ or blowing out a match to form vowel sounds).

Once the patient becomes successful in producing a volitional /a/ sound, the characteristics of pitch, duration, and loudness become the goals of intervention. Subsequently, other vowel sounds (e.g., /i/, /u/, /ou/) can be worked on in the same manner. According to Darley et al. (1975), singing and completing automatic phrases (e.g., "a cup of _____," "grass is _____") can also be useful techniques for initiating phonation. They further suggested the use of everyday expressions such as "Hello," "How are you," "Thank you," and "Goodbye" and the use of overlearned material such as the Lord's Prayer, the Pledge of Allegiance, the 23rd Psalm, nursery rhymes, and TV advertising jingles as means of eliciting full speech activities.

DiSimoni (1989) reviewed the use of augmentative or alternative systems that may be used with severely involved patients with apraxia, either to augment or supplant the use of oral communication. These approaches include communication boards, mechanical communication systems, finger spelling, sign language, pantomine and gesture, writing, and picture drawing. Kangas and Lloyd (2006), Shane and Sauer (1986), and Silverman (1989) offered additional reviews of augmentative or alternative systems that can be used with the patient with severe apraxia of speech.

Traditional Therapy for the Patient with Moderate and Mild Apraxia of Speech

Taking into account the previously described phonetic conditions that affect articulatory accuracy, additional phonemic therapy techniques involve working on individual vowels in the manner described in the "Traditional Therapy for the Patient with Severe Apraxia of Speech" section. When the patient has command of the vowel sounds (e.g., /i/, /u/, /ou/), the production of consonants can become the focus of therapeutic activity. For example, the /m/ sound, which is easily seen, might be a suitable consonant with which to begin therapy. The clinician produces the /m/ sound and then has the patient close the lips. The patient unable to perform this task should then be directed to imitate the clinician in closing and shaping the lips with the index finger and thumb. With the lips closed, the patient makes a humming sound.

Sometimes the patient will feel the clinician's larynx while the clinician produces this sound. The patient is encouraged to hum a familiar melody and receives feedback from the clinician concerning its correctness. The patient then reproduces the /m/ sound and subsequently changes mouth position by opening the lips. This change in mouth position is used to overcome patient fear of being unable to produce a particular articulatory posture again. Thus, the clinician works on changing from /m/ to open mouth posture, or from /m/ to a vowel that is already in the patient's phonemic repertoire.

Once the /m/ can be produced in isolation, it can be used in the initial position with the vowels that were learned (e.g., /ma/, /mu/, /mi/, /mou/). If other vowels are developed spontaneously or in response to therapy, they can also be used. Next, /m/ is produced in the final position in one-syllable words (e.g., "am, I'm, arm"), two-syllable words (e.g., "mama, memo"), and then in word lists with /m/ in all positions (e.g., "madam, omen").

From there one can proceed to simple phrases (e.g., "my man, my mama, my money"), to longer phrases (e.g., "miles from Montana, music man, made men are mean"), and to sentences (e.g., "The mailman will get the mail. A memo was sent to the milkman. The marmalade came from Memphis"). This can be followed by working on differentiating similar sounding words with /m/ in the initial position (e.g., "man–pan, mail–pail, make–bake, mat–bat"), /m/ in the final position (e.g., "come–cub, dumb–dub"), and progressively longer words ("measure–measured–measurable, mean–meaning–meaningful"). More examples of progressively longer words can be found in Keith and Thomas (1989).

Patients with mild apraxia of speech can now forego many of the imitative tasks that were presented in the earlier forms of therapy. With self-monitoring skills (e.g., slowing down their rate of speaking), they can attempt full conversational activities. For examples of tasks that range from the formulation of simple sentences (e.g., clinician says, "What barks?" and patient answers using a sentence) to explaining the meaning of metaphors (e.g., "She's the apple of his eye") and similes (e.g., "happy as a clam"), see therapy suggestions OED 7 through OED 11 in the "Therapy" portion of the section on aphasia.

Facilitators in Apraxia of Speech Therapy

DiSimoni (1989) reviewed the facilitators in apraxia of speech therapy that have proven successful. They include the following:

1. Procedures that pace the patient, such as metronomes, palilalia board, walk and talk, manual gesture for each word or syllable, finger tapping, reading aloud using a blind (usually a 3" × 5" card with a rectangular hole in it, placed over copy to be read so that only one word at a time is visible), pointing to words while reading, stressing underlined words, stressing different colored words, reading with print upside down or sideways, visualizing each word, visualizing a geometric figure, visualizing the first letter of each word
2. Procedures that relax the patient, such as biofeedback, progressive relaxation
3. Other procedures, such as standing while speaking, phonemic prompts, hypnosis

Additional reviews and therapeutic techniques for apraxia of speech have been described by Freed (2000) and Wambaugh and Shuster (2008).

The third goal of therapy is to encourage the patient and the caretaker(s) to continue the rehabilitative process outside of the clinical setting.

The ability to achieve carryover for the patient with apraxia of speech would follow guidelines similar to those described for the patient with dysarthria (see the section on dysarthria).

Advanced Study: Augmentative-Alternative Communication (AAC)

Initial interventions for individuals with apraxia of speech usually focus on articulatory intelligibility and verbal expression. Ultimately, interventions may shift to implementing compensatory strategies, such as augmentative-alternative communication, to facilitate functional communication. Improved verbal output is sometimes an outcome associated with AAC training and use, so clients and caregivers should be told that vocal speech will not be ignored. AAC interventions have traditionally focused on the individual, rather than the speaking partners or family members. More recently, professionals have been investigating the role of facilitators or family members working with AAC systems (for an overview see Beukelman, Fager, Ball, & Dietz, 2007). Numerous studies have reported on the success of including the spouse in aphasia treatment (Avent, 2004; Boles, 1998; Kagan, Black, Duchan, Simmons-Mackie, & Square, 2001), and these may also apply to treatment for apraxia of speech. For example, the spouse of an adult with nonfluent aphasia and apraxia of speech was trained (Hough & Johnson, 2009) in the use of a light technology, aided AAC device (see below for a description of these terms). The treatment protocol involved identifying each symbol on the display, navigating to category, choosing a symbol requested by the clinician, and answering questions about everyday activities and interests with short phrases, using symbols.

Use of AAC devices should focus on a particular treatment plan. For example, using Garrett & Beukelman's (1992) Assessment of Capabilities and Communication Type, a participant may be identified as a "specific-need communicator" with the primary goals of requesting basic daily needs and saying names of family members.

Augmentative communication is defined (Arroyo, Goldfarb, & Sands, in press) as a system that supports or enhances currently existing language and communication abilities. *Alternative communication* refers to a system that replaces the communication of nonvocal individuals (Nicolosi, Harryman, & Kresheck, 2005). According to the American Speech-Language-Hearing Association (ASHA, 2005, p. 1):

> AAC refers to an area of research, clinical, and educational practice. AAC involves attempts to study and, when necessary, compensate for temporary or permanent impairments, activity limitations, and participation restrictions of individuals with severe disorders of speech-language production and/or comprehension.

Modes of AAC

Unaided AAC. Unaided AAC methods, such as sign language or gestural cueing systems, require no external device. American Sign Language (ASL) is a complex visual-spatial language that is used by the Deaf community in the United States and the English-speaking parts of Canada (Humphries & Padden, 2004). It is a linguistically complete and natural language. ASL encompasses hand gestures, facial expression, and the use of the space surrounding the signer to aid in the description of places and persons. Many signs represent ideas and are therefore iconic, using a visual image to represent a specific idea (Riekehof, 1987). A number of manual sign systems, including ASL, also have been used by individuals with severe communication disorders, but no hearing impairment (Beukelman & Mirenda, 2005).

American Indian Hand Talk (Amer-Ind) is a basic hand signal code developed as long ago as the Asian migration to the Americas, in order to accommodate the lack of a common tongue among the hundreds of Native American tribes (Skelly, 1979). Nearly all signals can either be performed one-handed or adapted for one-handed execution. According to Santo Pietro and Goldfarb (1995), Amer-Ind may be useful for adults with apraxia of speech who retain typical symbolism, intact auditory reception of language, and adequate motoric competence.

Raymer, McHose, and Graham (2010) reviewed literature examining the effects of gesture as a modality to promote reorganization to improve verbal production in AOS and anomia. They found that gestural facilitation effects are strongest in individuals with moderate AOS. Several factors appear to mitigate the effects of gestural facilitation for verbal production, including severe AOS and semantic anomia. Severe limb apraxia, which often accompanies severe AOS, appears to be amenable to gestural treatment, providing improvements in gesture use for communication when verbal production gains are not evident.

Unaided AAC requires a certain level of motor control to produce signs or gestures, which may contraindicate its use for individuals with limb apraxia. This method of AAC has the advantage of speed, portability, and access to a wide number of messages.

Aided AAC—Light Technology. Aided AAC involves an external component for communication, using symbols or voice output. Light technology involves little to no technology or electronic output, but requires external aids. These may include alphabet boards, communication books, and programs such as the *Picture Exchange Communication System* (PECS) (Frost & Bondy, 1998, 2002). Light technology does not provide voice output, and requires a communication partner to interpret the messages that the AAC user selects.

Aided AAC—High Technology. Devices classified as high technology may range from a stand-alone device with voice output to a computer operating with communication software. A dedicated communication device may also be able to interface with a computer and perform environmental control functions. The voice output provided by high technology has advantages over light technology, especially for individuals with more severe disabilities or gestural impairment. Improvements in memory capacity, processing speeds, and battery life yield new generations of lighter and more powerful devices.

Types of displays. There are two primary methods of displaying symbols for communication on AAC devices: fixed (or static) and dynamic displays. In fixed displays, pages or overlays containing symbols or photographs are set up on a board or on a simple voice output communication aid. Simple fixed-display AAC devices are relatively inexpensive, and permit recording a variety of voices easily. Disadvantages include the dependence on others to create and change the symbol overlays, the limited number of symbols available at one time, and the limited number of possible messages (Wilkinson & Hennig, 2007).

In dynamic displays, a modified computer runs communication software. Symbols correspond to words, phrases, and sentences via digitized voice. There can be links to different pages of symbols, activated via a navigation button on the device. The AAC user is not reliant on someone else to change an overlay to access additional vocabulary or messages (Wilkinson & Hennig, 2007).

Roles of AAC as a Communication Mode. The primary role of AAC is to enhance or augment the expressive language skills of individuals who have severe communication impairments. The range of available AAC options makes it useful for a variety of language impairments. AAC may also serve to reduce challenging behaviors such as aggression, self-injurious behaviors, or behaviors resulting from frustration.

CASE DESCRIPTION 1

A patient with apraxia of speech who also had mild aphasia was a retired chemist who, along with thousands of other professionals, worked on the making of the first atomic bomb during World War II (the Manhattan Project). His assignment was to select, from books already in his possession, material relating to the Manhattan Project, rehearse it with his wife at home, and then present it orally to the author during the therapy session. In this way, he was practicing with his wife's help, away from the clinical setting, to help overcome his articulation and prosody problems resulting from the apraxia of speech and his word-finding difficulty caused by the aphasia.

To boot, the author learned a great deal from this erudite gentleman in the process of the assignment. For example, the patient mentioned that although he sensed that his specific area of chemistry was making a contribution to something of major importance, he did not know the nature of the finished product. He had learned about the A-bomb via a memo circulated after the bomb was dropped on Hiroshima. In this way, the Manhattan Project, with thousands of people involved, was able to maintain its secrecy and prevent leaks. To the end, only a handful of people knew its ultimate goal. Throughout this entire narrative, the patient maintained a consistent and considerable improvement in articulation, prosody, and word-finding.

CASE DESCRIPTION 2

A gregarious and generous man invited the author to visit at any time, indicating that he had a "Scandro consterble." His attempt to say, "Castro convertible," which is now a part of our informal battery to differentiate apraxia of speech from dysarthria, reveals some preserved phonological rules, as well as ways to differentiate two motor speech disorders. Replacing a consonant singleton (e.g., the /k/ in "Castro") with a consonant cluster (/sk/) occurs in apraxia of speech, but not in dysarthria, where consonant clusters are likely to be simplified. In addition, changing the "str" in "Castro" to "ndr" in "Scandro" indicates that alveolar placement (for both /st/ and /nd/) and manner features (/st/ sounds are both voiceless and /nd/ sounds are both voiced) are observed in his phonemic approaches to the target sound.

CASE DESCRIPTION 3

(Arroyo, Goldfarb, & Sands, in press) GR, a 63-year-old left-handed native English-speaking man with a high school education, presented with severe aphasia and apraxia of speech. He had a cerebral hemorrhage and seizures following aortic valve replacement and removal of an aortic aneurysm 2 years and 8 months before the current treatment. His hearing, bilaterally, and vision with corrective lenses were assessed as within normal limits. Speech and language assessment indicated unintelligible utterances with some appropriate gestures, and severely limited reading and writing abilities. Auditory comprehension was moderately impaired, but adequate for indicating basic needs with gestures and facial expressions.

Clinical intervention focused on caretaker (GR's wife) training in the use of an augmentative-alternative communication device at the clinic and at home. The AAC device selected for intervention was the LEO, manufactured by Tobii ATI. The LEO was selected for its portability (since the participant was ambulatory) and ease of use and programming. The LEO uses recorded, digitized voice output, and is accessed via direct selection by pressing on picture overlays designed for the individual user. Using Garrett and Beukelman's (1992) Assessment of Capabilities and Communicator Type, the participant was identified as a "specific-need communicator" with the primary need of saying names of family members. Two overlays were designed for the AAC device, one with basic messages such as "coffee please" and one with family members' names, with photographs accompanying the written names and messages.

The goals of caretaker training were to provide opportunities for GR to use AAC to initiate conversation and to help him to use AAC to respond, by pausing long enough, focusing his attention, and using such nonvocal cues as an expectant facial expression. The clinicians also instructed the caretaker to limit yes/no questions and to ask open-ended questions wherever possible. For example, she was to ask, "What do you want to drink?" instead of, "Do you want coffee?" The caretaker used data sheets to record initiations and responses using the AAC device, as well as any vocalized attempts that accompanied the use of the device. We met with GR and his spouse weekly to collect data sheets, review procedures, and address any questions or concerns.

We learned that it is important to persevere with the program, even if early indications are not encouraging. In the first 14 of the 20 data collection dates, we did not observe much change in the number of times GR initiated or responded using the AAC device. However, beginning with recording session 15 and for the 5 sessions that followed, GR's successful attempts to initiate and respond increased from an average of about 5 to an average of more than 30. He also used the AAC device, independently and without instruction, to press on the photos of family members and repeat the recorded name.

Discussion Questions: Theory

1. What are the stages of planning and programming for speech?

2. Take and justify the position that apraxia of speech is a speech disorder or that it is a language disorder.

3. How is apraxia of speech different from literal or phonemic paraphasia?

4. How is apraxia of speech different from dysarthria?

5. What is the timing problem in apraxia of speech?

Discussion Questions: Therapy

1. How can the same informal test be used for apraxia of speech and dysarthria, and how will the responses differ?

2. What general principles underlie therapy for apraxia of speech?

3. Does therapy for apraxia of speech work? For whom?

4. Describe one specific therapy in detail.

5. What are some facilitators used in treating apraxia of speech?

Assignment: Write a multiple-choice question with five options. Explain why the key option is correct, and why the distractors or decoys are incorrect. Avoid using forms such as, "All of the following are (in)correct *except*" in the stem, and "All (or none) of the above" in the options.

Example: Which of the following characterizes apraxia of speech more than dysarthria?

a. Affects respiration, phonation, resonation, articulation, and prosody
b. Influenced by automaticity, communicative context, or linguistic variables
c. Distortion errors
d. Errors of simplification
e. Consistent errors

The correct answer is *b*: Severity of apraxia of speech can vary according to linguistic criteria. *a* is incorrect because dysarthria, not apraxia, affects all aspects of the speech effector system; *c* is incorrect because apraxia of speech results in substitution, not distortion errors; *d* is incorrect because consonant clusters may replace consonant singletons in apraxia, but clusters will be reduced in dysarthria; *e* is incorrect because errors are consistent in dysarthria and inconsistent in apraxia of speech.

References

Aichert, I., & Ziegler, W. (2008). Learning a syllable from its parts: Cross-syllabic generalisation effects in patients with apraxia of speech. *Aphasiology, 22*, 1216–1229.

Ardila, A. (1992). Phonological transformations in conduction aphasia. *Journal of Psycholinguistic Research, 21*, 473–484.

Aronson, A. (1990). *Clinical voice disorders*. New York, NY: Thieme.

Arroyo, C., Goldfarb, R., Cahill, D., & Schoepflin, J. (2010). AAC interventions: Case study of in-utero stroke. *Journal of Speech-Language Pathology and Applied Behavior Analysis, 5*, 32–47.

Arroyo, C., Goldfarb, R., & Sands, E. (in press). Caregiver use in an AAC intervention for severe aphasia. *Journal of Speech-Language Pathology and Applied Behavior Analysis*.

American Speech-Language-Hearing Association. (2005). Roles and responsibilities of speech-language pathologists with respect to augmentative and alternative communication: Position statement. Retrieved January 7, 2011 from http://www.asha.org/docs/html/PS2005-00113.html.

Aten, J., Johns, D., & Darley, F. (1971). Auditory perception of sequenced words in apraxia of speech. *Journal of Speech and Hearing Research, 14*, 131–143.

Austermann, H., Shannon, N., Robin, D., Maas, E., Ballard, K., & Schmidt, R. (2008). Effects of feedback frequency and timing on acquisition, retention, and transfer of speech skills in acquired apraxia of speech. *Journal of Speech, Language, and Hearing Research, 51*, 1088–1113.

Avent, J. (2004). Reciprocal scaffolding treatment for aphasia. *Neurophysiology and Neurogenic Speech and Language Disorders, 14*(2). (Special Interest Division 2 Newsletter, 15–18). Rockville, MD: American Speech-Language-Hearing Association.

Ballard, K. J., Varley, R., & Kendall, D. (2010). Promising approaches to treatment of apraxia of speech: Preliminary evidence and directions for the future. *Neurophysiology and Neurogenic Speech and Language Disorders, 20*(3). (Special Interest Division 2 Newsletter, 87–93). Rockville, MD: American Speech-Language-Hearing Association.

Bartle, C., Goozee, J., & Murdoch, B. (2007). Preliminary evidence of silent articulatory attempts and starters in acquired apraxia of speech: A case study. *Journal of Medical Speech-Language Pathology, 15*, 207–222.

Bartle-Meyer, C., Carly, J., Goozee, J., & Murdoch, B. (2009). Kinematic investigation of lingual movement in words of increasing length in acquired apraxia of speech. *Clinical Linguistics and Phonetics, 23*, 93–121.

Benson, D. F., & Ardila, A. (1996). *Aphasia: A clinical perspective*. New York, NY: Oxford University Press.

Beukelman, D., Fager, S., Ball, L., & Dietz, A. (2007). AAC for adults with acquired neurological conditions: A review. *Augmentative and Alternative Communication, 23*, 230–242.

Beukelman, D., & Mirenda, P. (2005). *Augmentative and alternative communication: Management of severe communication impairments* (3rd ed.). Baltimore, MD: Brookes.

Boles, L. (1998). Conducting conversation: A case study using the spouse in aphasia treatment. *Neurophysiology and Neurogenic Speech and Language Disorders, 8*(3). (Special Interest Division 2 Newsletter, 24–31). Rockville, MD: American Speech-Language-Hearing Association.

Burns, M., & Canter, G. (1977). Phonemic behavior of aphasic patients with posterior cerebral lesions. *Brain and Language, 4*, 492–507.

Dabul, B. (1979). *Apraxia battery for adults*. Tigard, OR: CC Publications.

Dabul, B., & Bollier, B. (1976). Therapeutic approaches to apraxia. *Journal of Speech and Hearing Disorders, 41*, 268–276.

Darley, F. (1964). *Diagnosis and appraisal of communicative disorders*. Englewood Cliffs, NJ: Prentice-Hall.

Darley, F. (1982). *Aphasia*. Philadelphia, PA: Saunders.

Darley, F., Aronson, A., & Brown, J. (1975). *Motor speech disorders*. Philadelphia, PA: Saunders.

Davis, C., Farias, D., & Baynes, K. (2009). Implicit phoneme manipulation for the treatment of apraxia of speech and co-occurring aphasia. *Aphasiology, 23*, 503–528.

Deal, J. (1974). Consistency and adaptation in apraxia of speech. *Journal of Communication Disorders, 7*, 135–140.

Deal, J., & Darley, F. (1972). The influence of linguistic and situational variables on phonemic accuracy in apraxia of speech. *Journal of Speech and Hearing Research, 15*, 639–653.

Deal, J., & Florance, C. (1978). Modification of the eight-step continuum for treatment of apraxia of speech in adults. *Journal of Speech and Hearing Disorders, 43*, 89–95.

Deutsch, S. (1981). Oral form identification as a measure of cortical sensory dysfunction, in apraxia of speech and aphasia. *Journal of Communication Disorders, 14*, 65–73.

Deutsch, S. (1984). Prediction of site of lesion from speech apraxic error patterns. In J. Rosenbek, M. McNeil, & A. Aronson (Eds.), *Apraxia of speech: Physiology, acoustics, linguistics management* (pp. 113–134). San Diego, CA: College Hill Press.

DiSimoni, F. (1989). *Comprehensive apraxia test* (CAT). Dalton, PA: Praxis House.

DiSimoni, F., & Darley, F. (1977). Effect on phoneme duration control through utterance-length conditions in an apractic patient. *Journal of Speech and Hearing Disorders, 42*, 257–264.

Duffy, J. R. (2005). *Motor speech disorders: Substrates, differential diagnosis, and management* (2nd ed.). St. Louis, MO: Elsevier Mosby.

Duffy, J., Peach, R., & Strand, E. (2007). Progressive apraxia of speech and a sign of motor neuron disease. *American Journal of Speech-Language Pathology, 16*, 198–208.

Dunlop, J., & Marquardt, T. (1977). Linguistic and articulatory aspects of single word production in apraxia of speech. *Cortex, 13*, 17–29.

Dworkin, J. (1991). *Motor speech disorders: A treatment guide.* St. Louis, MO: Mosby.

Dworkin, J., Abkarian, G., & Johns, D. (1988). Apraxia of speech: The effectiveness of a treatment regimen. *Journal of Speech and Hearing Disorders, 53*, 280–294.

Freed, D. (2000). *Motor speech disorders: Diagnosis and treatment.* Clifton Park, NY: Delmar Cengage Learning.

Frost, L. A., & Bondy, A. S. (1998). The picture exchange communication system. *Seminars in Speech and Language, 19*, 373–389.

Frost, L. A., & Bondy, A. S. (2002). *The picture exchange communication system training manual* (2nd ed.). Newark, NJ: Pyramid Education Products.

Garrett, K. L. & Beukelman, D. L. (1992). Augmentative communication approaches for persons with severe aphasia. In K. M. Yorkston (Ed.), *Augmentative communication in the medical setting* (pp. 245–337). Tuscon, AZ: Communication Skill Builders.

Goldfarb, R. (2006). An atheoretical discipline. In R. Goldfarb (Ed.), *Ethics: A case study from fluency* (pp. 117–137). San Diego, CA: Plural Publishing, Inc.

Halpern, H., Darley, F., & Brown, J. (1973). Differential language and neurologic characteristics in cerebral involvement. *Journal of Speech and Hearing Disorders, 38*, 162–173.

Hardison, D., Marquardt, T., & Peterson, H. (1977). Effects of selected linguistic variables on apraxia of speech. *Journal of Speech and Hearing Research, 20*, 334–345.

Hecaen, H. (1972). *Introduction a la neuropsychologie* [Introduction to neuropsychology]. Paris, France: Larousse.

Helm, N., & Barresi, B. (1980). Voluntary control of involuntary utterances: A treatment approach for severe aphasia. In R. Brookshire (Ed.), *Clinical aphasiology conference proceedings* (pp. 308–315). Minneapolis, MN: BRK Publishers.

Hill, A., Theodoros, D., Russell, T., & Ward, E. (2009). Using telerehabilitation to assess apraxia of speech in adults. *International Journal of Language and Communication Disorders, 44*, 731–747.

Hillis, A., Work, M., Barker, P., Jacobs, M., Breese, E., & Maurer, K. (2004). Re-examining the brain regions crucial for orchestrating speech articulation. *Brain, 127*, 1479–1487.

Hough, M., & Johnson, R. K. (2009). Use of AAC to enhance linguistic communication skills in an adult with chronic severe aphasia. *Aphasiology, 23*, 965–976.

Hough, M., & Klich, R. (1998). Lip EMG activity during vowel production in apraxia of speech: Phrase context and word length effects. *Journal of Speech-Language-Hearing Research, 41*, 786–801.

Humphries, T., & Padden, C. (2004). *Learning American Sign Language* (2nd ed.). Boston, MA: Pearson Education, Inc.

Jacks, A. (2008). Bite block vowel production in apraxia of speech. *Journal of Speech, Language, and Hearing Research, 51*, 898–913.

Jacks, A., Mathes, K., & Marquardt, T. (2010). Vowel acoustics in adults with apraxia of speech. *Journal of Speech, Language, and Hearing Research, 53*, 61–74.

Johns, D., & Darley, F. (1970). Phonemic variability in apraxia of speech. *Journal of Speech and Hearing Research, 13*, 556–583.

Kagan, A., Black, S., Duchan, J., Simmons-Mackie, N., & Square, P. (2001). Training volunteers as conversation partners using "supported conversation for adults with aphasia" (SCA): A controlled trial. *Journal of Speech, Language, and Hearing Research, 44*, 624–638.

Kahn, H. J., Stannard, T., & Skinner, J. (1998). The use of words versus nonwords in the treatment of apraxia of speech: A case study. *Neurophysiology and Neurogenic Speech and Language Disorders, 8*(3). (Special Interest Division 2 Newsletter, 5–10). Rockville, MD: American Speech-Language-Hearing Association.

Kangas, K., & Lloyd, L. (2006). Augmentative and alternative communication. In N. Anderson & G. Shames (Eds.), *Human communication disorders: An introduction* (pp. 436–470). Boston, MA: Allyn & Bacon.

Katz, W. F., & McNeil, M. R. (2010). Studies of articulatory feedback treatment for apraxia of speech based on electromagnetic articulography. *Neurophysiology and Neurogenic Speech and Language Disorders, 20*(3). (Special Interest Division 2 Newsletter, 73–79). Rockville, MD: American Speech-Language-Hearing Association.

Keith, R., & Aronson, A. (1975). Singing as therapy for apraxia of speech and aphasia: Report of a case. *Brain and Language, 2*, 483.

Keith, R., & Thomas, J. (1989). *Speech practice manual for dysarthria, apraxia, and other disorders of articulation.* Philadelphia, PA: Decker.

Keller, E. (1984). Simplification and gesture reduction in phonological disorders of apraxia and aphasia. In J. Rosenbek, M. McNeil, & A. Aronson (Eds.), *Apraxia of speech: Physiology, acoustics, linguistics, management* (pp. 221–256). San Diego, CA: College Hill Press.

Kent, R., & Rosenbek, J. (1983). Acoustic patterns of apraxia of speech. *Journal of Speech and Hearing Research, 26*, 231–249.

Klich, R., Ireland, J., & Weidner, W. (1979). Articulatory and chronological aspects of consonant substitution in apraxia of speech. *Cortex, 15*, 451–470.

Laganaro, M. (2008). Is there a syllable frequency effect in aphasia or in apraxia of speech or both? *Aphasiology, 22*, 1191–1200.

LaPointe, L., & Horner, J. (1976). Repeated trials of words by patients with neurogenic phonological selection-sequencing impairment (apraxia of speech). In R. Brookshire (Ed.), *Clinical aphasiology conference proceedings* (pp. 261–277). Minneapolis, MN: BRK Publishers.

LaPointe, L., & Johns, D. (1975). Some phonetic characteristics in apraxia of speech. *Journal of Communication Disorders, 8*, 259–269.

LaPointe, L., & Katz, R. (1998). Neurogenic disorders of speech. In G. Shames, E. Wiig, & W. Secord (Eds.), *Human communication disorders: An introduction* (pp. 434–471). Needham Heights, MA: Allyn & Bacon.

LaPointe, L., & Wertz, R. (1974). Oral-movement abilities and articulatory characteristics of brain-injured adults. *Perceptual and Motor Skills, 39*, 39–46.

Li, E., & Williams, S. (1990). Repetition deficits in three aphasic syndromes. *Journal of Communication Disorders, 23*, 77–88.

Ludlow, C., Connor, N., & Bassich, C. (1987). Speech timing in Parkinson's and Huntington's disease. *Brain and Language, 32*, 195–214.

Maas, E. (2010). Conditions of practice and feedback in treatment for apraxia of speech. *Neurophysiology and Neurogenic Speech and Language Disorders, 20*(3). (Special Interest Division 2 Newsletter, 80–86). Rockville, MD: American Speech-Language-Hearing Association.

Marquardt, T., Reinhart, J., & Peterson, H. (1979). Markedness analysis of phonemic substitution errors in apraxia of speech. *Journal of Communication Disorders, 12*, 481–494.

Marquardt, T., & Sussman, H. (1984). The elusive lesion—Apraxia of speech link in Broca's aphasia. In J. Rosenbek, M. McNeil, & A. Aronson (Eds.), *Apraxia of speech: Physiology, acoustics, linguistics, management* (pp. 91–112). San Diego, CA: College Hill Press.

McNeil, M., Liss, J., Tseng, C., & Kent, R. (1990). Effects of speech rate on the absolute and relative timing of apraxic and conduction aphasic sentence production. *Brain and Language, 38*, 135–158.

McNeil, M., Weismer, G., Adams, S., & Mulligan, M. (1990). Oral structure nonspeech motor control in normal, dysarthric, aphasic, and apraxic speakers: Isometric force and static position control. *Journal of Speech and Hearing Research, 33*, 255–268.

Nicolosi, L., Harryman, E., & Kresheck, J. (2005). *Terminology of communication disorders* (5th ed.). Baltimore, MD: Williams & Wilkins.

Odell, K., McNeil, M. R., Rosenbek, J. C., & Hunter, L. (1990). Perceptual characteristics of consonant production by apraxic speakers. *Journal of Speech and Hearing Disorders, 55,* 345–359.

Odell, K., McNeil, M. R., Rosenbek, J. C., & Hunter, L. (1991). Perceptual characteristics of vowel and prosody production in apraxic, aphasic, and dysarthric speakers. *Journal of Speech, Language, and Hearing Research, 34,* 67–80.

Ogar, J., Willock, S., Baldo, J., Wilkins, D., Ludy, C., & Dronkers, N. (2006). Clinical and anatomical correlates of apraxia of speech. *Brain and Language, 97,* 343–350.

Porch, B. (1981). *Porch index of communicative ability.* Palo Alto, CA: Consulting Psychologists Press.

Raymer, A. M., McHose, B., & Graham, K. (2010). Gestural facilitation treatment of apraxia of speech. *Neurophysiology and Neurogenic Speech and Language Disorders, 20*(3). (Special Interest Division 2 Newsletter, 94–98). Rockville, MD: American Speech-Language-Hearing Association.

Rickchof, L. L. (1987). *The joy of signing* (2nd ed.). Springfield, MO: Gospel Publishing House.

Robin, D., Bean, C., & Folkins, J. (1989). Lip movement in apraxia of speech. *Journal of Speech and Hearing Research, 32,* 512–523.

Robin, D., Jacks, A., Hageman, C., Clark, H., & Woodworth, G. (2008). Visuomotor tracking abilities of speakers with apraxia of speech or conduction aphasia. *Brain and Language, 106,* 98–106.

Rosenbek, J. (1984). Treatment for apraxia of speech in adults. In W. Perkins (Ed.), *Dysarthria and apraxia* (pp. 49–56). New York, NY: Thieme-Stratton.

Rosenbek, J. (1985). Treating apraxia of speech. In D. Johns (Ed.), *Clinical management of neurogenic communicative disorders* (pp. 267–312). Boston, MA: Little, Brown.

Rosenbek, J., Hansen, R., Baughman, C., & Lemme, M. (1974). Treatment of developmental apraxia of speech: A case study. *Language Speech and Hearing Services in the Schools, 5,* 13–22.

Rosenbek, J., Kent, R., & LaPointe, L. (1984). Apraxia of speech: An overview and some perspectives. In J. Rosenbek, M. McNeil, & A. Aronson (Eds.), *Apraxia of speech: Physiology, acoustics, linguistics, management* (pp. 1–72). San Diego, CA: College Hill Press.

Rosenbek, J., Lemme, M., Ahern, M., Harris, E., & Wertz, R. (1973). A treatment for apraxia of speech in adults. *Journal of Speech and Hearing Disorders, 38,* 462–472.

Rosenbek, J., Wertz, R., & Darley, F. (1973). Oral sensation and perception in apraxia of speech. *Journal of Speech and Hearing Research, 16,* 22–36.

Santo Pietro, M. J., & Goldfarb, R. (1995). *Techniques for aphasia rehabilitation generating effective treatment* (TARGET). Vero Beach, FL: The Speech Bin.

Schuell, H., Jenkins, J., & Jimenez-Pabon, E. (1964). *Aphasia in adults: Diagnosis, prognosis, and treatment.* New York, NY: Hoeber Medical Division, Harper.

Seddoh, S., Robin, D., Sim, H., Hageman, C., Moon, J., & Folkins, J. (1996). Speech timing in apraxia of speech versus conduction aphasia. *Journal of Speech and Hearing Research, 39,* 590–603.

Shane, H., & Darley, F. (1978). The effect of auditory rhythmic stimulation on articulatory accuracy in apraxia of speech. *Cortex, 14,* 444–450.

Shane, H., & Sauer, M. (1986). *Augmentative and alternative communication.* Austin, TX: Pro-Ed.

Shankweiler, D., & Harris, K. (1966). An experimental approach to the problem of articulation in aphasia. *Cortex, 2,* 277–292.

Silverman, F. (1989). *Communication for the speechless.* Englewood Cliffs, NJ: Prentice-Hall.

Skelly, M. (1979). *Amer-Ind gestural code based on universal Americal Indian hand talk.* New York, NY: Elsevier North-Holland.

Skenes, L., & Trullinger, R. (1988). Error patterns during repetition of consonant-vowel-consonant syllables by apraxic speakers. *Journal of Communication Disorders, 21,* 263–269.

Sparks, R. (2008). Melodic intonation therapy. In R. Chapey (Ed.), *Language intervention strategies in aphasia and related neurogenic communication disorders* (5th ed.) (pp. 837–851). Baltimore, MD: Lippincott Williams & Wilkins.

Sparks, R., & Deck, J. (1994). Melodic intonation therapy. In R. Chapey (Ed.), *Language intervention strategies in adult aphasia* (pp. 368–379). Baltimore, MD: Williams & Wilkins.

Sparks, R., & Holland, A. (1976). Method: Melodic intonation therapy for aphasia. *Journal of Speech and Hearing Disorders, 41,* 287–297.

Square, P. (1981). *Auditory perceptual abilities of patients with apraxia of speech* (Unpublished doctoral dissertation). Kent State University, Kent, Ohio.

Square, P., & Martin, R. (1994). The nature and treatment of neuromotor speech disorders in aphasia. In R. Chapey (Ed.), *Language intervention strategies in adult aphasia* (pp. 467–498). Baltimore, MD: Williams & Wilkins.

Square-Storer, P., Darley, F., & Sommers, R. (1988). Nonspeech and speech processing skills in patients with aphasia and apraxia of speech. *Brain and Language, 33*, 65–85.

Square-Storer, P., & Hayden, D. (1989). Prompt treatment. In P. Square-Storer (Ed.), *Acquired apraxia of speech in aphasic adults* (pp. 190–219). London, UK: Erlbaum.

Staiger, A., & Ziegler, W. (2008). Syllable frequency and syllable structure in the spontaneous speech production of patients with apraxia of speech. *Aphasiology, 22*, 1201–1215.

Stevens, E. (1989). Multiple input phoneme therapy. In P. Square-Storer (Ed.), *Acquired apraxia of speech in aphasic adults* (pp. 220–238). London, UK: Erlbaum.

Strand, E., & McNeil, M. (1996). Effects of length and linguistic complexity on temporal acoustic measures in apraxia of speech. *Journal of Speech and Hearing Research, 39*, 1018–1033.

Trost, J. (1970). *Patterns of articulatory deficits in patients with Broca's aphasia* (Unpublished doctoral dissertation). Northwestern University, Chicago, Illinois.

Trost, J., & Canter, G. (1974). Apraxia of speech in patients with Broca's aphasia: A study of phonemic production accuracy and error patterns. *Brain and Language, 1*, 63–79.

Varley, R., Whiteside, S., Windsor, F., & Fisher, H. (2004). Moving up from the segment: A comment on Aichert and Ziegler's syllable frequency and syllable structure in apraxia of speech, *Brain and Language, 88*, 148–159.

Wambaugh, J. (2006). Treatment guidelines for apraxia of speech: Lessons for future research. *Journal of Medical Speech-Language Pathology, 14*, 317–321.

Wambaugh, J. (2010). Sound production treatment for acquired apraxia of speech. *Neurophysiology and Neurogenic Speech and Language Disorders, 20*(3). (Special Interest Division 2 Newsletter, 67–72). Rockville, MD: American Speech-Language-Hearing Association.

Wambaugh, J., Duffy, J., McNeil, M., Robin, D., & Rogers, M. (2006). Treatment guidelines for acquired apraxia of speech: Treatment descriptions and recommendations. *Journal of Medical Speech-Language Pathology, 14*, 35–67.

Wambaugh, J., Kalinyak-Flisger, M., West, J., & Doyle, P. (1998). Effects of treatment for sound errors in apraxia of speech and aphasia. *Journal of Speech-Language-Hearing Research, 41*, 725–743.

Wambaugh, J., & Shuster, L. (2008). The nature and management of neuromotor speech disorders accompanying aphasia. In R. Chapey (Ed.), *Language intervention strategies in aphasia and related neurogenic communication disorders* (pp. 1009–1042). Baltimore, MD: Lippincott Williams and Wilkins.

Warren, R. (1977). Rehearsal for naming in apraxia of speech. In R. Brookshire (Ed.), *Clinical aphasiology: Conference proceedings* (pp. 80–90). Minneapolis, MN: BRK Publishers.

Wertz, R. (1984). Response to treatment in patients with apraxia of speech. In J. Rosenbek, M. McNeil, & A. Aronson (Eds.), *Apraxia of speech: Physiology, acoustics, linguistics, management* (pp. 257–276). San Diego, CA: College Hill Press.

Wertz, R. (1985). Neuropathologies of speech and language: An introduction to patient management. In D. F. Johns (Ed.), *Clinical management of neurogenic communicative disorders* (pp. 1–96). Boston, MA: Little, Brown.

Wertz, R., LaPointe, L., & Rosenbek, J. (1984). *Apraxia of speech in adults.* New York, NY: Grune & Stratton.

Wilkinson, K. & Hennig (2007). The state of research and practice in augmentative and alternative communication for children with developmental/intellectual disabilities. *Mental Retardation and Developmental Disabilities Research Reviews, 13*, 58–69.

Wolk, L. (1986). Marked analysis of consonant error productions in apraxia of speech. *Journal of Communication Disorders, 19*, 133–160.

Yoss, K., & Darley, F. (1974). Therapy in developmental apraxia of speech. *Language, Speech and Hearing Services in the Schools, 5*, 23–31.

Ziegler, W., Aichert, I., & Staiger, A. (2010). Syllable- and rhythm-based approaches in the treatment of apraxia of speech. *Neurophysiology and Neurogenic Speech and Language Disorders, 20*(3). (Special Interest Division 2 Newsletter, 59–66). Rockville, MD: American Speech-Language-Hearing Association.

Ziegler, W., Thelen, A-K., Staiger, A., & Liepold, M. (2008). The domain of phonetic encoding in apraxia of speech: Which sub-lexical units count? *Aphasiology, 22*, 1230–1247.

Glossary

Abstract reasoning: the process of looking at evidence, making inferences, and drawing conclusions

Acetylcholine: the primary neurotransmitter of the PNS and also important in the CNS; cholinergic neurons are concentrated in the reticular formation, the basal forebrain, and the striatum

Action potential: results from charged particles (ions) moving through the cell membranes.

Adequacy: appropriateness of use of the semantic component of language

Afferent: sensory; toward the brain

Agnosia: the inability to recognize people or objects, sounds or voices, even when basic sensory modalities, such as vision and hearing, are intact

Agrammatism: impaired syntax in nonfluent aphasia, characterized by omission of function words and grammatical morphemes

Agraphia: an acquired impairment in the formulation of written language due to brain damage

Alexia: an acquired impairment in reading comprehension due to brain damage

Alternating attention: the capacity for mental flexibility that allows one to shift focus of attention and move between tasks that have different cognitive requirements or require different behavior responses; controls which information will be selectively attended to and incorporates the concept of shifting an established set easily

Alzheimer disease: a dementia identified by problems in language, cognition, visuospatial abilities, behavior, and motor problems in the latter stages

Amyotrophic lateral sclerosis (ALS): progressive degeneration of both upper and lower motor neurons

Aneurysm: swelling or ballooning of an artery

Angular gyrus: lies directly behind the supramarginal gyrus and plays a major role in reading comprehension

Anomia: impairment in naming and word finding; a symptom of all aphasias, not to be confused with the syndrome (collection of symptoms) of anomic aphasia

Anomic aphasia: characterized by fluent, well-articulated, mildly paraphasic, grammatically intact, and somewhat empty speech; outstanding symptom is a naming or word-finding problem that can affect any of the modalities; no difficulty with repetition of words, phrases, and sentences

Anosognosia: lack of awareness of illness and deficits

Aphasia: a multimodality language disturbance (of the person's regular language of communication) due to brain damage; modalities involved are auditory comprehension, reading comprehension, oral expression, and written expression

Apraxia of speech: an articulation and prosody disorder that results from impairment, due to brain damage, of the capacity to order the positioning of the speech musculature and the sequencing of muscle movements for volitional production of phonemes and sequences of phonemes; not accompanied by significant weakness, slowness, or incoordination of these same muscles in reflex and automatic acts

Arcuate fasciculus: connects the association area of the temporal lobe with that of the frontal lobe, that is, Wernicke's area to Broca's area

Arousal: an aspect of consciousness and is the next step above coma, which is a loss of consciousness

Artereovenous malformation (AVM):   congenital communication between arteries and veins, which tend to bleed and cause subarachnoid hemorrhage

Arteries: carry blood away from the heart

Articulation disorder: the atypical production of speech sounds characterized by substitutions, omissions, additions, or distortions that may interfere with intelligibility

ASHA: the American Speech-Language-Hearing Association

Astrocytes: function as connective tissue, providing skeletal support for the brain cells and their processes; contribute to the *blood–brain barrier* by contacting capillary surfaces with their end feet and using tight junctions

Ataxic dysarthria: occurs because of bilateral or generalized damage to the cerebellum; affected muscles tend to be hypotonic, voluntary movements are slow, and the force, range, timing, and direction of movements are inaccurate; for speech production, the important features of cerebellar disease are inaccuracy of movement, slowness of movement, and hypotonia

Attention: observing stimuli in space and holding objects, events, words, or thoughts in one's consciousness

Auditory comprehension deficit: difficulty in the comprehension of spoken language

Automatic speech: verbal stereotypes

Autonomic nervous system (ANS):   contains a sympathetic division and a parasympathetic division

Axon hillock: a cone-shaped region of the cell

Axons: efferent (motor) structures that transmit neural impulses away from the cell body

Basal ganglia: a mass of gray matter that lies deep within the cerebrum and below the cerebral cortex; consist of the caudate nucleus, the globus pallidus, and the putamen; responsible for controlling and stabilizing motor functions and for interpreting sensory information so as to guide and influence motor behavior

Basilar artery: ascends and divides into two *posterior cerebral arteries*; through its branches, the basilar artery also supplies portions of the spinal cord, medulla, pons, midbrain, and cerebellum

BDAE: Boston Diagnostic Aphasia Examination, an aphasia examination using a neuropsychology framework

Bilingual (polyglot) aphasiology: study of whether patients with aphasia who are bilingual or polyglot (multilingual) show equal impairment in the different languages, or better recovery in just one of them

Binswanger disease: infarcts involving the subcortical white matter of both hemispheres

Biopsies: used for analyzing samples of tissue

Bipolar cells: have two processes, one extending from each pole of the body; a peripheral process (dendrite) and a central process (axon)

Blocking: interruption of a train of thought (speech) before completion of the thought or idea; after a period of silence, the patient indicates an inability to recall what he meant to say

Blood: composed of a liquid component called plasma, and solid components made up primarily of red corpuscles, white corpuscles, and platelets

Blood–brain barrier: restricts the movement of certain substances from the blood to the brain through selective permeability

B-mode carotid imaging: used for observing extracranial blood vessels with ultrasound

Borderzone (or extrasylvian area or watershed area):   area of the dominant hemisphere located outside the perisylvian area, in the vascular borderzone between the territory of the middle cerebral artery and the territory of the anterior or posterior cerebral artery; aphasias caused by lesions in the borderzone area include transcortical motor aphasia, transcortical sensory aphasia, and mixed transcortical aphasia (isolation of the speech area)

Brain: composed of the cerebral hemispheres, the basal ganglia, the cerebellum, and the brainstem

Brainstem: an upward extension of the spinal cord as it thrusts upward into the brain between the cerebral hemispheres; in ascending order, consists of the medulla oblongata, the pons, the midbrain (mesencephalon)

Broca's aphasia: nonfluent aphasia characterized by a sparse output of words and sentences, misarticulations, and impaired expressive syntax; speech is laborious and filled with many pauses, and is telegraphic

Broca's area: third frontal convolution of the language-dominant hemisphere (areas 44/45)

Brodmann (1868–1918): a German neurologist who established the numbering system for 52 areas of the cerebral cortex, which remains the universal standard (called Brodmann areas) used today

Bulbar palsy: damage to Cranial Nerves IX, X, XI, and XII; *bulbar* refers to the brainstem

Capillaries: connect the arteries to the veins

Catatonic behavior: marked motor abnormality; either immobility or non-goal-directed excitement, resistance to being moved, posturing, echopraxia, and stereotypical movement

Cell body (also called *perikaryon* or *soma*): consists of protoplasm and cytoplasm; intracellular fluids contain a high concentration of potassium and low concentrations of sodium and chloride; concentrations are reversed in the extracellular fluids, thus creating an electrical current for transmission of neural impulse

Central nervous system (CNS): contains the brain, spinal cord, meninges, ventricles, and blood supply

Central sulcus: divides the brain into anterior and posterior regions

Cerebellar disease: characterized by inaccuracy of movement, slowness of movement, and hypotonia

Cerebellum: located just behind the pons and the medulla at the base of the occipital lobe; right and left hemisphere are connected by the vermis

Cerebral angiography: used for observing the veins and arteries of the brain and brainstem

Cerebral cortex: covers the cerebrum and is composed of many prominent sulci or fissures and gyri; in each hemisphere is partitioned into the frontal, parietal, temporal, and occipital lobes

Cerebral hemispheres: composed of a left and a right hemisphere and connected by the corpus callosum

Cerebrospinal fluid: produced by the choroid plexus within each ventricle, fills all the ventricles

Cerebrovascular accident (CVA): commonly known as a stroke; depriving the brain of oxygen and circulation, thus causing brain damage

Cerebrum: the largest part of the brain; made up of the two cerebral hemispheres and the basal ganglia

Circle of Willis: formed in the brainstem by the joining together of the two internal carotid arteries and the two vertebral arteries

Circumlocutions: can be empty speech, a description of the use or function of the item to be named, or use of a word that is correct semantically and syntactically but is not in common usage

Circumstantiality: speech that is very indirect and delayed in reaching its goal; includes the intrusion of many tedious details; differs from poverty of content and derailment in that the goal of the communication is eventually reached by the speaker

Clanging: speech in which sounds govern word choice, so that intelligibility is impaired; includes rhyming and puns

Closed head injury: a nonpenetrating injury where the meninges remain intact

Cognitive functioning: orientation, arousal, attention, speed of processing, memory, abstract reasoning, and visuospatial perception

Collagen fibers: compose connective tissue throughout the body, and in the brain form *fibroblasts* and other cells that form an *endoneurial membrane*

Coma: a state of profound unconsciousness

Common subclavian arteries: have branches called the vertebral arteries, which ascend into the brain

Communication disorder: an impairment in the ability to receive, send, process, and comprehend concepts of verbal, nonverbal, and graphic symbol systems

Comprehensibility: listener understanding of speech in a communicative setting

Computed tomography (CT):   relies on the penetration of X-ray beams processed through computerized mathematics, which provides a tomographic (pictures of body section) image of the brain without physical invasion of the body

Conduction aphasia: fluent, verbal, and phonemic paraphasic speech, usually less severe than that in Wernicke's aphasia; auditory and reading comprehension are relatively good, written expression is defective; repetition of words, phrases, and sentences is disproportionately severely impaired

Confabulation: telling tall tales; associated with confused language

Constraint-induced language therapy: requiring only verbal responses, with all compensating measures such as gesturing or drawing suppressed

Constructional impairment: impaired visuospatial ability associated with dementia

Contact injury: occurs when the head collides with another object

Context: the information received or expressed within the whole communicative setting

Contrecoup: injury to the brain on the opposite side from the point of impact

Convergent circuit: has two patterns of connections; postsynaptic neuron receives impulses from several diverged fibers of the same presynaptic nerve cell, or impulses from different nerve cells converge on one postsynaptic nerve cell

Convergent semantic behavior: logical conclusions or necessities

Corpora quadrigemina: located in the midbrain; synapses for vision (two superior colliculi) and hearing (two inferior colliculi)

Corpus callosum: a mass of white matter; passes neuronal information from one cerebral hemisphere to the other

Corpus striatum: consists of the caudate nucleus and the lentiform nucleus

Cortical dementia: language components affected according to stage of the disorder; mild stage—phonologic, morphologic, and syntactic components are all intact, while the semantic and pragmatic components begin to deteriorate; moderate stage—phonologic component is intact, while the morphologic and syntactic components begin to deteriorate, and the semantic and pragmatic components further deteriorate; advanced stage—phonologic component begins to deteriorate, along with a further deterioration of the morphologic and syntactic components, and a still greater deterioration of the semantic and pragmatic components; language impairment does not stand out in relation to other abilities

Coup: brain trauma at the point of impact

Creutzfeldt-Jacob disease: a transmissible spongiform encephalopathy, resulting in cortical and subcortical abnormalities; the bovine form is known as "mad cow" disease

Crossed aphasia: a language disorder that follows damage to the nondominant cerebral hemisphere

Cyst: formed when astrocytes seal the cavity after large lesions

Cytoplasm: composed of a watery substance and protein molecules, and is enclosed within the cell membrane

Delusion: acute confusional state

Dementia: etiology is brain damage involving both hemispheres; mostly progressive; cognitive abilities affected in direct proportion to mild, moderate, and advanced stages

Dendrites: numerous short projections that carry neural impulses to the cell body

Derailment (loss of goal):   a pattern of spontaneous speech in which ideas slip off the track in an obliquely related manner or in an unrelated manner; errors are similar to tangentiality, but occur in the spontaneous conversational mode

Diadochokinesia: ability to perform rapidly alternating movements

Diencephalon: composed of the epithalamus, dorsal thalamus, subthalamus, and hypothalamus

Diffuse: involving both hemispheres of the brain

Diffuse axonal injury: shearing, stretching, or tearing of nerve fibers

Distractible speech: a tendency to change topic inappropriately in response to extraneous stimuli present in the environment, an object in the room, and so forth

Divergent circuit: amplifies an impulse when an impulse from a single presynaptic cell activates several postsynaptic cells

Divergent semantic behavior: logical alternatives or possibilities

Divided attention: the ability to respond simultaneously to multiple tasks or multiple task demand; two or more behavioral responses may be required, or two or more kinds of stimuli may need to be monitored

Dominant frontal (anterior) agraphia: associated with the nonfluent aphasias and hemiplegia; output is limited to single, substantive words with spelling errors; short grammatical words are omitted in sentences; mechanics of writing are large and messy

Dominant parietal-temporal (posterior) agraphia: associated with the fluent aphasias; output contains many spelling errors and verbal paragraphia (semantic); sentences are wordy, empty; mechanics of writing are adequate; no hemiplegia

Dopamine: projections are the mesostriatal (midbrain and striatum) and mesocortical (midbrain to cortex) systems (we are more interested in the first group); mesostriatal projections are dopaminergic cells from the substantia nigra to the putamen and caudate nucleus of the basal ganglia; degeneration of the substantia nigra reduces production and transmission of dopamine and is associated with Parkinson disease

Dorsal spinal cord: posterior portion; conducts sensory neurons

Dysarthria: a collective name for a group of speech disorders that result from disturbances in muscular control over the speech mechanism due to damage of the central or peripheral nervous system

Dysphagia: pain or difficulty in the act of swallowing

Echolalia: echoing what is heard

Edema: swelling

Efferent: motor nerves; going from the brain or spinal cord to the muscles

Electroencephalogram (EEG):   used for obtaining a graphic record of the electrical activity of the cerebral cortex

Electromyography: used for recording the electrical activities of muscles

Embolism (cerebral):   occlusion of an artery by a fragment of a blood clot or foreign substance carried in the bloodstream

Emotion: includes mood and affect, where mood indicates the inner and subjective feelings of the patient, and affect is the outward expression of emotion

Endoneurium: wraps around a peripheral axon and merges with *neurilemma*

Ependymal cells: form the inner surface of the ventricles; the choroid plexus, which secretes cerebrospinal fluid, consists of vascular pia surrounded by an epithelial layer of ependymal cells

Event-related potential (ERP):   a stimulus played into a participant's ear will evoke a response at the cortex that will be recorded by these electrodes; each resulting waveform shows the averaged electrical activity recorded for one second after the presentation of a word; the response to a given stimulus is described in terms of the negative and positive peaks and their latencies

Excitability: a cell's response to various stimuli and conversion of this response into a nerve impulse or action potential

Excitatory postsynaptic potential (EPSP):   refers to a lowered membrane potential in the postsynaptic neuron, which creates an environment for a new impulse; the opposite is true for *inhibitory postsynaptic potential (IPSP)*

Executive dysfunction: difficulty in setting a goal, planning a course to achieve it, holding the plan in working memory while executing it, sequencing the steps in the plan, initiating taking those steps and shifting between them, monitoring progress for both pace and quality, regulating attention and emotional responses to challenges that arise, making flexible changes in the plan as needed, and evaluating the outcome for use of the plan in a subsequent similar activity

Extrapyramidal system: responsible for regulating the muscle tone required for posture and for changing position

Facial nerve: CN VII, Motor, Sensory, and Special Sensory; receives sensory impulses from the anterior two-thirds of the tongue (taste), soft palate (taste), and nasopharynx (taste), and sends motor impulses to the face, lips, and the stapedius muscle of the middle ear

Fissures (sulci):   grooves in the surface of the cerebrum

Fluency disorder: an interruption in the flow of speaking characterized by atypical rate, rhythm, and repetitions in sounds, syllables, words, and phrases; may be accompanied by excessive tension, struggle behavior, and secondary mannerisms

Fluent aphasia: usually caused by damage to posterior portions of the language-dominant side of the brain

Focal: involving one hemisphere of the brain or any part of one hemisphere

Focused attention: the ability to respond discretely to specific visual, auditory, or tactile stimuli; does not imply purposefulness of response

Foramen magnum: a large opening at the base of the skull that serves as a boundary between the medulla oblongata and the spinal cord

Formants: peaks of resonance in the vocal tract

Friedreich ataxia: characteristics include ataxic dysarthria as the most frequently occurring type, followed by spastic dysarthria, and then by scattered other types; the most common mixture includes ataxic and spastic components

Frontal alexia: associated with nonfluent aphasia; ability to understand single words more easily than sentences

Frontal association area: responsible for initiation and integration of purposeful behavior and for planning and carrying out sequences of volitional movement

Frontal lobe: bounded in the back by the central sulcus and below by the lateral fissure

Functional magnetic resonance imaging (fMRI):   magnetic properties of oxygenated blood are different from those of deoxygenated blood; changes in brain function or physiology are detected and are associated with performance on language, cognitive, sensory, and motor tasks

GABA, or γ-aminobutyric acid: a major neurotransmitter for the CNS, just as acetylcholine is in the periphery; serves as the inhibitory neurotransmitter from the striatum to the globus pallidus and substantia nigra, from the globus pallidus and substantia nigra to the thalamus, and from the Purkinje cells to the deep cerebellar nuclei

Glial cells: means "glue"; support and protect the nerve cells; found in the gray and white matter of the brain, there are 40 to 50 times as many glial cells as nerve cells; do not generate or transmit nerve impulses

Glioma: a rare and slowly growing neoplastic growth that can affect production of myelin (oligodendroglioma)

Global aphasia: severe impairment in auditory and reading comprehension, and oral and written expression; communication may be limited to verbal stereotypes and automatic speech; lesion involves a widespread area of the perisylvian zone of the dominant hemisphere, affecting all areas whose damage correlates with the aphasias

Glossopharyngeal nerve: CN IX, Motor, Secretomotor, Special Sensory, and Sensory; receives sensory impulses from the posterior one-third of the tongue (taste and sensation) and from the pharynx, and sends motor impulses to the pharynx for dilation, contributing to the elevation and closure of the pharynx and larynx during the act of swallowing

Golgi complexes: responsible for protein secretion and transportation

Golgi type I: nerve cells whose axons leave the gray matter of which they form a part

Golgi type II: cells with short axons which ramify in the gray matter

Granulovacuolar degeneration: fluid-filled cavities containing granular debris that appear within nerve cells

Gyri: elevations or ridges on the surface of the cerebrum

Hematoma: accumulation of blood

Hemiparesis: weakness on one side of the body (less severe than hemiplegia)

Hemiplegia: paralysis on one side of the body (more severe than hemiparesis)

Hemorrhage (cerebral): the rupture of a blood vessel with subsequent bleeding into the brain

Heschl's gyrus: primary auditory cortex; located on the lateral fissure, two-thirds of the way back on the upper surface of the temporal lobe; the cortical center for hearing, responsible for appreciating the meaning of sound (area 41)

Homeostasis: the body's tendency to maintain itself in an essentially healthy state

Huntington disease: a hereditary degenerative disorder affecting movement and cognition

Hyperkinesia: abnormal involuntary movements, usually due to damage in the basal ganglia control circuit, or occasionally in the cerebellar control circuit or other parts of the extrapyramidal system; abnormal involuntary movements are excessive, and their speed can be fast (e.g., chorea) or slow (e.g., dystonia)

Hypoglossal nerve: CN XII; receives sensory and taste impulses from the tongue, and sends motor impulses to the tongue

Hypokinesia: reduction of movements, slowness of movement, limited range of movement, immobility and paucity of movement, rigidity, loss of automatic aspects of movement, and rest tremor

Hypoperfusion: decreased blood flow through an organ

Hypophonia: decreased voice volume

Hypothalamus: controls aspects of emotional behavior (rage and aggression) and aids in the regulation of body temperature, food and water intake, and sexual and sleep behavior

Hypotonia: low muscle tone; flaccidity

Hypoxia: lack of oxygen

Illogicality: speech in which conclusions reached do not follow logically; includes *non sequiturs*, faulty inductive references; does not include delusions

Incoherence: speech that is essentially incomprehensible; at times includes paragrammatism (syntactic confusions, random word choice); this disorder is rare

Indirect activation pathway: the extrapyramidal system

Inertial injury: occurs when the head accelerates and then rapidly decelerates

Infarction: cell death due to lack of oxygen in the brain

Inhibitory postsynaptic potential (IPSP): see *Excitatory postsynaptic potential (EPSP)*

Institutional neurosis: characterized by apathy and sometimes a stereotyped posture and gait; may affect individuals who are institutionalized for two years or longer

Insula: also called Island of Reil, is in the paralimbic area; can be seen if the two borders of the lateral fissure are pulled apart; function of the insula is not clearly defined, but a lesion there can result in aphasia or apraxia of speech

Intelligence: an innate capacity to use one's thought processes

Ischemia: deficient circulation in the brain

Isotope brain scan: involves an injection of an isotope followed by counts of radioactivity over brain areas

Jargon: can be unintelligible words that usually follow the phonological rules of our language (e.g., "freach") or unintelligible words that bear no relationship to the stimulus

Lacunar state: infarcts involving the basal ganglia, thalamus, and internal capsule

Language disorder: impaired comprehension and/or use of spoken, written, and/or other symbol systems; may involve the form of language (phonology, morphology, syntax)

Lateral inhibition: the signal or cellular message is sharpened by inhibiting the adjacent nerve cells

Lee Silverman Voice Treatment (LSVT): a therapy program for Parkinson disease that centers around techniques for improving loudness

Lentiform nucleus: consists of the globus pallidus and putamen

Limb apraxia: motor programming disorder affecting the limbs; different from a language disorder affecting gestural ability

Limbic lobe: situated on the medial surface of the cortex and contains the orbital frontal region, the cingulate gyrus, and the medial portions of the temporal lobe; regulates emotions and behavior

Linguistic competence: the knowledge of syntax, meaning, and sound that makes linguistic performance possible

Linguistic performance: actual acts of speaking and listening, with temporal limitations, and subject to a variety of distractions

Longitudinal cerebral fissure: runs from the front to the back of the brain, separates the two hemispheres

Lower motor neuron disorder: lesions in motor units of the cranial nerves involved in speech (V, VII, IX–X, XII) that innervate the respiratory musculature or to the cranial nerves that innervate the speech musculature; can result in a flaccid dysarthria

Lumbar punctures: used for analyzing a sample of cerebrospinal fluid

Lysosomes: contain enzymes that participate in intracellular digestion

Magnetic resonance imaging (MRI):   uses a powerful magnetic field to alter electrical fields in the brain, which can then be monitored electronically to produce computerized images (slices) of brain tissues; MRI does not use X-ray and does not introduce radioactive material into the patient's body

Medulla: contains nuclei for several of the cranial nerves, and ascending and descending tracts to and from the cortex that are important for the control of speech production

Memory: the mental faculty or power that enables one to retain and to recall, through unconscious associative processes, previously experienced sensations, impressions, ideas, and concepts, and all information that has been consciously learned

Meninges: three layers of tissue (dura, arachnoid, pia) that cover the brain

Microglial cells: multipotential, because they sometimes act as phagocytes (which remove dead neural tissue debris), and at other times as astrocytes or oligodendrocytes; the scavengers of the CNS

Midbrain, or mesencephalon: serves as a way station in the auditory and visual nervous systems; prominent cell groups include the motor nuclei of the trochlear and oculomotor nerves, the red nucleus, and the substantia nigra

MIT: Melodic Intonation Therapy; most effective when used to treat moderate nonfluent aphasia, where language comprehension is better than production

Mitochondria: contain enzymes involved with cellular metabolic energy

Mixed transcortical aphasia (or isolation syndrome):   similar to global aphasia, but these patients can repeat and show echolalia of words, phrases, and sentences; relatively rare

Morphology: the system that governs the structure of words and the construction of word forms

Motor programming (motor planning):   a set of muscle commands that are structured before a movement sequence begins

MTDDA: Minnesota Test for Differential Diagnosis of Aphasia, one of the earliest aphasia batteries

Multiple sclerosis (MS):   most frequent characteristics include a mixture of ataxic and spastic dysarthric components, although each component can be present alone because of the unpredictability of MS

Multipolar cells: have many dendrites and one axon; most are in the CNS; most common examples are spinal interneurons and cerebellar Purkinje cells

Myelin: a fatty sheath that insulates the larger axons; can increase the speed of neural transmission and also reduce interference with the neural message

Myelography: used for observing the spinal cord and spinal nerves

Necrosis: cell death; an island of dead tissue surrounded by normal tissue

Neglect: also known as hemispatial inattention; difficulty in receiving sensory stimuli (auditory, visual, tactile) in the field opposite to the involved hemisphere; follows damage to the parietal lobe or occasionally because of damage to other cortical or subcortical areas; neglect problems are far greater after right rather than left hemisphere damage

Neologisms: new word formations that can render language unintelligible

Nerve conduction studies: used for measuring stimulation and response points along the nerve fiber

Nerve fiber: an axon and its covering sheath

Neurilemma: the most external layer of the multilayered myelin, which contains the nucleus of the Schwann cell; the neurilemma is important in the regeneration of injured axonal fibers in the PNS

Neuritic plaques: minute areas of tissue degeneration consisting of granular deposits and remnants of neuronal processes

Neurofibrillary tangles: filamentous structures in the nerve cell body, dendrites, axon, and synaptic endings, which become twisted or tangled

Neurofibrils: serve as channels for intracellular communication; tend to become tangled in Alzheimer disease

Neuroleptics: first-generation antipsychotic medications

Neurologic evaluation: includes those procedures used in determining the type of pathology and the location of the brain lesion

Neuron: nerve cell; consists of a cell body, dendrites, and an axon; can transmit neural impulses to other neurons, glands, or muscles

Neurotransmitters: chemical substances released at a synapse to transmit signals across neurons

Neurotrophils: the scavenger white blood cells, which release a growth factor

Nigrostriatal area: the parts of the brain that are rich in dopamine receptors

Nodes of Ranvier: intervals between the segments of the myelin sheath

Nonfluent aphasia: usually caused by damage to anterior portions of the language-dominant side of the brain

Norepinephrine-containing (noradrenergic) neurons: occur in the pons and medulla, with most in the reticular formation; noradrenergic neurons project to the thalamus, hypothalamus, limbic forebrain structures, and the cerebral cortex; descending fibers project to other parts of the brainstem, cerebellar cortex, and spinal cord

Nucleus: a membrane-enclosed organelle that contains most of a cell's genetic material

Nystagmus: abnormal eye movements

Occipital alexia: not associated with other language problems; inability to comprehend through reading, while other language modalities are normal; written expression is preserved, but the patient cannot understand through reading what was just written correctly

Occipital (visual) association area: Brodmann areas 18 and 19; primary visual cortex is area 17

Occipital lobe: located at the back of the cerebral hemisphere, includes the primary visual cortex and visual association areas; bounded in the front by the parietal and temporal lobes and in back by the longitudinal fissure

Oligodendroglia: cells that form and maintain the myelin sheath in the CNS

Olivopontocerebellar atrophy: characteristics include ataxic, spastic, or flaccid dysarthric components, or various mixtures of all three; atrophy also may be associated with Parkinsonian features, so there is a possibility that a hypokinetic dysarthric component may be present

Open head injury: a penetrating head injury where the skull is fractured or perforated and the meninges are torn or lacerated

Operativity: a stimulus that can involve other senses

Oral (also nonverbal or buccofacial) apraxia: a difficulty in performing voluntary movements with the muscles of the lips, tongue, mandible, and larynx in nonspeech tasks (coughing, chewing, sucking, or swallowing), although automatic movements of the same muscles are preserved

Oral expression deficit: difficulty in the formulation of spoken language

Orientation: the ability to locate oneself in one's environment with reference to time (year, month, day, date, hour, etc.), place (thinking where one is at the moment), and person (the identification of self and other people)

PACE: Promoting Aphasics' Communicative Effectiveness; may be used in individual or group therapy

Palilalia: the involuntary repetition of words and phrases with increasing rate and decreasing loudness

Paragrammatism: substitution of function words (e.g., prepositions, pronouns); associated with fluent aphasia

Parasympathetic division (ANS):   responsible for such activities as slowing down the heart rate, increasing contractions of the intestines, increasing salivation, and increasing secretions of the glands in the gastrointestines

Parietal association area: also called somesthetic area; responsible for the discrimination and integration of tactile information

Parietal lobe: bounded in the front by the central sulcus and below by the back end of the lateral fissure

Parietal-temporal alexia: also called alexia with agraphia; associated with the fluent aphasias; characteristics are the almost total loss of reading comprehension and written expression

Parkinson disease: a degenerative disorder that affects movement and produces the majority of all subcortical dementias

Perception: the ability to organize incoming sensory stimuli by recognizing features and their relationships and then combining them with previous knowledge of these features (memory); the level above basic vision or hearing, and the level below reading or auditory comprehension

Perfusion: injection of fluid into a blood vessel; the purpose to supply nutrients or oxygen to an organ or to tissues

Peripheral nervous system (PNS):   composed of the spinal peripheral nerves and the cranial nerves

Perisylvian area: located around the lateral fissure in the dominant hemisphere and contains the major language areas used for comprehension and expression; aphasias caused by lesions in the perisylvian area include Broca's, Wernicke's, and conduction

Perseveration: persistent repetition of words, phrases, ideas that are no longer appropriate

Personality: an aspect of emotion that refers to the total behavior over time and to the person's immediate emotional state

Phagocytosis: engulfing cellular debris, leaving a cavity

Phonemic paraphasia: also called literal paraphasia (e.g., saying *corned beef and garbage,* or saying *fable, sable,* or *cable* for *table*); typically found in patients with conduction or Wernicke's aphasia

Phonology: the sound system of a language and the rules that govern the sound combinations

PICA: Porch Index of Communicative Ability, which uses a multidimensional scoring system to assess aphasia

Pick disease: a dementia involving the appearance of neuronal abnormalities called Pick bodies (dense globular formations) and Pick cells (enlarged neurons); personality and language impairment have an early onset, whereas cognitive problems come later

Polarized: positive and negative ions on each side of a cell membrane are unequal

Polytypic nature of aphasia: virtually all aphasias involve reduction of available vocabulary, linguistic rules, and verbal retention span, as well as impaired comprehension and production of messages

Pons: contains nuclei for several of the cranial nerves, has major connections to the cerebellum, and has other connections to the cortex that are important for speech production

Positron emission tomography (PET):   cerebral blood flow and metabolism studies which involve the use of positron isotopes; provide relatively precise neuroanatomical delineation based on variations in glucose metabolism

Postcentral gyrus: located within the parietal lobe in back of the central sulcus; a mirror image to the "motor strip" area of the frontal lobe and is a primary sensory cortical area ("sensory strip") having to do with temperature, pain, touch, and proprioception

Posterior cerebral arteries: (one for each hemisphere); supply the inferior lateral surface of the temporal lobe, and the lateral and medial surfaces of the occipital lobe

Poverty of content of speech: speech that is adequate in amount, but conveys little information

Poverty of speech: restriction in the amount of spontaneous speech

Pragmatics: the system that combines the above language components into functional and socially appropriate communication; involves eye contact with the listener, topic maintenance, turn-taking, modulation of loudness, proper decorum in the communicative setting, facial and bodily gestures that reflect the mood proper use of register, and providing relevant information to the listener

Precentral gyrus: lies immediately anterior to the central sulcus; also known as the primary motor cortex or "motor strip" area; controls voluntary muscular movement on the opposite side of the body

Pressured speech: an increase in the amount of speech; the patient speaks rapidly and is difficult to interrupt; speech tends to be loud and emphatic

Primary damage: a traumatic injury caused by the actual impact to the brain

Primary progressive aphasia (PPA):   an ongoing cerebral atrophy in a language area of the brain resulting in progressive language deterioration; nonverbal memory and intellect remain intact

Primary visual cortex: responsible for basic vision; a lesion in this area can produce degrees of blindness

Prognosis: indicators or predictors of who would make a good candidate for therapy

Progressive supranuclear palsy: characteristics include hypokinetic and spastic dysarthric components alone or as a mixture; ataxic dysarthric components, typically in combination with hypokinetic or spastic components, can also be present in some patients

PROMPT (prompts for restructuring oral musculature phonetic targets):   an approach that stresses the patient's kinesthetic awareness of speech movements or their prevention

Proprioception: includes the senses of movement, vibration, pressure, position, equilibrium, and deep pain; enables one to realize exactly where the individual parts of the body are in space, and the relationship of one body part to another

Prosody: refers to rate, stress, and melodic intonation of speech

Prosopagnosia: facial recognition impairment

Protoplasm: the nucleus and cytoplasm

Pseudobulbar palsy: bilateral spastic paralysis affecting the bulbar musculature and most commonly caused by multiple or bilateral strokes, and head trauma

Pyramidal system: supplies the voluntary muscles of the head, neck, and limbs; neurons of this tract originate in the postcentral gyrus or primary motor cortex

Receptive sites: in the connecting nerve cells, they are chemically activated to generate the electric impulses that stimulate the nerve cell body

Reflex arc: shortcut where a motor response avoids going through the higher centers of the cortex for interpretation

Regional cerebral blood flow (rCBF):   an indirect measure of metabolism, based on the assumption that neural activity in a cortical region causes an increased demand for nourishment; the corresponding increase in blood flow rate indicates increased metabolic activity

Replacement gliosis: in smaller lesions, astrocytes fill the space with a glial scar

Resting potential: the tug-of-war where opposite ions attract, and identical ions repel, which forms an electrochemical gradient along the cell membrane

Reverberating circuit: a self-propagating system between cells that, if activated, can discharge the signal continuously until its operation is blocked by an external source

Ribosomes: protein granules involved in synthesis of RNA

Right hemisphere damage: etiology is a brain lesion in the right hemisphere (nondominant for language); mostly chronic; cognitive abilities can be affected

Schizophasia: a form of schizophrenia characterized primarily by disorganized language

Schizophrenia: a thought disorder that affects the total personality in all aspects of its functioning

Schwannoma: also called neurofibroma; a moderately firm, benign, nonencapsulated tumor resulting from proliferation of Schwann cells in a disorderly pattern that includes portions of nerve fibers (sometimes observed as an acoustic neuroma)

Secondary damage: such consequences of brain injury as infection, hypoxia, edema, elevated intracranial pressure, infarction, and hematoma

Selective attention: the ability to maintain a behavioral or cognitive set in the face of distracting or competing stimuli; incorporates the concept of freedom from distractibility

Self-reference (egocentric speech):   the patient repeatedly refers the topic back to himself and refers neutral topics to himself (personalizes)

Semantic paraphasia: also called verbal paraphasia; confusion with closely associated words (e.g., *driving range* for *parking lot*)

Semantics: the system that governs the meanings of words and sentences; probably the most common error found in all of the neurogenic adult language disorders

Serotonin neurons: found at most levels of the brainstem, with terminals in the reticular formation, hypothalamus, thalamus, septum, hippocampus, olfactory tubercle, cerebral cortex, basal ganglia, and amygdala

Sheath of Schwann: also called neurolemma or *neurilemma*; in the peripheral nervous system (PNS), the myelin sheath is produced by Schwann cells that lie along the axons

Shy-Drager syndrome: characteristics include ataxic, hypokinetic, and spastic dysarthric components in different mixtures, although each component can be present alone in some patients

Single-photon emission-computed tomography (SPECT):   uses relatively stable isotope products to demonstrate cerebral blood flow and, to a lesser degree, perfusion of metabolites

Small-molecule transmitters: include acetylcholine and the following five monoamines, which are derived from amino acids: dopamine, norepinephrine, serotonin, glutamate, and γ-aminobutyric acid (GABA)

Somatic pathways: the route that signals for touch, pressure, temperature, and pain take when they are delivered to the brain

Somatosensory cortex: in the dominant hemisphere, appears to play a part in motor speech programming, especially in the integration of sensory information in preparation for motor activity

Speech disorder: an impairment of the articulation of speech sounds, fluency, and/or voice

Speed of processing: the amount of time it takes for a person to absorb information

Spinal accessory nerve: CN XI; spinal portion sends motor impulses to the neck and the shoulder; unilateral or bilateral damage to the motor function can cause neck turning and shoulder elevation problems, which may indirectly affect respiration, phonation, and resonance; cranial portion sends motor impulses to the soft palate, pharynx, and larynx

Spinal cord: extends from the skull through the foramen magnum down to the lower back; encased in the vertebral column

Spinal nerves: 31 pairs of nerves; sensory information from the receptor (e.g., skin) to the cortex for evaluation of the sensations of pain, temperature, touch, and vibration; motor information from the CNS to the effector (e.g., muscles)

Spontaneous recovery: the body healing itself without any therapy; most likely due to a reduction of edema or swelling in the damaged hemisphere, a return to normal blood flow or circulation in the undamaged hemisphere, and collateral or compensatory blood circulation in the damaged hemisphere

Stenosis: narrowing of blood vessels

Stilted speech: speech with an excessively formal quality, overly pompous

Strain injuries: deformation of brain tissue, with three subtypes: tensile strain indicates pulling apart; compressive strain involves pushing together; and shear strain involves parallel deforming forces

Stunning: occurs when neural connections are severed and areas of the brain that have not been destroyed cease to function; some cells that are not seriously damaged may respond to the natural recovery process and survive

Subcortical dementia: a gradual decline in cognitive abilities without appreciable loss in associational cortical areas affecting language

Substantia nigra: responsible for the production of dopamine

Sulci or fissures: grooves on the surface of the brain or spinal cord

Supplementary motor areas: receive information from other regions of the brain, and integrate, refine, and plan or program motor speech output

Supramarginal gyrus: curves around the back end of the lateral fissure and is responsible for the formulation of written language and possibly for phonological storage

Suprasegmental features: rate, stress, and melodic intonation

Sustained attention: the ability to maintain a consistent behavioral response during continuous and repetitive activity; incorporates concepts of vigilance

Sympathetic division (ANS):   responsible for such activities as speeding up the heart rate, constricting the peripheral blood vessels, elevating blood pressure, raising the eyelids, redistributing blood, dilating the pupils, and decreasing contractions of the intestines

Synapse: the juncture at which neural impulses are transmitted

Synaptic cleft: the space between the axon of the presynaptic nerve cell and the receptive ends of the postsynaptic cell; nerve impulses do not cross the synapse, but are communicated through the neurotransmitter released from the bouton terminals

Synaptic knobs: filaments of dendrites that contain neurotransmitters

Synaptic vesicles: subdivisions of embryonic neural tubes; filled with neurotransmitters

Syntax: the system governing the order and combination of words to form sentences, and the relationships among the elements within a sentence

Tangentiality: replying in a tangential, irrelevant manner; refers only to immediate replies to questions (stimulus-response mode) and not to transitions in spontaneous speech

Tangential speech: also called disorganized speech; difficulty in maintaining a specific topic

Tardive dyskinesia: a movement disorder, often affecting the tongue and mandible, caused by long-term ingestion of antipsychotic medications

Telodendria: ends of dendrites that branch into smaller multiple filaments

Temporal (auditory) association area: needed for the discrimination and integration of auditory information

Temporal lobe: bounded on top by the lateral fissure and in the back by the front border of the occipital lobe

Terminal bouton: end knob that contains neurotransmitters

Thalamus: a relay station for sensory information going to and from the sensory areas of the cortex, with direct ties to cortical language and motor speech systems

Thrombosis (cerebral):   an occlusion of an artery to the brain by a clot

Transcortical motor aphasia: similar to Broca's aphasia, but these patients have the ability to repeat words, phrases, and sentences; relatively rare syndrome

Transcortical sensory aphasia: similar to Wernicke's aphasia, but these patients have the ability to repeat and show echolalia of words, phrases, and sentences; relatively rare syndrome

Traumatic brain injury: occurs when a swiftly moving object hits the head or when the moving head strikes a stationary object

Trigemina nerve: CN V, Sensory and Motor; receives sensory impulses from the jaw, lips, face, and tongue, and sends motor impulses to the jaw

Type I error: rejecting the null hypothesis when it should have been the accepted alternative

Type II error: accepting the null hypothesis when it should have been the rejected alternative

Unipolar cells: T-shaped with one process that extends from the body; divide into central (axonal) and peripheral (dendritic) portions; found in spinal dorsal roots

Upper motor neuron disorder: involving combined damage to the pyramidal system and to a portion of the extrapyramidal system, both of which arise from the same motor cortex areas; lesions to upper motor neurons produce spastic muscles that are stiff, move sluggishly through a limited range, and tend to be weak

Vagus nerve: CN X, Motor, Sensory, and Special Sensory; receives sensory impulses from the larynx, pharynx, soft palate, and thoracic and abdominal viscera, and sends motor impulses to the larynx, pharynx, soft palate, and visceral organs

Vascular dementia: also called fronto-temporal dementia, and formerly, multi-infarct dementia; can involve multiple infarcts in cortical, subcortical, or both areas

Veins: carry blood toward the heart

Ventral spinal cord: anterior portion; conducts motor neurons

Ventricles: a network of cavities within the brain

Verbal stereotype: automatic speech or a noncommunicative utterance, for example, "thrill, thrill, thrill," or "I come over there"; associated with nonfluent aphasia

Verbigeration: use of words in a repetitive manner

Vertebral artery: branches (one from each side) join together to form the *basilar artery*

Vestibulocochlear nerve: CN VIII; vestibular branch receives sensory impulses from the vestibular apparatus of the inner ear (responsible for equilibrium or balance) and forwards those impulses to the cerebellum and other areas to help maintain balance cochlear branch receives sensory impulses from the cochlea of the inner ear (responsible for sound sensitivity) and forwards those impulses to the cochlear nuclear complex in the CNS

Visual association area: needed for integrating and organizing incoming visual stimuli; a lesion here can result in visual perception problems, which in turn can influence reading comprehension

Visuo-spatial perception: can include the ability to copy two- and three-dimensional drawings (e.g., circle, red cross, cube, cylinder, etc.), connect a series of numbers, draw on command a house or clock face, or reproduce figures that an examiner makes out of matches

Voice disorder: characterized by the abnormal production and/or absence of vocal quality, pitch, loudness, resonance, and/or duration, which is inappropriate for an individual's age and/or sex

WAB: Western Aphasia Battery, an aphasia examination using a neuropsychology framework, similar to the BDAE

Wallerian degeneration: degeneration of the axonal part that is separate from its cell body

Wernicke's aphasia: fluent aphasia characterized by fluent, well-articulated speech; jargon, neologisms, and empty speech; auditory and reading comprehension and written expression are impaired; repetition of words, phrases, and sentences is poor

Wernicke's area: posterior–superior portion of the temporal lobe of the dominant hemisphere (area 22)

Wilson disease: characteristics include ataxic, spastic, and hypokinetic dysarthric components in different mixtures, although each component can be present alone in some patients

Word approximations: words used in a new and unconventional way or actual new words that are developed by conventional rules of word formation

X-rays: used for observing the skull and/or spine

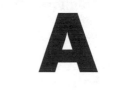
Time-Altered Word Association Tests (TAWAT): Functional Specifications Document

© Robert Goldfarb and Harvey Halpern, 2009–2011

Introduction

Time-Altered Word Association Tests (TAWAT) is based on 30 years of research with adults with aphasia, adults with chronic undifferentiated schizophrenia, institutionalized elderly with and without dementia, neurotypical elderly, and neurotypical young adults. The computerized version of TAWAT is available at this text's companion website. Instructions and a listing of the most frequent associations produced by healthy young adults are also available on the website.

The professional who intends to use TAWAT should be familiar with the theory and development and administration and scoring sections in the appendix that follows this one. After gaining this competence, the functional specifications documented in this section will guide the clinician in implementing, scoring, and printing responses to the test. Always begin with the pretest, to allow the examinee to calibrate to the selected modality and speed. Because Tests A and B are parallel or equivalent forms, one can be randomly selected for baseline, and the other for baseline recovery. Results should help guide the initial stages of clinical intervention, as follows:

1. Modality: auditory or visual
2. Speed: fast (20 milliseconds for visual, 10 phonemes per second for auditory) or slow (250 milliseconds for visual, 5 phonemes per second for auditory)
3. Word characteristics:
   a. length (long or short)
   b. frequency of occurrence (frequent, infrequent)
   c. grammatical class (noun, verb, adjective)
   d. abstraction level (high, medium, low)

The examiner is counseled to avoid assigning a diagnostic category based solely on TAWAT. Scores obtained from an individual client are likely to deviate from those garnered from the population. Although we disagree with television's Dr. House, who says that the patient always lies (the patient has no reason to lie when taking TAWAT), more information is necessary before making a differential diagnosis.

Site Objective

To allow an examiner to test a participant's word association responses to various words flashed on the screen or presented auditorily at varying intervals and to analyze these responses.

Features

Before Test

- Allows the examiner to enter the personal information of the test participant.
- Allows the examiner the option to choose where on the screen (left, center, right) the word appears (visual modality only).
- Allows the word to be played from a sound file (auditory modality only).
- Allows examiner to choose auditory or visual modality of stimulus presentation.
- Allows the examiner to choose how long each word appears on screen (20 milliseconds or 250 milliseconds) for the visual presentation.
- Allows the examiner to choose the speed of stimulus presentation (5 phonemes per second or 10 phonemes per second) for the auditory modality.
- Allows examiner to decide which of two word lists (A or B) the main test will show.

During Test

- Shows a Pretest before the main (scored) test with static words.
- Allows the examiner to grade each response (P, S, R, A, U).
- Allows examiner to write the word association produced for each word.

After Test

- Indicates what percentage of questions were graded P, S, R, A, or U.
- Breaks down each grade into categories (grammatical class, abstraction level, word length, and word frequency), and indicates what percentage of each grade matched a certain aspect of that category (Word Length: long or short; Word Frequency: frequent or infrequent; Grammatical Class: noun, verb, or adjective; Abstraction Level: high, medium, or low).
- Lists each word and its corresponding association for further analysis.
- Permits the test and responses to be printed.

Page Components

The computerized test has four pages (or stages), all of which are loaded dynamically.

Stage 1: Information. The examiner enters information about the participant. Alternatively, the examiner can click on "Fill" at the top of the page, and all fields will fill. The examiner can then key in changes to any field. The examiner then clicks on "Continue" at the bottom of the page.

Stage 2: Setup. The examiner sets which word list will be used, at what speed the words will be shown (visual modality) or played (auditory modality), and at what location the words will appear on the screen (visual modality only).

Stage 3: Pretest and test. The pretest is shown first and then the actual test is loaded. A comments box as well as a grade selector appears under each word, and these responses are saved once the examiner clicks the next button.

Stage 4: Analysis. Total percentages of each grade are shown, as well as the percentages of each grade broken up into category attributes (e.g., Word length: 10% long, 90% short). Additionally, each word is shown next to the examiner's comments on it. Responses to the pretest are not analyzed.

Navigation Requirements

The test is set up linearly, so that the test can only move forward at each stage and there are few options, in order to reduce confusion. The first stage requires all the input fields to be filled in. If some are not filled in, the examiner is alerted regarding which inputs still need to be filled before advancing to the next stage. For a quick start, click the "Fill" box at the top of the page. All fields will be automatically filled, and the demographic fields required by the examiner can be erased and re-entered. Then the examiner scrolls to the bottom of the page and clicks "Continue."

In Stage 2, the examiner is given drop-down menu options to select the speed of each word to be shown (20 milliseconds or 250 milliseconds) or played (5 phonemes per second or 10 phonemes per second), where it will be shown (left, right, or center of the screen), and which word list to use (List A or List B). The drop-down menu is initially set to a default value.

In Stage 3, the examiner writes the association in the response box, assigns a score (P, S, R, A, or U) from the drop-down menu (set at default to P), and clicks the "Next" button, and the response and grade will be stored for the relevant word. Clicking "Next" also triggers presentation of the following word. To review scoring, using the stimulus word GLEE as an example:

Paradigmatic response: HAPPINESS (an appropriate response of the same grammatical class).

Syntagmatic: CLUB (a grammatical continuation) or HAPPY (an appropriate association, but of a different grammatical class).

Repetitious: GLEEFUL (a repetition of the stimulus word + or − a prefix or suffix).

Anomalous: YELLOW (even if it appears that the participant saw or heard a different word, e.g., *green* instead of *glee*, the response is an anomalous association for *glee*).

Unclassifiable: No response, variations of "I don't know," or a long phrasal response. If the response lacks intelligibility, but the examiner can interpret the intention, then treat the response as if it were produced with accurate articulation and score as (usually) P or S. If the articulation is unintelligible, score the response as U.

After the test, the examiner is immediately taken to Stage 4, where there is a large printout option with information and the analyses and examiner entries for all words.

Manual for Time-Altered Word Association Tests (TAWAT): Theory and Development; Administration and Scoring

Use and Abuse of TAWAT

1. *Diagnostic.* Our data are based on population norms, with severity indices available only for institutionalized elderly with and without senile dementia. To diagnose an individual as, say, having aphasia or the language of schizophrenia, or to specific severity of impairment based solely on TAWAT, is unwarranted.

2. *Therapeutic.* Results of TAWAT offer guidance for the initial stages of language rehabilitation. We caution against overdependence on any test results, including ours. The clinician should also avoid "teaching the test" if TAWAT is to be used for collection of baseline and baseline recovery data.

3. *Professional preparation.* Although graduate students, under appropriate professional supervision, may use TAWAT, it is imperative that they understand the "Theory and Development" and "Administration and Scoring" sections before administering the test. In addition we strongly advise several "dry run" practice sessions for familiarity before using TAWAT with clinical or experimental participants.

Part One: Theory and Development

Word Association Tests

Since the last century, researchers have employed word association tests to generate psychoanalytic data. For example, although adults with schizophrenia do not differ from typical adults in their associations to neutral words, they give significantly more associations to affective (pleasant and unpleasant) words (Buss, 1966). Several studies (Gordon, Silverstein, & Harrow, 1982; Merten, 1992; and Shean, 1999) were conducted to see whether responses to word association tests can reflect the underlying aberrant associative processes of individuals with schizophrenia. Their results indicated that word association tests, while valuable, cannot be used alone in exploring the underlying aberrant associative processes. Other factors such as natural language situations, length of hospitalization, and the course of the disease must be considered in explaining the underlying processes.

Summerall, Timmons, James, Ewing, and Oehlert (1997) used the *Controlled Oral Word Association Test* (COWAT), which measures the person's ability to make verbal associations to specified letters (i.e., C, F, and L) to detect changes in word association fluency in a neurotypical elderly population. Information regarding total numbers of words produced as well as frequency of perseverations, breaking set, using the same word stem, and using a proper noun is provided.

The COWAT, as a component of a neuropsychological battery for differentiating various disorders, has been used in testing participants with schizophrenia (Friedman, Kenny, Jesberger, Choy, & Meltzer, 1995), Alzheimer disease, subcortical ischemic vascular dementia (Tierney et al., 2001), and Machado-Joseph disease (Zawacki, Grace, Friedman, & Sudarsky, 2002).

Word association tests have also been used for linguistic analyses. The production of a word association response has been described (Collins & Loftus, 1975) as a process that involves decoding through word retrieval, lexical search, and encoding. To test for word association, lists of stimulus words are compiled (Goldfarb & Halpern, 1984; Kent & Rosanoff, 1910; Palermo & Jenkins, 1964; Russell & Jenkins, 1954) and presented to typical adults. Results showed that specific response classes could be predicted. Furthermore, when children undertook word association tests, the results differed from those obtained with adults (Woodrow & Lowell, 1916).

Studying this discrepancy more closely, Ervin (1961) and Brown and Berko (1960) found that responses to word association tests correlated with age and linguistic development. Young children tend to give responses that are not the same part of speech (noun, verb, adjective, etc.) but that follow the stimulus in syntax. These are completion or "syntagmatic" responses. For example, to the word *tall*, a child might say "boy" and "tree." Older children and adults tend to give responses within the same grammatical class (as *tall*), such as "short" or "high." These responses are "paradigmatic." The shift from syntagmatic to paradigmatic (McLaughlin, 1998; Owens, 2005; Pan, 2005) occurs between six and eight years of age (McNeill, 1970), at which time children also are able to distinguish anomalous from fully grammatical sentences. Ervin-Tripp (1970) noted that children and uneducated adults have fewer paradigmatic responses that may be related to social class, and that these responses may be increased by education. She added that the most common form of paradigmatic response is the antonym.

According to Vygotsky (1934), "The meanings of words are not constant. They change as the child develops; they change also in accordance with the different ways in which thought functions. Word meaning is a dynamic, not a static function" (p. 514). Indeed, the word associations of children often involve similarity of word sound ("tall" → "ball"), a type of association that is reduced in frequency later in life (Posner, Lewis, & Conrad, 1972).

Word association techniques used by investigators of child language (Brown & Berko, 1960; Ervin, 1961; Ervin-Tripp, 1970; McNeill, 1970) have presented evidence dealing with two basic hypotheses: horizontal development and vertical development. These two hypotheses are not mutually exclusive, and may both be true regarding the enlargement of dictionaries (sometimes called *lexicon*, or vocabulary). They differ in when, earlier or later, a semantic feature spreads through the dictionary. A semantic feature is a distinction that separates one class of words from another. For example, four-leggedness separates animals that stand upright from those that do not.

In horizontal development, a word enters the dictionary even though not all the semantic features associated with the word are present. Thus, a word can be in a child's vocabulary, but the same word may have different semantic properties in the vocabularies of an older child or adult. Sentences that adults and older children regard as anomalous, such as "My father shouts fast," may be regarded as acceptable by younger children. Semantic development will then consist of horizontally completing the dictionary entries of words already acquired as well as acquiring new words.

McNeill's (1970) horizontal development hypothesis neglects to suggest an order, if any, of the acquisition of the semantic properties that will result in the word having "adult" semantic properties. Clark (1973a, 1973b) addressed herself to questions concerning the nature of semantic features. In the early stages of language development, a child, having learned the word *dog*, may call a cat, cow, sheep, and goat "dog" since only the feature of four-leggedness has been learned. This feature is, obviously, not adequate to identify a dog in the same way as an adult does. Later on, the child would be expected to experience difficulty with such antonym pairs as *more* and *less*. These terms refer, respectively, to the positive and negative poles of "amount." If the child learns the positive pole of "amount" first, then, for a time, both the words *more* and *less* will actually mean "more." Examples similar to the above have been noted in the verbal behavior literature under the classification of "response generalization" (Skinner, 1957). Here the rationale for the child's use of the word *dog* to refer to four-legged creatures lies in the reinforcement supplied by the verbal community and not in cognitive development.

In vertical development most of all of the semantic features of a word enter the dictionary when the word does. At first, however, dictionary entries are separated from each other so that semantic features appear at unrelated places in the dictionary. That is, the same semantic features may or may not be recognized as being the same in different entries within the dictionary. Words would then have the same meaning for a young child as for an older child or an adult. Semantic development, in this case, would consist of vertically collecting these separate occurrences of semantic features in the dictionary into unified semantic features.

Evidence supporting vertical development may be found in the work of Schlesinger (1974). In addition to instances of overextension, as previously cited, children also demonstrate overrestricted use of words. For example, a child may use the word *hot* to describe hot objects but not hot weather, or *white* for snow but not for other white things. Schlesinger noted that examples of overrestriction are less common than overextension, and would provide an inadequate basis for a theory of semantic development.

McNeill (1970) considered syntagmatic (e.g., *throw → ball*) responses that, because of the size of the semantic categories available to young children, fall outside the grammatical class of the stimulus. That is, the greater breadth of the semantic categories available to young children can accommodate an association of *fast → shout* in a single grammatical class. For an older child or an adult, the words *fast* and *shout* belong to different semantic categories and different grammatical classes (*fast* is an adverb; *shout* is a verb). A paradigmatic R matches its S semantically, and a syntagmatic R is a grammatical continuation.

In a study testing both frequency of occurrence and grammatical class, Deese (1962) hypothesized that paradigmatic and syntagmatic associations would vary by part of speech. A word association test was administered to undergraduates at Johns Hopkins University. A word list was presented using nouns, verbs, and adjectives ranging from 100+ occurrences per million words to 1 or 2 occurrences per million. Results showed that largely paradigmatic responses occurred only for nouns and frequently used adjectives.

Abeysinghe, Bayles, and Trosset (1990) studied the nature of semantic memory impairment in 23 persons with dementia of the Alzheimer type (DAT). They used three semantic tasks: word association (which replicated the study using TAWAT stimuli reported by Santo Pietro & Goldfarb, 1985), definition, and associate rank ordering. Analyzing the responses to the word association task, participants with DAT were more likely than typical control participants to give multiword, repetitious, or unrelated responses. Additionally, the ratio of paradigmatic to syntagmatic responses was significantly decreased in individuals with DAT.

Surprisingly, participants with DAT were able to provide definitions for many stimulus words for which they were unable to provide meaningful associates. This finding suggests the need for caution in interpreting a decrease in the number of paradigmatic responses as indicative of a loss of conceptual knowledge.

More recently, Colangelo, Stephenson, Westbury, and Buchanan (2003) used auditory and visual word association tasks to test the integrity of the semantic system in two patients with deep dyslexia (an acquired reading disorder). The data support the notion that semantics remain intact and that the disorder and associated errors arise through a selection impairment related to failure of inhibiting connections in the phonological lexicon.

Psycholinguistic considerations of word association have been joined by cybernetic models. In discussing analogue networks of word association, Guiliano (1969) indicated the need for a means of automatically recognizing associations present among words. In such a network, requests with roughly equivalent meaning would retrieve roughly the same documents. Unfortunately, this task represents an overwhelming challenge.

It is difficult (if not impossible) to find two words that are synonymous under all interpretations. What is more surprising is that it is difficult to find two words with completely disjoint meanings. In fact, all substantive words in natural language are more or less associated; the real question is how much or less (Guiliano, 1969, pp. 167–168).

In his review of cybernetic theories of word association Norman (1969, p. 175) considered Guiliano's proposal for using an electrical network to determine the associations among words and contexts. An electrical model would appeal to those who consider human memory to be only an interconnected network of information links. However, statistical associations probably do not tell us much about the organization of the information storage system. Word association behavior necessitates the use of a broad search of episodic and semantic memory, so that multiple possible solutions to a problem can be formulated. It may also involve ecphory, or the conversion of information from two sources, the engram and the retrieval cues, into a state in which the remember would be conscious of it (Tulving, 1983). A final argument against Guiliano's model is that the foundation of language lies in the application of rules, rather than in the relative frequency with which words are used.

Studies in psycholinguistics have been prone to stamp dichotomous labels (syntagmatic–paradigmatic, heterogeneous–homogeneous) on responses to word association tasks. A useful measure of word association should consider yet another dichotomy, described as synonymy (similarity) and contiguity (see, for example, Jakobson, 1961).

Synonymy refers to similarity of meaning among such terms as *canine* and *dog*, or *lamp* and *light*. There are two problems with word association modeling synonymy. When it is found, synonymy is almost always partial and extremely difficult to measure; there is rarely such a thing as complete synonymy. A wolf is a canine but not a dog; some lamps are not lights and some lights are not lamps. In addition, synonymy is not the only kind of association present among words. In fact, for many applications it may not even be the most important kind of association. This is because synonymous expressions are readily constructible of nonsynonymous components or parts, which are nonetheless associates; that is, the expressions are synonymous, but the parts are not. An example is *Equal Rights Amendment* and *Women's Liberation Movement*. Although the two expressions are synonymous in that they focus on the same political issues, a comparison of the individual words—*women's–equal, liberation–rights, movement–amendment*—does not demonstrate synonymy.

A second type of word association should be considered: association that is primarily due to real-word relationships among the objects or actions that the words designate. Examples are: *table–top, hammer–nail, bank–money.* These are called *contiguity associations,* because the objects or properties denoted by the words are presumed to be contiguous in some sense in the real world.

In summary, the linguistic analyses of word association test data have led to theories of semantic development in children as well as to descriptions of the lexical retrieval behavior of both children and adults. In addition, these normative data provide a model with which pathological language behavior may be compared.

Temporal Manipulation of Stimuli

Auditory Stimuli

In his review of the models of linguistic processing, Owens (2005), noted that an individual will originate, analyze, and synthesize incoming linguistic information according to the specific task. Information processing represents the voluntary problem-solving strategy of each individual. He further states that information processing can be divided into the cognitive processes of attention and discrimination, organization, memory, and transfer.

Attention includes both awareness of a learning situation and active cognitive processing. The individual does not attend to all stimuli. Discrimination is the ability to identify stimuli differing along some dimension. Especially for language decoding, discrimination requires a special type of memory called *working memory,* which holds the message during processing.

The organization of incoming sensory information is important for later retrieval. Information is organized or "chunked" according to category. Words may be stored in various locations based on meaning, word class, sound pattern, and various associational categories.

Memory is the ability to recall information that has been learned previously. The three types of memory are working, short-term, and long-term. Working memory holds new input while the brain discriminates this information for further processing. During linguistic decoding, sentences are held in short-term memory while they are compared and analyzed for meaning. This step is quite important because speech is quick, and sometimes once said it fades away. Information is retained in long-term memory by rehearsal or repetition, and organization.

The ability to apply previously learned material in solving similar but novel problems is called *transfer* or *generalization.* The greater the similarity between the two, the greater the transfer.

Studies of temporal auditory acuity have attempted to determine the shortest time interval within which the ear can discriminate the order of auditory events. The limitations of temporal resolution may relate to the ear's minimum time-constant. In a system such as the hearing mechanism it is important to know how much of the past affects the present output. If hearing represented a simple linear system, recent values of the input would be given greater weight and more remote values of the input would be given less weight. The parameter of this exponential decay is called the time constant of the ear. Even though auditory processing probably represents a more complex linear system, the present output can still be measured as a weighted function of past outputs. However, the weighting function would be more complicated (Green, 1971).

The time constant for typical listeners is extremely short, when making both same–different judgments (Ronken, 1970) or identifying soft–loud and loud–soft click pairs (Green, 1971). We may postulate that the short time constant is disrupted in listeners with auditory processing disorders. Because of the sluggish response of the long time-constant device, the order in which the clicks arrive would probably not create a noticeable difference in the overall response. This postulate is indirectly supported by Green (1971), to whom it seems likely that studies of temporal acuity are, in effect, studies of how quickly the peripheral nervous system can respond to changes in auditory waveforms.

Much of the evidence from psychology evolved from studies of perceptual processing, or the identification of acoustic information that is probably stored sequentially. A visual image prolongs the stimulus in its correct spatial pattern (Sperling, 1969). If the auditory image does something analogous to the visual image, it must preserve the stimulus in its original sequential pattern for perceptual processing.

Perceptual units and perceptual processing time are important for auditory perception (Massaro, 1970, 1972; Studdert-Kennedy et al., 1970). In identification of two syllables with dichotic presentation, the second syllable was lowest if it led the second by 20 milliseconds and improved with increases in lead time. Identification of the first syllable was still only 80% correct when it led the second syllable by 120 milliseconds. Further increases in lead time would have increased identification of the first syllable. Therefore presentation of the second syllable should interfere with identification of the first. This follows from the assumption that a second input that cannot be integrated with the first terminates perceptual processing of the first (Massaro, 1972).

A rather different model of perceptual processing is offered by Lockhead (1972). The alternative suggested was that a stimulus is first processed or perceived holistically. The resultant holistic configuration was called a *blob*. If the task can be performed on the basis of just this processing, as in an identification task, a response is accessed. If not, blob processing is followed, as necessary, by serial processing. This is a dynamic model in the sense that the organism employs only those processes necessary for the task. Mere identification or recognition of an item takes less time than abstraction of an aspect of it. In the first instance blob processing alone is required; in the second instance serial processing must be added. The models cited above seem to suggest that the auditory processing and auditory comprehension of linguistic events are enhanced by a slower presentation of stimuli.

Visual Stimuli

Ely (2005) has identified the major components involved in skilled reading as letter recognition, grapheme-phoneme correspondence rules, word recognition, semantic knowledge, and comprehension and interpretation.

Letter recognition involves the ability to extract the defining features of a letter even though the typeface or font may be a little different for the same letter.

Grapheme-phoneme correspondence rules define the relationship between a letter (grapheme) or combination of letters, and the sound (phoneme) they represent. In a perfect rules system, each letter (grapheme) of the alphabet would be pronounced (phoneme) the same way all the time. According to the grapheme-phoneme correspondence rules of a language like English, a skilled reader would know that the alphabet letter "c" is pronounced in different ways (e.g., c̲at, c̲ity, c̲ello).

Word recognition is the identification of letter strings as representing conventional words in the spelling portion of the language. True words (e.g., *king*) are words that follow the accepted correct spelling and are not part of the language. Nonsense words are words that do not exist in the language (e.g., *gink*), although they are possible words because they follow some conventional spelling rules. False words are words that violate the accepted spelling rules (e.g., *nkgi*) and would unlikely be found in the language. In lexical decision tasks, true words are identified more quickly than nonsense words or false words.

Semantic knowledge pertains to all the information about a word, its possible meanings, and its relations to other words and to real word referents. Incomplete sentence knowledge interferes with understanding or written text.

Comprehension and interpretation is the final component of the reading process. Successful comprehension and interpretation rely on several developing skills and knowledge including the automaticity of word recognition, vocabulary, the extent of working memory, and overall word knowledge.

One of the major difficulties in assessing comprehension of visual stimuli lies in developing a means to measure what has been seen in one brief exposure. Sperling (1969) identified the inadequacies of instructing an observer of a brief presentation to repeat what he has seen:

> When complex stimuli consisting of a number of letters are tachistoscopically presented, observers enigmatically insist that they have seen more than they can remember afterwards, that is, report afterwards (Sperling, 1969, p. 61).

Certainly there is a limit on the memory report. This information has been known for some time and has been widely disseminated by Miller (1956) using such terms as *span of attention*, *apprehension*, or *immediate-memory*. Sperling's contribution is his deduction that more information is available during, and possibly for a short time after, the presentation of the stimulus than can be reported. After indicating all the letters (or numbers) they had seen, Sperling's subjects noted that they knew more information was presented, but were unable to remember it. This new description of memory expanded the traditional conception of short-term and long-term memory. First, according to Sperling, is the memory of events occurring at the present time, which is complete. Second is an immediate or short-term (working) memory containing the limited information extracted from the rapidly decaying sensory image. Third is the small part of the image that may be stored in permanent, long-term memory. One requirement not mentioned by Sperling for what may be termed *just-occurring memory* to take place is that the visual stimulus have sufficient size, clarity and duration to impress a sensory image upon the viewer.

Time-altered visual stimuli studies of neurotypical participants by Sperling (1969), Gough (1972), and Educational Developmental Laboratories (EDL) (1968, 1972) have indicated that the visual processing and comprehension of linguistic events are enhanced by a slower presentation of stimuli.

A 10-millisecond exposure was demonstrated (Gough, 1972) to be enough time for the eyes to sweep 1–4 degrees of visual angle (or 10–12 letter spaces). Competence at the 5th-grade level required correct recognition of 5 letters and 5 numbers following a 10-millisecond exposure (EDL, 1968, 1972). Gough found that, preceding and following a sweep, the reader's eyes remain in a fixation for approximately 250 milliseconds. "The Reader's initial fixation yields an icon containing materials corresponding to the first 15 to 20 letters and spaces of the sentence" (Gough, 1972, p. 333). The icon may be defined as a relatively direct representation of a visual stimulus that persists for a brief period after the stimulus vanishes.

Part Two: Administration and Scoring

Materials

The stimuli in TAWAT are 72 words chosen from the Darley, Sherman, and Siegel (1959) list of single words scaled according to abstraction levels (low, medium, and high). These words also are classified by grammatical class (noun, verb, adjectives) as defined by a standard dictionary. Word length was established by a criterion involving number of letters and number of syllables. "Long" words contained two or more syllables and six or more letters. "Short" words contain one syllable of four or fewer letters. All words were checked against graded word lists (Buckingham & Dolch, 1936; Gates, 1935) and were classified as being no higher than 5th-grade reading level.

Halpern (1965a, 1965b) reported the frequency of occurrence in written English language usage of these words with the Thorndike and Lorge (1944) word list. The 200 most frequently occurring words constituted the "frequent" level. The 72 words in the Halpern list consisted of the following: 24 words at each of the three levels of abstraction (low, medium, high); 24 nouns, 24 verbs, 24 adjectives; 36 short and 36 long words; and 36 frequent and 36 infrequent words. Halpern's list of 72 words actually represents two equivalent lists of 36 words balanced for abstraction, grammatical class, length and frequency.

For TAWAT, the Halpern list was modified to control for possible ambiguity of words presented through the auditory modality. For example, the word *be*, a verb in the Halpern list, might elicit the associate *sting* (for *bee*, a noun) when presented auditorily. The following substitutions were made without jeopardizing the integrity of Halpern's balancing: *joy* for *soul*, *zone* for *ware*, *tub* for *ant*, *fail* for *ail*, *let* for *know*, *try* for *be*, *bake* for *sew*, and *mid* for *mum*. The substituted words were equivalent to the originals in Halpern's list for frequency of occurrence in written English language usage, abstraction level, grammatical class, and word length (see **Table 1**).

TABLE 1

The 72 Words Classified and Counterbalanced According to Their Abstraction Level, Part of Speech, Word Length (L = long, S = short), and Frequency of Occurrence in Written English Usage (F = frequent, I = infrequent)

Abstraction	Nouns		Verbs		Adjectives	
High	goblin	LI	behave	LI	adorable	LI
	scholar	LI	disappoint	LI	dreadful	LI
	heaven	LF	forget	LF	happiest	LF
	problem	LF	understand	LF	wonderful	LF
	glee	SI	fail	SI	cute	SI
	goal	SI	heal	SI	pert	SI
	art	SF	let	SF	mere	SF
	joy	SF	try	SF	nice	SF
Medium	brownie	LI	explore	LI	rotten	LI
	helper	LI	celebrate	LI	selfish	LI
	country	LF	prepare	LF	central	LF
	family	LF	arrange	LF	several	LF
	gap	SI	tore	SI	mid	SI
	zone	SI	gape	SI	slim	SI
	news	SF	keep	SF	tall	SF
	game	SF	join	SF	loud	SF
Low	banana	LI	salute	LI	woolen	LI
	cabbage	LI	awaken	LI	chilly	LI
	dollar	LF	arrive	LF	silent	LF
	children	LF	tremble	LF	southern	LF
	tub	SI	bake	SI	bald	SI
	oat	SI	hum	SI	deaf	SI
	mile	SF	jump	SF	sick	SF
	cat	SF	pour	SF	ill	SF

Temporal Manipulation of Stimulus Materials

For auditory stimuli, words spoken by one of the authors at approximately 10 phonemes per second were digitally recorded into a Dell desktop computer with a Pentium 4 microprocessor, using an omnidirectional ElectroVoice Dynamic Cardioid microphone, model N/D257A. Word stimuli were stored in Sound Forge 7.0 (Sony, 2004), and were recorded a second time at 5 phonemes per second (half-speed), using the "time stretch" software program. A male speech-language pathologist experienced in these recording procedures read the word list.

The optimal rate of speaking is 165 words per minute (wpm) (Fairbanks, 1960, p. 115). The "Amplifier Passage" used by Fairbanks (p. 114) to train optimal rate of speech contains 300 words. Transcribed into phonetic form, the same passage contains 1167 phonemes. Conversion of optimal rate from wpm to phonemes per second results in an optimal speaking rate of about 10 (10.7) phonemes per second.

For visual stimuli, a 10-millisecond exposure did not permit some computers to refresh in time for the exposure of the next word at 10 milliseconds in pilot studies of the program. Accordingly, the length of exposure was increased to 20 milliseconds for the fast speed, which can run on all computers.

In summary, the following presentation speeds are used in TAWAT:

Auditory

Normal speed: 10 phonemes per second; Half-speed: 5 phonemes per second

Visual

Fixation speed: 250 milliseconds; Sweep speed: 20 milliseconds

Procedure

The directions given to all participants are identical to those in the Goldfarb and Halpern (1981) study: *I am going to say a word and I want you to say the first word you think of. For example, if I say* sky *you may say* blue; *if I say* up *you may say* down. *Just say the first word you think of, whatever it is. There aren't any wrong answers.*

There is no limit on the number of times these instructions can be given, but there is a 20-second maximum response latency before a rating of "No Response" is scored. Presentation of the word lists should be counterbalanced to control for effect of order of presentation. That is, the examiner should randomly select which modality (auditory or visual) and speed (fast or slow) is to be presented first. Only oral responses are accepted, and these are to be keyed in by the examiner.

Scoring

The five categories for scoring were modified from the Palermo and Jenkins (1964) classification system used in the Sefer and Henrickson (1966) study. According to Ervin (1961), *paradigmatic* refers to two words belonging to the same grammatical class (e.g., "up–down," where both words are adverbs); *syntagmatic* refers to two words of different grammatical classes (e.g., "throw–ball," where "throw" is a verb and "ball" is a noun). TAWAT applies a broader definition of *syntagmatic* to account for contiguous real-world relationships of words in the same grammatical class. An association of *paper* for the word *news* is scored as syntagmatic, even though both words are nouns. Consult **Table 2** for typical responses for all stimulus words.

When distortions, neologisms, phonemic reversals, or phonemic paraphasias occur, all involving less than accurate articulation, the procedure described by Halpern, Darley, and

TABLE 2

Most Frequent Word Association Responses (See Goldfarb & Halpern, 1984)

1. Adorable: cute, baby, lovable
2. Arrange: fix, order, flowers, organize, set, prepare
3. Arrive: come, late, leave, depart, here, home, on time
4. Art: painting, picture, music, work, paint, gallery, museum
5. Awaken: sleep, arise, morning, asleep, up, get up, rise
6. Bake: cake, cook, bread, cookies
7. Bald: head, hair, hairy, man, eagle, old, hairless
8. Banana: fruit, yellow, peel, monkey, split, cake, apple
9. Behave: good, well, act, yourself, child(ren), bad(ly), misbehave
10. Brownie: cake, chocolate, cookie, girl scout, fudge, mix
11. Cabbage: stuffed, lettuce, vegetable, corn beef, patch, green, food
12. Cat: dog, mouse
13. Celebrate: party, birthday, happy, holiday, rejoice
14. Central: middle, park, mid, station, main
15. Children: kid, young, adult, little, play, baby, small
16. Chilly: cold, warm, cool, night, weather
17. Country: city, club, U.S.A., mountain, nation, state
18. Cute: adorable, ugly, pretty, baby, sweet, girl, nice, child
19. Deaf: mute, hear, dumb, blind, ear, hearing
20. Disappoint: sad, let down, upset, unhappy, sorrow
21. Dollar: bill, money, cent
22. Dreadful: horrible, awful, terrible, bad
23. Explore: find, discover, look, adventure, cave, search, seek
24. Fail: pass, succeed, class, course, test
25. Family: friend, home, tree, together, unit, parents, affair, people, group
26. Forget: remember, me not, it
27. Game: play, fun, Monopoly, win, show
28. Gap: space, hole, generation
29. Gape: stare, look, hole, open
30. Glee: happy, club, job, happiness
31. Goal: aim, achieve, hockey, reach, post, score
32. Goblin: ghost, Halloween, witch
33. Happiest: saddest, sad, day, person, moment, best
34. Heal: wound, cure, fix, shoe, well, doctor, sick, better, toe
35. Heaven: hell, sky, earth, angel, clouds, god
36. Helper: aid, assistant, aide, friend, mother's, worker
37. Hum: sing, song, tune, whistle, drum
38. Ill: sick, well
39. Join: together, club, in, help, group, up, hands, belong
40. Joy: happy, happiness, joyful, world
41. Jump: up, rope, hop, skip, leap, high, fall, down
42. Keep: hold, save, give, take, up, going, have, lose, out, quiet
43. Let: me, go, allow
44. Loud: soft, noise, noisy, quiet, mouth
45. Mere: only, small, little, slight, just, pittance
46. Mid: night, way, middle, century, center, central
47. Mile: run, walk, yard, long, distance, high, kilometer, inch
48. News: paper, good, bad, bulletin, cast

TABLE 2

Most Frequent Word Association Responses (See Goldfarb & Halpern, 1984) (Continued)

49. Nice: good, sweet, mean, kind, bad, person, pleasant
50. Oat: meal, wheat, horse, cereal, grain
51. Pert: cute, awake, alert, lively
52. Pour: spill, milk, out, water, liquid, spout
53. Prepare: make, dinner, ready, food, fix, work, cook
54. Problem: solve, math, child, solution, trouble
55. Rotten: apple, egg, bad, spoiled
56. Saluted: flag, army, soldier, attention
57. Scholar: smart, student, school, professor, teacher, intelligent
58. Selfish: greedy, mean, generous, stingy, person, self-centered
59. Several: many, few, people
60. Sick: ill, well, healthy, cold
61. Silent: quiet, night, noisy, loud, movie
62. Slim: fat, thin, skinny, Jim, trim, slender
63. Southern: northern: belle, accent, state, chicken, bell
64. Tall: short, small
65. Tore: rip, ripped, up, paper, apart
66. Tremble: shake, scared, shiver, fear, nervous, cold
67. Try: hard, succeed, again, try again, attempt
68. Tub: bath, shower, soap, wash, clean
69. Understand: comprehend, know, me
70. Wonderful: great, good, happy, fantastic, terrific, marvelous, nice, person
71. Woolen: sweater, socks, scarf, mittens, gloves, hat, itchy, cotton, coat
72. Zone: area, zip code, number, parking

Keith (1976) is used. The above responses are each placed into the categories of recognizable or unrecognizable distortions. The examiner transcribes a recognizable distortion (e.g., *pasghetti* in response to *noodle*) in the correct form of the presumed target word, and scores an unrecognizable distortion as a jargon (unintelligible) response. When reapproaches (repeated attempts to produce the target word) occur, the final attempt is recorded. The examiner does not score responses that do not include the vocal production of a word. Gesture, pantomime and spelling—either aloud or "written" in the air with one's finger—are not scored but are encouraged if they result in a spoken word.

Responses are scored as the following:

1. Paradigmatic: words belonging to the same grammatical class (*short* for *tall*)
2. Syntagmatic: words belonging to different grammatical classes or a grammatical continuation (*boy* for *tall*; *paper* for *news*)
3. Repetitious: repeating the stimulus words, or the stimulus word ± a prefix or suffix (*taller* for *tall*)
4. Anomalous: actual, intelligible words showing no obvious relationship between stimulus and response (*earth* for *tall*)
5. Unclassifiable: a long phrase, jargon (unintelligible), or no response

The examiner experiencing difficulty in classifying a response should consult Table 2. In most instances, the difficulty will involve a choice between paradigmatic and anomalous, or syntagmatic and anomalous. If the examinee's response is listed among the typical responses indicated in Table 2, it is *not* anomalous. Be sure to remember, though, that many perfectly acceptable paradigmatic and syntagmatic responses to the word stimuli are not listed in Table 2.

We recommend that the first letter of each classification category (i.e., P, S, R, A, U) be used to save time in scoring responses. The program uses P as the default score, and includes a drop-down list of the other scores. Although it is desirable to administer the complete battery of four stimulus presentations (two speeds through the auditory modality and two speeds through the visual modality), useful information may be gleaned from even a single stimulus presentation. If a participant refuses to, or is unable to, respond to stimuli presented at a faster speed, responses to the slower speed may be analyzed. Similarly, if the participant refuses to, or is unable to, respond to visually-presented stimuli, then responses to auditory presentations may be analyzed.

Each of the 4 possible stimulus presentations consists of 36 words. Ideally, the examiner should present 2 word lists (List A and List B) during a single examination session for a total of 72 words presented. The examiner should then wait one week before the second 2 presentations to avoid the possibility of a practice effect. There are three random choices that may be made by coin toss to select modality (e.g., heads = auditory, tails = visual), first list presented (e.g., heads = List A, tails = List B), and speed (e.g., heads = fast, tails = slow). The following may serve as an example:

Examination Session #1 (8/14/11): List B, Auditory, 5 phonemes per second, followed by List A, Auditory, 10 phonemes per second.

Examination Session #2 (8/21/11): List A, Visual, 20 milliseconds, followed by List B, Visual, 250 milliseconds.

Response classifications (i.e., P, S, R, A, U) should be noted where appropriate on the response screen. The first group of analyses will yield data about total responses as a function of both modality and speed of stimulus presentation. The second group of analyses will provide information about word characteristics (grammatical class, abstraction level, frequency of occurrence, and word length), also as a function of both modality and speed of stimulus presentation.

Validity and Reliability

We have considered *validity* to mean generalizability of the data, and have addressed factors that affect both internal and external validity. Our goal was to eliminate alternative explanations that might account for the treatment effects. The fewer the alternative explanations, the greater the internal validity of the experiments (Schiavetti & Metz, 2002).

By presenting the complete TAWAT in one session, three threats to internal validity are avoided. The first threat, *history*, refers to events that occur between the first and second measurements in addition to the experimental variable. If one were to administer, say, the auditory portion of TAWAT and the individual with a language disorder receives speech-language therapy focusing on word association, then this history might affect the individual's performance on the visual portion of TAWAT when given at a later date. Similarly, there is a threat of *maturation*, similar to history, which refers to changes in the individuals themselves that cannot be controlled by the experimenter. When working with individuals with aphasia, particularly those within six months postonset of cerebrovascular accident (CVA), spontaneous recovery may be a factor of maturation. Aphasia is a disorder that may migrate, say, from jargon to Wernicke to anomic forms. Finally, there is no effect of *mortality*, or differential loss of participants in comparison groups, when TAWAT is given in a single session.

We have controlled for *practice effects* in the construction of TAWAT by using pseudorandom ordering of the stimulus variables, so that there are no three consecutive occurrences of any of the word parameters of grammatical class, abstraction level, frequency of occurrence, and length. It is important that, in administering TAWAT, the clinician vary presentation of Lists A and B, as well as auditory and visual modalities and speed of presentation.

Regarding *instrumentation*, the compact disc that accompanies this manual has been calibrated to present visual stimuli at 20-millisecond (sweep speed) and 250-millisecond (fixation speed) exposures. Similarly, the auditory stimuli have been prepared, using Sony Sound Forge 7.0, to play at 10–14 phonemes per second (normal speed) and at 5–7 phonemes per second (half-speed). Clinicians administering TAWAT must be sure to gain facility and confidence in the ability to score the five parameters of *paradigmatic*, *syntagmatic*, *repetitious*, *anomalous*, and *unclassifiable* by practicing administration and scoring on typical adults before attempting to test individuals with language impairments. Changes in scorers or observers may produce changes in the obtained measurements, but this is minimized by the strict definitions of the five parameters for classification.

One use of the pretest is to reduce the possibility of *statistical regression* or outlier scores. Atypically high or low scores tend to regress to a more typical mean score. By using the ceiling and floor cutoffs on the pretest as exclusionary criteria, the likelihood of atypical scores will be reduced.

Part Three of this manual, "Research and TAWAT," indicates the efforts the authors made to minimize *differential selection of participants*, where the goal is to avoid differences between comparison groups with the exception of the classification variable (e.g., individual who is typical or has aphasia, dementia, or the language of schizophrenia) under study.

The *Hawthorne effect* obtains when an individual is aware of participating in an experiment. This effect is minimized by carefully reciting the instructions, as indicated in the "Procedure" section.

Remember to minimize factors that affect internal validity, because two or more jeopardizing factors interacting can magnify the threat that each might pose individually.

Among the factors that affect external validity, *reactive or interactive effects of pretesting* is important to TAWAT. Participants exposed to a pretest may react differently to the experimental treatment from those who receive the treatment without the pretest. Do not try to save time by skipping the pretest. Everyone who is given TAWAT must also be given the pretest.

We have normed the stimuli for TAWAT and have studied its effect on various typical and atypical populations. However, the relationships we have reported relate to populations and not necessarily to individuals. There may be a threat of *subject selection* to the external validity of TAWAT, as we cannot make predictions about the language behavior of an individual participant.

It is possible for the Hawthorne effect to operate as a threat to external validity, a phenomenon called *reactive arrangements*. Presenting TAWAT as a therapy task, and not as a test, minimizes the Hawthorne effect.

Reliability and Validity of Tests and Measurements

The term *reliability* means precision of measurement; it also refers to consistency. A butcher's scale may be fraudulently set to overcharge each customer two ounces. The scale is reliable, but not valid. On the other hand, *validity*, or the degree to which a test measures what it purports to test, the truth or correctness or reality of the measurement, depends on its also being reliable.

There are three typical ways to check the reliability of a test or measurement (Schiavetti & Metz, 2002): test-retest reliability, parallel or equivalent form, and split-half. A form of TAWAT presented to institutionalized elderly, with and without dementia, who resided in New Jersey (Santo Pietro & Goldfarb, 1985) was replicated by an independent group in

Arizona (Abeysinghe, Bayles, & Trosset, 1990), whose results with an independent population of individuals with dementia were similar.

The total of 72 words in List A and List B of TAWAT are equivalent forms, with both including the 36 words needed to represent 1 instance each of 3 parts of speech (noun, verb, adjective), 3 levels of abstraction (high, medium, low), 2 frequencies of occurrence (frequent, infrequent) and 2 lengths (long, short): $3 \times 3 \times 2 \times 2 = 36$.

There are also three typical ways to establish the validity of a test or measure. *Content validity* is a subjective procedure for evaluating items on a test to see how well they measure what the tester claims. By counterbalancing the items in the TAWAT word list, as noted above, the authors have a reasonable claim to be measuring these four word parameters. Claiming content validity for modality of stimulus presentation is less secure, as the visual modality involves serial processing and the auditory modality requires parallel resonance processing, so the two should not be compared.

There are two types of *criterion validity*, one of which has been addressed in TAWAT, but only in part. There is no *predictive validity* in TAWAT, as the test will not predict some future behavior. However, the word association responses of institutionalized elderly demonstrated *concurrent validity* with the *Mini-Mental Status Questionnaire* (Kahn et al., 1960) in nearly identically tracking severity of dementia.

Finally, *construct validity* refers to the degree to which a test reflects a theory of the characteristics to be measured. If the test is valid and the theory is correct, the test should confirm the theory. The section below addresses our research in relation to the received wisdom about the paradigmatic shift.

Part Three: Research and TAWAT

Young Adults

Goldfarb and Halpern (1984) standardized the word stimuli in TAWAT using 316 undergraduates at Queens College in Flushing, New York. The ages of the participants ranged from 18 to 24 years, with a mean of 19.9 years; educational level ranged from 13 to 16 years, with a mean of 14.9 years.

Paradigmatic and syntagmatic responses accounted for approximately 90% of the total. The greatest percentage of responses was paradigmatic (48.1%), followed by syntagmatic (41.6%), unclassifiable (4.7%), anomalous (4.5%), and repetitious (1.1%). More paradigmatic responses were observed for words of a medium level of abstraction than for words of high or low levels of abstraction. In terms of grammatical class, the most paradigmatic responses occurred for adjectives, followed by nouns and verbs. Long words elicited more paradigmatic responses than short words, and frequent words more than infrequent.

Adults with Aphasia

Goldfarb and Halpern (1981) presented TAWAT auditorily to 32 adults with aphasia and 32 matched controls, and visually to 20 adults with aphasia and 20 matched controls. For auditory stimulation, control participants were 27 men and 5 women free of aphasia and who reported no neuropathology. For visual stimulation, control participants were 17 men and 3 women. Both control groups were matched to the aphasic samples for age, sex, and educational level.

The following are responses to TAWAT presented through the auditory modality:

Regarding temporal manipulation of word stimuli, the results indicate that adults with aphasia produce significantly more paradigmatic word association responses when stimuli are presented at a slower speed. The number of these responses produced by neurotypical adults was not affected by the temporal manipulation.

Regarding abstraction level of words, results showed that for paradigmatic responses, the group with aphasia behaved more consistently than the control group. That is, for the participants with aphasia, the percentage of paradigmatic word association responses increased as the level of word abstraction decreased. This pattern was affected by speed of stimulus presentation. No clear pattern emerged from the control group. The order of abstraction level that corresponded to the order of greatest-to-least number of paradigmatic associates was medium, high, low for words presented at normal speed; and medium, low, high for words presented at half-speed.

Regarding grammatical class, the largest percentage of paradigmatic responses was produced for adjectives, followed closely by nouns, with responses to verbs clearly diminished. Without exception, this pattern occurred for participants with and without aphasia at normal speed and half-speed.

Regarding word length, a greater percentage of paradigmatic responses generally occurred following presentation of long words than short words. A greater percentage of paradigmatic responses resulted when the speed of stimulus presentation was expanded to half-speed.

Regarding frequency of occurrence, frequent words produced a greater percentage of paradigmatic associates than did infrequent words. Participants with and without aphasia reacted similarly to the frequency of occurrence variable; that is, frequent words elicited more paradigmatic responses than did infrequent ones. Furthermore, the results apparently are not affected by speed of stimulus presentation or by presence or absence of aphasia.

The following are responses to TAWAT presented through the visual modality:

Regarding temporal manipulation of word stimuli, when stimuli were presented at a slower speed, the adults with aphasia produced significantly more paradigmatic responses. No differences existed in the number of paradigmatic responses of the neurotypical participants relative to speed of presentation.

Regarding abstraction level for the group with aphasia, the number of paradigmatic associates varied inversely with abstraction level. That is, regardless of speed of stimulus presentation, significantly more paradigmatic word association responses followed the presentation of concrete rather than abstract words. No clear pattern emerged from the control group relative to abstraction level.

Regarding grammatical class, the order of greatest-to-least number of paradigmatic associates was adjectives, nouns, and verbs. This was true for both populations, regardless of temporal manipulation.

Regarding word length for the group with aphasia, no significant difference was found between short and long words and the number of paradigmatic responses produced.

Regarding frequency of occurrence, more paradigmatic responses were produced to frequent than to infrequent words, regardless of speed of stimulus presentation or existence of aphasic impairment.

Adults with the Language of Schizophrenia

Halpern, Goldfarb, Brandon, and McCartin-Clark (1985) presented TAWAT through the visual and auditory modalities to 49 adults with chronic undifferentiated schizophrenia. The participant pool of 35 men and 14 women was drawn from a large state psychiatric center. Their ages ranged from 21 years, 2 months to 81 years, 1 month with a mean age of 49 years, 2 months.

The following are responses to TAWAT presented through the auditory modality:

Regarding temporal manipulation of word stimuli, adults with chronic undifferentiated schizophrenia produced significantly more unclassified word association responses when stimuli were presented at a slower speed. All other response differences were not significant.

Regarding abstraction level of words, the percentage of paradigmatic word association responses tended to increase as the level of word abstraction decreased. The order of abstraction level that corresponded to order of greatest-to-least number of paradigmatic responses was low, medium, high for words presented at normal speed (10 phonemes per second); and medium, low, high for words presented at half-speed (5 phonemes second).

Regarding grammatical class, the largest percentage of paradigmatic responses was produced for nouns, followed closely by adjectives, with responses to verbs clearly diminished. Without exception, this pattern occurred at normal speed and half-speed.

Regarding word length, a greater percentage of paradigmatic responses occurred following presentation of long words rather than short words.

Regarding frequency of occurrence, frequent words resulted in a greater percentage of paradigmatic responses than did infrequent words. The results were not affected by speed of stimulus presentation.

The following are responses to TAWAT presented through the visual modality:

Regarding temporal manipulation of word stimuli, significantly more paradigmatic, syntagmatic, and unclassified responses occurred on stimuli presented at 1000 milliseconds. Speed differences were not significant for repetitious and anomalous responses.

Regarding abstraction level of words, regardless of speed of stimulation, significantly more paradigmatic word association responses followed the presentation of concrete rather than abstract words.

Regarding grammatical class, the order of greatest-to-least number of paradigmatic responses was nouns, adjectives, verbs at both 10-millisecond and 1000-millisecond speeds. Results also indicated that the effects of speed varied from one part of speech to another.

Regarding word length, paradigmatic responses to short and long words differed only slightly.

Regarding frequency of occurrence, paradigmatic responses to frequent and infrequent words differed only slightly.

Institutionalized Elderly with and Without Dementia

Santo Pietro and Goldfarb (1985) presented the fast auditory portion of TAWAT to 91 institutionalized elderly participants with and without dementia, to determine characteristic patterns of word association responses. The sample included 79 women and 12 men. Participants ranged in age from 60 to 96 years with a mean of 82.1 years.

The following are responses to 36 items from TAWAT presented through the auditory modality at fast speed.

Institutionalized elderly with dementia demonstrated a unique pattern of word association responses characterized by a marked reduction in paradigmatic responses, an increase in unclassifiable responses, and the presence of up to 45% multiword, short phrasal responses. This profile is distinct from that of neurotypical institutionalized elderly, as well as other groups previously tested with this tool. Word association response patterns do appear to change progressively with the degree of dementia (e.g., more anomalous, unclassifiable, and multiword responses as the condition worsens).

In terms of abstraction level, grammatical class, word length, and frequency of occurrence, this group produced significantly more anomalous and unclassifiable responses than neurotypical elderly in all categories. However, the relative percentages of responses falling into the various categories presented profiles remarkably similar to neurotypical except in relation to level of abstraction. Compared to neurotypical elderly in the same institution and typical young adults, the group with dementia showed a marked increase in syntagmatic responses and decrease in unclassifiable responses when stimulus words had a low level of abstraction.

References

Abeysinghe, S., Bayles, K., & Trosset, M. (1990). Semantic memory deterioration in Alzheimer's subjects: Evidence from word association, definition, and associate ranking tasks. *Journal of Speech and Hearing Research, 33,* 574–582.

Brown, R. W., & Berko. J. (1960). Word association and the acquisition of grammar. *Child Development, 31,* 1–14.

Buckingham, B., & Dolch, F. (1936). *A combined word list.* Boston: Ginn.

Buss, A. H. (1966). *Psychopathology.* New York: Wiley.

Clark, E. (1973a). How children describe time and order. In C. Ferguson & D. Slobin (Eds.), *Studies of child language development* (pp. 585–606). New York: Holt, Rinehart & Winston.

Clark, E. (1973b). What's in a word? On the child's acquisition of semantics in his first language. In T. Moore (Ed.), *Cognitive development and the acquisition of language* (pp. 65–110). New York: Academic Press.

Colangelo, A., Stephenson, K., Westbury, C., & Buchanan, L. (2003). Word associations in deep dyslexia. *Brain and Cognition, 53,* 166–170.

Collins, A. M., & Loftus, E. F. (1975). A spreading activation theory of semantic processing. *Psychological Review, 82,* 407–428.

Darley, F., Sherman, D., & Siegel, G. (1959). Scaling of abstract level of single words. *Journal of Speech and Hearing Research, 2,* 161–167.

Deese, J. (1962). Form classes and the determinants of association. *Journal of Verbal Learning and Verbal Behavior, 1,* 70–84.

Educational Developmental Laboratories. (1968). *Learning 100 instructor's manual.* New York: McGraw Hill.

Educational Developmental Laboratories. (1972). *Performance objectives for learning 100.* New York: McGraw Hill.

Ely, R. (2005). Language and literacy in the school years. In J. Berko Gleason (Ed.), *The development of language.* Boston, MA: Pearson Education.

Ervin, S. (1961). Changes with age in the verbal determinants of word association. *American Journal of Psychiatry, 74,* 361–372.

Ervin-Tripp. S. (1970). Substitution, context, and association. In L. Postman & L. Keppel (Eds.), *Norms of word association.* New York, NY: Academic Press.

Fairbanks, G. (1960). *Voice and articulation drillbook.* New York: Harper & Row.

Friedman, L., Kenny, J., Jesberger, J., Choy, M., & Meltzer, H. (1995). Relationship between smooth pursuit eye tracking and cognitive performance in schizophrenia. *Biological Psychiatry, 37,* 265–272.

Gates, A. I. (1935). *A reading vocabulary for the primary grades.* New York: Columbia University.

Goldfarb, R., & Halpern, H. (1981). Word association of time-altered auditory and visual stimuli in aphasia. *Journal of Speech and Hearing Research, 24,* 234–247.

Goldfarb, R., & Halpern, H. (1984). Word association responses in normal adult subjects. *Journal of Psycholinguistic Research, 13,* 37–55.

Gordon, R., Silverstein, M., & Harrow, M. (1982). Associative thinking in schizophrenia: A contextualist approach. *Journal of Clinical Psychology, 38,* 684–696.

Gough, P. (1972). One second of reading. In J. Kavanagh & I. Mattingly (Eds.), *Language by ear and by eye.* Cambridge, MA: MIT Press.

Green, D. (1971). Temporal auditory acuity. *Psychological Review, 78,* 540–551.

Guiliano, V. (1969). Analog networks for word association. In D. Norman (Ed.), *Memory and attention.* New York: Wiley.

Halpern, H. (1965a). Effect of stimulus variables on verbal perseveration of dysphasic subjects. *Perceptual and Motor Skills, 20,* 421–429.

Halpern, H. (1965b). Effect of stimulus variables on dysphasic verbal errors. *Perceptual and Motor Skills, 21,* 291–298.

Halpern, H., Darley, F., & Keith, R. (1976). The phonemic behavior of aphasic subjects without dysarthria or apraxia of speech. *Cortex, 12,* 365–372.

Halpern, H., Goldfarb, R., Brandon, J., & McCartin-Clark, M. (1985). Word-association responses to time-altered stimuli by schizophrenic adults. *Perceptual and Motor Skills, 61,* 239–253.

Jakobson, R. (1961). Aphasia as a linguistic problem. In S. Saporta (Ed.), *Psycholinguistics: A book of readings.* New York: Holt, Rinehart & Winston.

Kahn, R., Goldfarb, A., Pollack, M., & Peck, A. (1960). Brief objective measures for the determination of mental status in the aged. *American Journal of Psychiatry, 117,* 326–328.

Kent, G., & Rosanoff, A. (1910). A study of association in insanity. *American Journal of Insanity, 67,* 37–96.

Lockhead, G. (1972). Processing dimensional stimuli: A note. *Psychological Review, 79,* 410–419.

Massaro, D. (1970). Perceptual images. *Journal of Experimental Psychology, 85,* 411–417.

Massaro, D. (1972). Perceptual images, processing time, and perceptual units in auditory perception. *Psychological Review, 79,* 124–145.

McLaughlin, S. (1998). *Introduction to language development.* San Diego, CA: Singular.

McNeill, D. (1970). *The acquisition of language.* New York: Harper & Row.

Merten, T. (1992). Word association and schizophrenia: An empirical study. *Nervenarzt, 63,* 401–408.

Miller, G. (1956). The magical number seven, plus or minus two: Some limits on our capacity for processing information. *Psychological Review, 63,* 81–97.

Norman, D. (1969). *Memory and attention.* New York: Wiley.

Owens, R. (2005). *Language development: An introduction.* Boston, MA: Pearson Education.

Palermo, D., & Jenkins, J. (1964). *Word association norms: Grade school through college.* Minneapolis, MN: University of Minnesota Press.

Pan, B. (2005). Semantic development: Learning the meanings of words. In J. Berko Gleason (Ed.), *The development of language.* Boston, MA: Pearson Education.

Posner, M., Lewis, J., & Conrad, C. (1972). Component processing in reading: A performance analysis. In J. Kavanagh & I. Mattingly (Eds.), *Language by ear and by eye.* Cambridge, MA: MIT Press.

Ronken, D. (1970). Monaural detection of a phase difference between clicks. *Journal of the Acoustical Society of America, 47,* 1091–1099.

Russell, W., & Jenkins, J. (1954). *The complete Minnesota norms for responses to 100 words from the Kent-Rosanoff word association tests* (Tech. Rep. 11, Contract N 8-ONR-66216). Office of Naval Research, University of Minnesota.

Santo Pietro, M. J., & Goldfarb, R. (1985). Characteristic patterns of word association responses in institutionalized elderly with and without senile dementia. *Brain and Language, 26,* 230–243.

Schiavetti, N., & Metz, D. E. (2002). *Evaluating research in communicative disorders* (4th ed.). Boston, MA: Allyn and Bacon.

Schlesinger, I. (1974). Relational concepts underlying language. In R. Schiefelbusch & L. Lloyd (Eds.), *Language perspectives—Acquisition, retardation, and intervention.* Baltimore, MD: University Park Press.

Sefer, J., & Henrickson, E. H. (1966). The relationships between word association and grammatical classes in aphasia. *Journal of Speech and Hearing Research, 9,* 529–541.

Shean, G. (1999). Syndromes of schizophrenia and language dysfunction. *Journal of Clinical Psychology, 55,* 233–240.

Skinner, B. F. (1957). *Verbal behavior.* New York, NY: Appleton-Century-Crofts.

Sperling, G. (1969). The information in brief presentations. In D. Norman (Ed.), *Memory and attention.* New York: Wiley.

Studdert-Kennedy, M., Shankweiler, D., & Schulman, S. (1970). Opposed effects of a delayed channel on perception of dichotically and nontically presented CV syllables. *Journal of the Acoustical Society of America, 48,* 599–602.

Sumerall, S., Timmons, P., James, A., Ewing, M., & Oehlert, M. (1997). Expanded norms for the controlled Oral Word Association Test. *Journal of Clinical Psychology, 53,* 517–521.

Thorndike, E., & Lorge, I. (1944). *The teachers wordbook of 30,000 words.* New York: Columbia University.

Tierney, M., Black, S., Szalai, J., Snow, W., Fisher, R., Nadon, G., & Chui, H. (2001). Recognition memory and verbal fluency differentiate probable Alzheimer disease from subcortical ischemic vascular dementia. *Archives of Neurology, 58,* 1654–1659.

Tulving, E. (1983). *Elements of episodic memory.* Oxford, England: Clarendon Press.

Vygotsky, L. (1934). Thought and speech. Translated in S. Saporta (Ed.), *Psycholinguistics: A book of readings* (1961). New York: Holt, Rinehart & Winston.

Woodrow, L., & Lowell, F. (1916). Children's association frequency tables. *Psychological Monographs, 22*(97).

Zawacki, T., Grace, J., Friedman, J., & Sudarsky, L. (2002). Executive and emotional dysfunction in Machado-Joseph disease. *Movement Disorders, 17,* 1004–1011.

Index